T0092785

Handbook for Registered Nurses

Handbook for Registered Nurses

Essential Skills

Edited by

CHRIS CARTER MEd, BSc (HONS), DIPHE, RN(A)
Birmingham City University
Birmingham, United Kingdom

JOY NOTTER PHD, MSc, PGDIP (SOC), PGCEA, RHV, CPT, SRN
Birmingham City University
Saxon University of Applied Sciences
Birmingham, United Kingdom

ELSEVIER

ISBN: 978-0-7020-7434-9

Content Strategist: Robert Edwards
Content Project Manager: Shubham Dixit
Design: Bridget Hoette
Marketing Manager: Belinda Tudin

Printed in Poland by Dimograf

Last digit is the print number: 9 8 7 6 5 4 3 2 1

Working together to grow libraries in developing countries

www.elsevier.com • www.bookaid.org

CONTENTS

FOREWORD

This handbook focuses on skills and procedures, as it is essential for Registered Nurses and students to have the knowledge and skills to deliver high-quality, safe, patient care in rapidly changing health settings, with increasing patient demand. The move to graduate entry in the UK has recognised the complexity and autonomy that nursing in all branches and sectors requires to deliver this. While the nursing profession has recognised the need for change to meet these needs, there needs to be a continued focus on research and evidence that supports improved care models led and delivered by Registered Nurses.

As a competency-based profession, at the centre of patient safety is the need for nurses to be able to make clinical decisions and coordinate care, this includes supervision of peers and junior staff as well other professional groups. The Nursing and Midwifery Council (UK) recognises the importance of fundamental nursing care; nurses and students need access to resources specifically designed to support their practice in both the community and hospital setting.

The new title, *Handbook for Registered Nurses: Essential skills*, reflects the changing face of nursing. It has been prepared by a team of experienced nurses from practice, education, and research to reflect the changing expectations of registered nurses and will help prepare the next generation of nurses for practice, by bridging the theory-practice gap.

Prof Mark Radford CBE, PhD, RN
Chief Nurse Health Education England
Deputy Chief Nursing Officer for England

Nursing is a dynamic and rapidly evolving profession and, since the publication of the forerunner to this book *Essential Nursing Skills*, there have been major advances in nursing and healthcare which are reflected in the complex care now required by patients. Nurses are now expected to have wide ranging knowledge and skills that they can translate to meet new clinical expectations. Therefore, this edition has been updated to reflect the wide ranging practice that nurses need to support patients throughout their individualised pathway. This new book, therefore, reflects these expectations and the content of the old Skills book has been expanded, updated and repositioned accordingly. A significant change has arisen due to the revised standards of proficiency for registered nurses, the introduction of the associate nurse role and revalidation (Nursing and Midwifery Council, 2018a, 2018b, 2019). The roles, responsibilities and accountability of registered nurses and associate nurses are now described as platforms, with additional annexes relating to communication and relationship management skills and procedures. These define the differences in professional roles (see table 1), and outline the expectations of a newly registered nurse at the start of their career.

TABLE 1 ■ NMC Revised Professional Roles

Platform 1:	Being an accountable professional	Being an accountable professional
Platform 2:	Promoting health and preventing ill health	Promoting health and preventing ill health
Platform 3:	Assessing needs and planning care	Provide and monitor care
Platform 4:	Providing and evaluating care	Working in teams
Platform 5:	Leading and managing nursing care and working in teams	Improving safety and quality of care
Platform 6:	Improving safety and quality of care	Contributing to integrated care
Platform 7:	Coordinating care	
Annex A	Communication and relationship management skills	Communication and relationship management skills
Annex B	Nursing procedures	Procedures to be undertaken by the nursing associate

The revised NMC standards help new graduates entering into the profession to understand the knowledge and skills they need at the point of registration. They need to accept that lifelong learning is a key component of professional development, and this book will enable them to build upon the knowledge and skills they have at the point of registration. *Handbook for Registered Nurses: Essential Skills* focuses on the clinical practice required by nurses caring for a range of adult patients. However, it is important to acknowledge that the skills themselves can be adapted to any clinical setting.

This book, written for nurses by nurses, has been compiled by a team from a variety of nursing backgrounds including clinical practice, and education. It reflects advances in practice, including the expanding role of the nurse and the recognition of complexity of care in both acute and community settings. The format provides a clear structure for nurses and student nurses to follow. *Handbook for Registered Nurses: Essential Skills* has been designed to act as a reminder for skills taught in education programmes as well as clinical settings, this will enable the learner to prepare for new skills. This book should be used to complement other nursing texts.

Supervised Practice and Preceptorship

All students and newly qualified nurses have to be supervised by a Registered Nurse until they have been assessed as competent to work unsupervised. As with all aspects of nursing, safety is paramount, and it is important to know the patient's diagnosis and the reason for carrying out the procedure before any skill is performed. For students and preceptors this book provides a practical resource which can be used in the clinical practice or as a teaching aid.

Nursing practice is subject to local policies and protocols, which refer to specific aspects of nursing practice that often vary between clinical areas, for example drug-checking procedures (e.g. intravenous drug therapy), cleansing solutions and skin preparation (e.g. prior to venepuncture or intramuscular injection). These must always be adhered to and nurses have a responsibility to regularly update themselves. National guidelines (e.g. resuscitation council guidelines) are also reviewed frequently and again it is the nurses responsibility to keep up to date with changes as they occur.

We hope that both learners and teachers will find this book helpful and that it will become a much-used resource to support and enhance clinical practice. Quality nursing care requires knowledge and competence but also compassion with respect for patients as individuals, underpinning every clinical skill. We hope that our passion and respect for nursing is evident throughout this book.

Chris Carter and Joy Notter
March 2023

References

Nursing and Midwifery Council, 2018a. Future Nurse: Standards of Proficiency for Registered Nurses. www.nmc.org.uk.
Nursing and Midwifery Council, 2018b. Standards of Proficiency for Nursing Associates. www.nmc.org.uk.
Nursing and Midwifery Council, 2019. Revalidation. www.nmc.org.uk.

Sarah Curr MSc, BA (Hons), BSc (Hons), RN, RNT, DTN, FHEA, AKC
King's College London
London, United Kingdom

Mary Raleigh DClin Pract, MSc, BSc (Hons), RN, RMN, RNT
King's College London
London, United Kingdom

Carolyne Stewart BA (Hons), PGCE, FHEA, RN, RNT
King's College London
London, United Kingdom

ACKNOWLEDGEMENTS

The editors and contributors wish to acknowledge the support from Dr Anne Jones, PhD, MSc, PGCAP, FHEA, RGN, King's College London, United Kingdom. The editors and contributors would also like to acknowledge the valuable contribution of Maggie Nicol, Carol Bavin, Patricia Cronin, Karen Rawlings-Anderson, Elaine Cole, Janet Hunter, and Shelagh Bedford-Turner.

The editors and contributors wish to dedicated this edition of the *Handbook for Registered Nurses: Essential Skills* to Sarah Curr who supported this revised edition from the beginning, however, sadly did not see it reach publication. Her commitment to students and colleagues will always be remembered.

CHAPTER 1

Bedside Clinical Teaching

While it may vary internationally, in the UK currently, preregistration nursing education programmes require students to spend up to 50% of the course in clinical practice (Nursing and Midwifery Council (NMC), 2018). Placements provide students with a rich experience and exposure to different healthcare care settings facilitating the development of the required levels of competency to enter professional registration (Wu et al., 2015). The practice learning environment also makes it possible for students to work alongside a range of professionals from across the four fields of nursing practice, enabling them to become proficient to deliver safe and effective care (NMC 2018a). Education programmes equip nurses for lifelong learning; the clinical environment provides an opportunity for a range of learning opportunities for different learners, for example, pre and post registration nurses, newly employed nurses completing preceptorship programmes, those returning to practice and those completing their statutory NMC revalidation.

However, it is a cause for concern that clinical teaching at the bedside has become more complex due to increasing patient dependency, nursing workloads, high numbers of students requiring placements and a focus on other teaching methods e.g. simulation (Qureshi, 2014; Reynolds et al., 2020). It is acknowledged that the clinical environment is unpredictable in terms of patient care, it does expose the student to different clinical experiences offering the opportunity to learn from a range of dynamic and innovative, solutions to patient needs. This provides students with the 'real world perspective', equipping them for their future roles as nurses and providing an opportunity to learn how to adapt and respond to changing patient care needs (National Health Service (NHS) Employers, 2020). The clinical learning environment and bedside teaching provides a rich opportunity for both planned and spontaneous learning and teaching.

Many of the skills covered in this book can be performed and assessed in either clinical practice or in other learning environments, including clinical skills centres and via clinical simulation. While simulation is an important component of clinical learning, it cannot completely replace supervised patient care. Therefore, to enhance the student experience, NHS Employers (2020) have developed a core set of recommendations for the clinical learning environment:

- Allow adequate time to utilise their skills and provide compassionate care.
- Provide time with patients and families to complete the episode of care, recognizing that they may be slower or require additional support while they are learning these new skills.
- Allow for time and space to reflect on the care they have given with other professionals.
- Provide an opportunity to contribute to team discussions and value their opinions.
- Allow students to work with staff who can take sufficient, dedicated time away from practice to spend with them.
- Expose students to a range of different experiences and procedures under supervision.
- Recognise students have individual learning needs and that no single approach fits all learning styles.

Practice assessors need to have:

- Support from peers, practice and academic assessors, Link Lecturers and organisational educational staff.
- Time to reflect on their own experiences of working with students.

- Training and education to develop their role as a teacher, mentor, coach and assessor.
- Access to a range of evidence-based learning resources within the clinical environment.
- Dedicated and protected time away from practice with students, to teach and complete any learning documentation.
- A flexible approach with students, recognising learning opportunities when they arise.
- Space to give effective and timely feedback.

Assessment

Assessments are outcome-focused, and should be evidence-based, robust and objective. Assessments can be formative or summative. Formative is an 'assessment for learning' and summative is an 'assessment of learning' (Harlen, 2015). Assessments are used to confirm the student's proficiency and are based on their understanding of both theory and practice. Assessments and confirmation of proficiency need to be timely, providing ongoing assurance of student achievements and competence. These assessments are often completed as part of a university programme. Formative assessments can be added if a student is unsure of a certain procedure, as this enables the student to practice in a safe environment. However, for this to be successful, the student and the practice assessor must be familiar with the assessment strategy and documentation.

T-Moments/Bite-size Teaching

Teachable moments (T-moments) are short individual learning opportunities incorporated with care delivery and education in the workplace (Reynolds et al., 2020). They allow students to build on their previous practice, with supervisors deciding the level and depth of content needed at that moment in practice, for that student.

Described as 'high-impact learning' experiences, bite-size teaching focuses on embracing all possible teaching opportunities and providing tutorials in the work environment. This approach is informal, does not require information technology (IT) equipment or specific resources and is accessible and flexible in meeting the needs of a particular clinical area. Bite size teaching can be used to support understanding of a specific clinical situation as it enables the student to focus on individualised care.

Top Tips for Teaching and Supervising Skills

When teaching and supervising skills, nurses may want to establish activities which support students relating theory to practice. The following are some examples of 'top tips' that can be used to facilitate learning.

When teaching and supervising skills first consider the learner's level of knowledge. Ask the learner to explain why the patient is having a specific procedure and to highlight the associated benefits and risks. Prior to the procedure, learners must be able to:

- Identify the relevant physiology.
- Identify potential complications, including any signs and symptoms, and what actions they would take.
- Provide opportunities for students to talk through procedures and practice in a safe environment (e.g. using a cannulation arm or observing the procedure first).
- Ask the student to provide a rationale for the procedure.
- Ask the student to research a condition or a situation and the professional, legal or ethical dilemmas that may occur when providing care.
- Discuss any special considerations that may be required to support a patient with a cognitive impairment.

- Involve the student in activities (e.g. performing drug calculations) so that they can build confidence and ask questions relating to the procedure.
- When supervising the skill, try to identify a patient who is stable to allow for adequate time to complete the procedure.
- When supervising a procedure, ask the student to explain why they are undertaking this training and how it will extend their practice

KEY POINTS

- As a competence based profession, bedside teaching is crucial as it enables the student to see excellence in practice and learn to follow evidence-based practice.
- Bedside clinical teaching provides an opportunity to bridge the theory-practice gap and enable students to develop the competence to enter registered practice.
- Clinical teaching must be structured, however, it is important to respond to opportunities as they arise. As that enables the student to see how changing patient status and condition is addressed in practice.
- A range of teaching strategies can be used, either of which can strengths and weaknesses, however, in combination this enable the student to integrate knowledge and skills into complex patient care.

References

Harlen, W., 2015. Assessment and the curriculum. In: Wyse, D., Hayward, L., Pandya, J. (Eds.), SAFE Handbook of Curriculum, Pedagogy and Assessment, vol 2. SAGE Publishing.

NHS Employers, 2020. What Makes A Good Placement? https://www.nhsemployers.org/your-workforce/plan/nursing-workforce/nursing-education-and-training/excellence-in-student-nursing-placements.

Nursing and Midwifery Council. (2018). Part 3: Standards for pre-registration nursing programmes. https://www.nmc.org.uk/globalassets/sitedocuments/standards-of-proficiency/standards-for-pre-registration-nursing-programmes/programme-standards-nursing.pdf

Nursing and Midwifery Council (NMC), 2018a. Realising professionalism: Standards for education and training Part 3: Standards for pre-registration nursing programme. www.nmc.org.uk.

Nursing and Midwifery Council (NMC), 2018b. Realising professionalism: Standards for education and training Part 2: Standards for student supervision and assessment. www.nmc.org.uk.

Qureshi, Z., 2014. Back to the bedside: the role of bedside teaching in the modern era. Perspect. Med. Educ. 3 (2), 69–72. doi:10.1007/s40037-014-0111-6.

Reynolds, L., Attenborough, J., Halse, J., 2020. Nurses as educators: creating teachable moments in practice. Nurs. Times [online] 116 (2), 25–28.

Wu, X.V., Enshar, J., Lee, C.C.S., et al., 2015. A systematic review of clinical assessment for undergraduate nursing students. Nurse Educ. Today. 35, 347–359.

CHAPTER 2

Infection Prevention and Control Principles

Standard Precautions

Hospital or healthcare acquired infections (HAI/HCAIs) are recognised globally as being of the most significant challenges facing healthcare service providers (Royal College of Nursing [RCN], 2019). Two essential approaches in infection prevention are standard precautions and aseptic non-touch technique (ANTT). Standard precautions are the specifically designed to prevent cross infection and reduce the risk of transmission of blood borne and other pathogens (RCN, 2017). They include the interventions required when contact with body fluids is likely. Previously referred to as universal precautions, they have been developed to protect both patients and staff and are the minimum standards for infection prevention control practices that should be applied to all patients regardless of suspected or confirmed infection (Centres for Disease Control and Prevention, 2019).

The standard precautions are:

- Hand hygiene (hand washing and/or hand decontamination with alcohol-based hand rubs)
- Safe clinical practice, includes, aseptic technique, risk assessment for the appropriate placement of patients, including isolation
- Management of invasive devices (e.g., urinary catheters; intravenous [IV] cannulas) to reduce the risk of infection as far as possible
- Appropriate use of protective protective equipment (PPE), including; aprons, gloves, masks, gowns and eye protection
- The promotion of respiratory hygiene and cough etiquette
- Safe infection prevention practices
- Safe disposal of waste using the national colour-coding system
- Appropriate decontamination of equipment
- Safe provision and storage of food
- Maintenance of a clean, safe environment
- Safe handling of contaminated linen.

Aseptic Non-Touch Technique (ANTT)

Nurses need to be aware that many of the procedures carried out have an inherent infection risk. For example, in wound care, any break to the continuity of the skin forms a wound which provides an entry point for microorganisms to enter and increases the risk of infection. Therefore, to reduce the risk of microorganisms entering the body, a range of measures should be taken. Aseptic technique is one of the most important method used to reduce the risk of introducing contamination to the wound or any insertion sites, to protect the patient from the risk of infection.

The ANTT refers to standardised guidelines for aseptic technique procedures and applies to all healthcare procedures where there is a risk of infection and a healthcare-associated infection (e.g. wound care, administration of IV medication and catheterisation (Fraise & Bradley, 2009;

National Institute for Health and Care Excellence [NICE], 2017). ANTT is designed to maintain asepsis and avoid contamination of wounds or vulnerable sites from microorganisms. It also means that you must avoid touching any part of the equipment that will come into contact with the patient (e.g. the centre of a sterile wound dressing, the tip of a needle or IV cannula). It is also essential to avoid touching the ends of equipment when connecting them (e.g. the spike of the IV giving set when inserting it into the IV fluids).

It is crucial element of ANTT is assessment of the risk of contamination before commencing the procedure, because the measures taken will vary depending on the procedure being carried out. For example, some procedures will require sterile gloves, sterile dressing pack, sterile towel and dressing (e.g. wound care); others may need only sterile equipment and nonsterile gloves (e.g. IV cannulation); both will require non-touch methods.

CONSIDERATIONS

There are several components for the use of ANTT, including:
1. Explanation of all procedures.
2. Give the patient the opportunity to wash his or her hands and bathe or shower; this is often possible even with a wound.
3. Use of sterile equipment when carrying out procedures wherever there is a risk of contamination (e.g. sterile dressing pack, IV cannula, syringe and needle).
4. Only handle the parts of equipment that are not in contact with the patient or other medical equipment.
5. Never place sterile equipment on to a non-sterile surface or touch sterile equipment without wearing sterile gloves. Remember, contamination will occur if you touch the outside of a sterile glove with a non-gloved hand or place a sterile item onto a non-sterile surface.
6. All items used for the procedure must be sterile; check that packaging is intact and within the expiration date.
7. Use of appropriate PPE, including gloves, aprons and face masks.
8. Use of hand hygiene to include hand washing and/or the use of an alcohol hand rub (p. 9).
9. All equipment must be cleaned prior to use. Some procedures will be carried out in a clean treatment room (e.g. wound dressing) and some in a ward environment (e.g. catheterisation). Surfaces (e.g. dressing trolley) should be cleaned according to local policy, before and after the procedure. It is essential to avoid carrying out sterile procedures (e.g. wound dressings) during bed making and at mealtimes.
10. All non-disposable equipment (e.g. blood pressure cuff or transfer hoist) must be decontaminated after each patient use, always follow local policy guidelines.

Hand Hygiene

Hand hygiene is the single most important intervention used to protect you and the patient, with effective hand hygiene internationally recognised as a way of significantly reducing HCAIs (Loveday et al., 2014).

Alcohol hand rub may be used instead of hand washing when the hands are 'socially' clean (i.e., not visibly soiled or likely to be contaminated). The alcohol must be applied to all areas of the hands and wrists and the hands then rubbed vigorously until dry. Alcohol effectively reduces microbial counts on clean hands, but it is ineffective if used on hands contaminated with body fluids or excreta. Alcohol-based hand rub is effective against methicillin-resistant *Staphylococcus aureus* (MRSA), however, you need to remember that the spores of *Clostridioides difficile* can survive in the

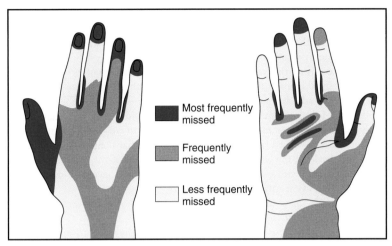

Fig. 2.1 Areas often missed when the hands are washed. (Nicol, M., Bavin, C., Cronin, P., Rawlings-Anderson, K., Cole, E., & Hunter, J. (2008). *Essential Nursing Skills*. Elsevier Ltd.)

environment and are not killed by alcohol. Therefore, hands must be washed with soap and water after contact with *C. difficile* patients or their environment (RCN, 2019a).

It is important to be aware that as research has demonstrated, hand washing techniques (including the alcohol hand rubs) are not always effective. Areas of the hands that are commonly missed are the thumbs, fingernails, fingertips, palms, backs of the hand and wrists (Fig. 2.1) (RCN, 2019b).

KEY POINTS

- Hands should be decontaminated before and after all patient contact
- Hand hygiene must be performed (RCN, 2019b):
  - before putting on personal protective equipment and after taking it off
  - before giving the patient food or drinks
  - after making the patient's bed
  - after helping the patient back from the toilet
  - after removing any waste from the patient's living area
  - before eating
  - after using the toilet
  - after covering your own mouth and nose while coughing or sneezing
  - after using a disposable tissue
  - when you start and finish work

EQUIPMENT

- A sink with elbow- or foot-operated mixer taps should be used where possible.
- Liquid soap or antiseptic detergent hand washing solution
- Disposable paper hand towels
- Foot-operated waste bins.

PROCEDURE

1. Arms must be kept bare below the elbows when delivering nursing care.

2. Remove rings, jewellery and wristwatches. Some local policies may permit the wearing of a wedding band. This should be a plain band and loose enough to allow washing and drying underneath it. Wristwatches must not be worn, because they prevent effective washing of the wrist area and are a potential contaminant.
3. Cuts or abrasions on the hands should be covered by waterproof, occlusive dressings.
4. Fingernails should be short with no nail polish or artificial fingernails.
5. Taps should be adjusted so that the water temperature is comfortable, the flow is steady and does not splash the surrounding area. Wet the hands.
6. Apply sufficient soap or antiseptic detergent solution to create a good lather.
7. Hands should be rubbed briskly together, make sure that the thumbs, fingernails, fingertips, palms, backs of the hands and the wrists are all thoroughly washed (Fig. 2.2).
8. Scrubbing the skin with a brush causes microabrasions so be avoided, unless the fingernails are visibly dirty, when a nailbrush may be used.
9. Wash the hands for at least 20 seconds, then rinse thoroughly until all traces of soap/antiseptic detergent are removed.
10. Turn off the taps with your foot or elbow, and allow the water to run off your hands by holding them with the fingers pointing upwards. Please note, if the taps are not elbow or foot operated, leave the water running until after drying your hands and then use a paper towel to turn off the taps.
11. Dry your hands thoroughly using disposable paper towels, always working in one direction from your fingertips towards the wrists. Use a separate towel for each hand. Thorough drying is essential to minimise the growth of microorganisms and to prevent the hands becoming sore. Avoid overfilling of paper towel dispensers, because this prevents the towels from being easily dispensed.
12. Discard the used paper towels according to local policy.
13. Hand cream should be provided to staff to help maintain good skin condition. Communal tubs should be avoided; instead, hand cream should be available from pump or wall-mounted dispensers.

Use of Non-Sterile Gloves

Latex-free nonsterile gloves are now considered an infection prevention and control measure for protecting both patients and staff (RCN, 2018). Wearing non-sterile gloves is an accepted part of hand hygiene but does not replace the need for hand washing. In addition, prolonged use of gloves can increase the risk of work related dermatitis due to the chemicals involved in their manufacture (Dean, 2019. RCN, 2018). Increasingly awareness programmes aim to highlight the appropriate use of gloves and to prevent overuse (RCN, 2019a).

KEY FACTS

- Gloves provide a physical barrier that prevents healthcare staff from becoming contaminated with blood and bodily fluids, non-intact skin or mucous membranes.
- Gloves may also be used when handling chemical hazards (e.g. disinfectants or cytotoxic drugs).
- Gloves do not replace the need for hand hygiene (e.g. hand washing or use of alcohol hand gel).
- Gloves are single-use items that must be removed and changed between each patient or nursing intervention.
- Latex gloves should not be used if the patient has a latex allergy.

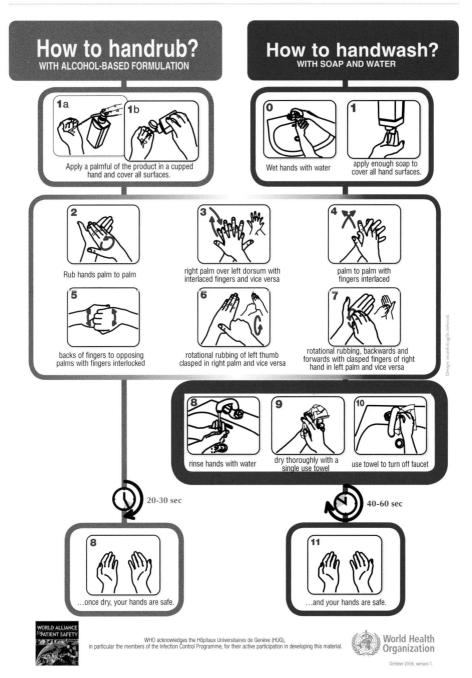

Fig. 2.2 Hand washing technique. (World Health Organization.)

EQUIPMENT

- Seamless, single-use gloves are recommended.

PROCEDURE

1. It is essential to choose the correct size of glove; otherwise, dexterity will be severely impaired.
2. If the gloves are required for a 'clean' procedure (e.g. blood glucose monitoring), they should be taken from a designated clean area where they are protected from dust.
3. Before and after glove use, appropriate hand hygiene must be performed.
4. Gloves should be put on only when the hands are thoroughly dry.
5. When used with an isolation gown, gloves must cover the wrist cuff.
6. Gloves should be changed if they are torn or become heavily contaminated.
7. Gloves should be removed when no longer required using the steps listed below.

TO REMOVE GLOVES

1. Grasp the outside of the glove with the opposite gloved hand, and peel the glove off.
2. Hold the removed glove in the gloved hand.
3. Slide the ungloved fingers under the remaining glove at the wrist.
4. Peel the second glove off over the first glove.
5. Gloves should be disposed of as clinical waste as per local policy and not left in the clinical environment.
6. Wash and dry the hands thoroughly.
7. Nurses should regularly assess their skin for early signs of dermatitis (e.g. itchy, dry or red skin). (Brown et al., 2019; Dean, 2019)

Putting on Sterile Gloves

Putting on sterile gloves differs from non-sterile gloves. The correct donning of sterile gloves can prevent the transmission of infection. Sterile gloves may be indicated for a variety of procedures, including wound dressings, insertion of a urinary catheter and cannulation. In some settings, sterile gloves may be included in the procedure pack.

EQUIPMENT

- Appropriately sized sterile gloves.

PROCEDURE

1. It is essential to choose the correct size of glove; otherwise dexterity will be severely impaired.
2. Before and after glove use, appropriate hand hygiene should be performed.
3. Gloves should be put on only when the hands are thoroughly dry.
4. Open the sterile glove package, and place the inner sterile pack on an appropriate surface (Fig. 2.3); open the pack, touching only the folded outer wrapper (Fig. 2.4).
5. Using your non-dominant hand, pick the glove up, touching only the inside of the glove cuff (i.e. the side that will be touching your skin) (Fig. 2.5) and insert your dominant

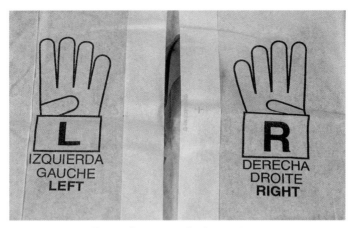

Fig. 2.3 Open the sterile glove package.

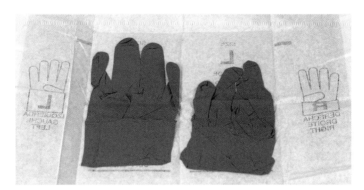

Fig. 2.4 Open the package, touching only the folded outer wrapper.

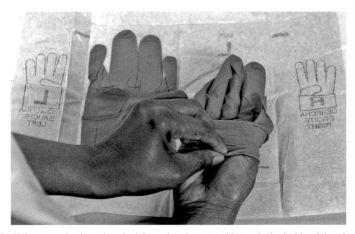

Fig. 2.5 Using your dominant hand, pick up the glove, touching only the inside of the glove cuff.

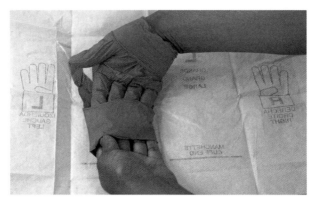

Fig. 2.6 Put on the second glove by putting the fingers of your gloved hand into the folded cuff of the glove.

hand. It is important to touch only the inside of the glove to prevent any potential contamination.

6. To put on the second glove, put the fingers of your gloved hand into the folded cuff of the other glove and lift it up (Fig. 2.6). Then pull the second glove over your hand.
7. Adjust your gloves as necessary. Avoid touching the skin and the cuff.

TO REMOVE GLOVES

1. Follow the same process as outlined on p. 10.
2. Nurses should regularly assess their skin for early signs of dermatitis (e.g. itchy, dry or red skin).

Use of Aprons

Aprons should be worn when there is direct patient contact or contact with body fluids and when handling bed linen, excreta, equipment, etc. from patients with infections such as MRSA or *C. difficile*. Plastic aprons may be available in a variety of colours. In some hospitals, different coloured aprons are used for specific purposes (e.g. for serving meals or performing aseptic dressings).

PROCEDURE

1. The apron should be put on after the hands have been washed (p. 9)
2. Wash and dry your hands thoroughly.
3. Pull the apron over your head; avoid touching your hair and clothing with your clean hands.
4. Tie the apron loosely at the back to avoid it becoming gathered at the waist, so that water splashes will run off easily.
5. If gloves are required, put them on after the apron and remove them before the apron is removed at the end of the procedure. Your gloves are likely to be more heavily contaminated

than your apron. Removing your gloves before the apron reduces the risk of contamination of your clothing when breaking the neckband and waist-ties to remove the apron.

6. To remove the apron, pull at the top to break the neckband and let the top fold down. Break the waist-ties and carefully fold the apron, touching only the 'clean' side, to prevent the spread of microorganisms. Folding the apron carefully as it is removed reduces the risk of shaking organisms into the air and your hands touch only the 'clean' side of the apron. Do not allow your hands to touch your uniform.
7. Discard the used apron into the clinical waste bag.
8. Wash and dry your hands thoroughly or use alcohol hand rub.

Use of Face Masks

When providing nursing care, it may be necessary to wear a face mask. The type of mask used depends on the situation (e.g. infectious case or working in the operating theatres). Consequently, nurses need to understand the different types of face masks used and select the most appropriate for the situation.

Fluid-resistant (type IIR) surgical masks (FRSMs) provide barrier protection against respiratory droplets reaching the mucosa of the mouth and nose (Public Health England, 2020). These types of masks are recommended for use in the operating theatre and if in contact with patients with pandemic flu. Surgical masks are worn by healthcare staff and patients, to prevent droplets being expelled from the mouth and nose into the environment. Eye protection (goggles or a visor) is added when there is a risk of splashing blood or body fluids into the mouth, nose or eyes (Public Health England, 2020).

Respirator masks are worn to protect healthcare workers from inhaling harmful respiratory particles. These masks are categorised according to their filtration efficiency (Table 2.1), and their use will be determined by your local policies and guidelines. Filtration face piece (FFP) masks are designed to allow expired air to escape via the valve in the mask and therefore will not prevent droplet or aerosol spread. They are worn in high-risk areas when dealing with highly virulent diseases (e.g. Covid-19) when aerosol-generating procedures (e.g. tracheal suctioning, intubation) are being performed.

When wearing an FFP 2 or 3 mask, the individual must be 'fit tested' and 'fit checked'. To make sure there is an adequate personal fit and seal, as only that way can individuals be protected.

TABLE 2.1 ▪ **Filtration Face Piece Protection Levels**

Filter Standard	Filter Capacity (Removal Percentage of All Particles ≥0.3 μm
FFP1	80%
FFP2	94%
N95	95%
FFP3	99%
N100	99.97%

FFP, Filtration face piece.
Sorbetto, M., El-Boghdadly, K., DiGiacinto, I., et al., 2020. The Italian corona virus disease 2019 outbreak: recommendations from clinical practice. Anaesthesia. doi:10.1111/anae.15049.

KEY POINTS

Patients may be required to wear a surgical face mask or FFP mask if they have a suspected or confirmed infectious respiratory condition (e.g. pulmonary tuberculosis or Covid-19). In consequence, nurses need to explain the rationale and how to wear the mask.

Face masks are used for different situations, nurses need to be able to select the appropriate mask for the situation.

All masks are single use only and cannot be reused once removed.

PROCEDURE

1. Before touching the mask, clean hands with an alcohol-based hand rub or soap and water.
2. If an apron or gown needs to be worn, this should be put on before the mask. Check carefully that you have the right type of mask.
3. Inspect the mask for tears or holes.
4. Orient which side is the top side (where the metal strip is).
5. Check the proper side of the mask faces outwards (the coloured side).
6. Place the mask to your face. Pinch the metal strip or stiff edge of the mask so it moulds to the shape of your nose.
7. Pull down the bottom of the mask so it covers your mouth and chin.
8. Secure the ties or stretch the elastic straps over the head. One tie should be above the ears in the middle of the head and the other below the ears at the neck.
9. Avoid touching the mask when it is being worn.
10. At the end of the care episode, remove the gloves, apron or gown and goggles (if worn) and then the mask. To remove the mask, remove the elastic loops from behind the ears while keeping the mask away from your face and clothes, to avoid touching potentially contaminated surfaces of the mask.
11. Discard the mask in a closed bin immediately after use.
12. Perform hand hygiene after touching or discarding the mask, using alcohol-based hand rub or, if visibly soiled, by washing your hands with soap and water.

References

Brown, L., Munro, J., Rogers, S., 2019. Use of personal protective equipment in nursing practice. Nurs. Stand. doi:10.7748/ns.2019.e11260.

Centres for Disease Control and Prevention, 2019. Standard Precautions. https://www.cdc.gov/oralhealth/infectioncontrol/summary-infection-prevention-practices/standard-precautions.html.

Dean, E., 2019. Correct use of gloves and how to protect the skin. Nurs. Stand. 34 (10), 67–88.

Fraise, A., Bradley, C., 2009. Ayliffe's Control of Healthcare-Associated Infection, fifth ed. Hodder Arnold, London.

Loveday, H.P., Wilson, J.A., Pratt, R.J., et al., 2014. epic3: National evidence-based guidelines for preventing healthcare-associated infections in NHS hospitals in England. J. Hosp. Infect. 86S1, S1–S70.

National Institute for Health and Care Excellence, 2017. Healthcare Associated Infections: Prevention and Control in Primary and Community Care. National Institute for Health and Care Excellence, London. www.nice.org.uk/guidance/cg139.

Public Health England, 2020. Guidance COVID-19 Personal Protective Equipment (PPE). Updated 21 May 2020. www.gov.uk.

Royal College of Nursing, 2017. Essential practice for infection prevention and control: guidance for nursing staff. Publication code: 005 940.

Royal College of Nursing, 2018. Tools of the trade: guidance for health care staff on glove use and the prevention of contact dermatitis. Publication Code: 006 922.

Royal College of Nursing, 2019. Essential practice for infection prevention and control guidance for nursing staff. Publication code: 005 940.

Royal College of Nursing, 2019a. Are You Glove Aware. https://www.rcn.org.uk/get-involved/campaign-with-us/glove-awareness.

Royal College of Nursing, 2019b. Hand Hygiene. https://rcni.com/hosted-content/rcn/first-steps/hand-hygiene.

Sorbetto, M., El-Boghdadly, K., DiGiacinto, I., et al., 2020. The Italian corona virus disease 2019 outbreak: recommendations from clinical practice. Anaesthesia. doi:10.1111/anae.15049.

CHAPTER 3

Patient Assessment

Nursing Assessment and Individualised Patient Care

RATIONALE

Assessing a patients' health needs is a core component of the role of the registered nurse (Nursing and Midwifery Council, 2019). Assessment, planning, decision-making and goal setting allows for the development of person-centred, evidence based, individual nursing care plan and goals. The type of assessment used will depend on the type of clinical setting and patient group. This approach supports objective evaluation of care delivery. In this chapter, the core elements of assessment are outlined and key definitions provided. This involves assessment of physical, mental, cognitive, behavioural, social and spiritual needs (NMC, 2018). The assessment consists of taking a detailed history and may include information on the patients' past medical history, travel history, allergies and information around the patients' presenting complaint. During the assessment, the nurse should gather objective and subjective information to analyse and develop the actual or potential problems to formulate the nursing diagnosis (Ballanytne, 2016; Peate, 2016). During the nursing process, you must provide clear, simple explanations appropriate to the patient's level of understanding.

> **KEY FACTS**
>
> - The clinical setting and patient status determine the type and nature of health assessment performed.
> - A range of assessment strategies and tools are available, with the Airway, Breathing, Circulation, Disability (neurological) and Exposure (A-E) approach being among the most commonly used.
> - Clinical assessment tools, care bundles and care pathways can all enhance patient care by providing evidence based, systematic approaches to specific conditions and clinical situations.

NURSING PROCESS

The nursing process is internationally recognised as an approach to identify the priorities and requirements for evidence based, person-centered, interventions and support (Peate, 2016). There are five stages involved in the nursing process, including assessment, nursing diagnosis, planning, implementation and evaluation (Ballantyne, 2016). However, since it's inception in the 1950's, there have been significant changes in the role and function of nurses (Toney-Butler & Thayer, 2022). As a result individual countries have developed their own process (based on the nursing processes) for nursing care (NMC, 2019).

In the UK, assessing needs and planning care is one of the seven platforms developed reflecting the expectations of Registered Nurses (NMC, 2019). However Stonehouse (2017) argues that as care is now delivered by a range of members of the multi-disciplinary team working in partnership, a more appropriate term would be the 'care planning process'.

CARE PATHWAYS

A care pathway is an interdisciplinary approach to a patient's condition, which uses patient centric clinical decision making strategies. This provides a standardised, evidence based approaches to care (NHS England, 2020). Documentation tends to be multiprofessional to aid communication and support the patient meeting specific predetermined goals and targets. Examples include Stroke Care Pathways, Fractured Neck of Femur Care Pathway, Chest Pain and Acute Coronary Syndrome Care Pathway.

CLINICAL ASSESSMENT TOOLS

Clinical assessment tools aid the nurses' decision making during the assessment, implementation and evaluation of care. Examples of clinical assessment tools include the National Early Warning Scoring (NEWS) tool and the Glasgow Coma Scale (GCS).

CARE BUNDLES

A care bundle differs from a care plan as it consisting of a series of evidence-based interventions that, when implemented together, have a more significant impact than when applied individually. The use of care bundles has resulted in a move away from the use of individualised patient-specific nursing care plans (Ballantyne, 2016; Healthcare Improvement Scotland, 2020). In many settings, both care plans and care bundles are used to guide patient care.

Care bundles are used for a specific intervention or situation and aim to provide patient safety, consistency and cost-effectiveness (Ballantyne, 2016). Examples include the 'Ventilator Care Bundle' to reduce ventilator-associated pneumonia and 'Sepsis Care Bundle' for the recognition and management of patients with confirmed or suspected sepsis.

Assessment of the Deteriorating Patient

Essential physiological observations for these patients are respiratory rate, oxygen saturations, pulse rate, blood pressure, temperature, conscious level using the Alert, Confused, Voice, Pain and Unresponsive (AVPU) assessment or the GCS scale, pain score and urine output (Carter et al., 2020). In many settings, an Early Warning Scoring (EWS) tool (sometimes known as Patient at Risk Scores) should be used to monitor all adult patients. EWS is a scoring system that uses the physiological measurements, routinely recorded, to identify acutely ill patients. In England, a nationally agreed upon tool has been developed, termed the NEWS (National Institute for Health and Care Excellence [NICE], 2020) (Fig. 3.1).

KEY POINTS

- Early Warning Score tools require full sets of vital signs to be performed.
- Physiological observations should be monitored at least every 12 hours, unless a decision has been made by a senior nurse or doctor to increase or decrease this frequency for an individual patient.
- Use of an EWS tool should not replace clinical acumen or the need for a comprehensive patient assessment; it should be used to support clinical decision making and not replace it.

Physiological parameter	Score						
	3	2	1	0	1	2	3
Respiration rate (per minute)	≤8		9–11	12–20		21–24	≥25
SpO$_2$ Scale 1 (%)	≤91	92–93	94–95	≥96			
SpO$_2$ Scale 2 (%)	≤83	84–85	86–87	88–92 ≥93 on air	93–94 on oxygen	95–96 on oxygen	≥97 on oxygen
Air or oxygen?		Oxygen		Air			
Systolic blood pressure (mmHg)	≤90	91–100	101–110	111–219			≥220
Pulse (per minute)	≤40		41–50	51–90	91–110	111–130	≥131
Consciousness				Alert			CVPU
Temperature (°C)	≤35.0		35.1–36.0	36.1–38.0	38.1–39.0	≥39.1	

Fig. 3.1 National early warning scoring tool. (Reproduced from Royal College of Physicians, 2017. National Early Warning Score (NEWS) 2: Standardising the Assessment of Acute-illness Severity in the NHS. Updated report of a working party. RCP, London.)

Each physiological observation is awarded a score. The overall score is calculated which then indicates the action required (Fig. 3.2) (e.g. more frequent observations or reporting to a doctor or senior nurse).

Abnormalities in physiological parameters of temperature, cardiovascular, respiratory or central nervous system observations and urine output are indicators that the patient may be deteriorating. EWS tools aim to predict which patients are in need of urgent attention, allow

NEW score	Clinical risk	Response
Aggregate score 0–4	Low	Ward-based response
Red score Score of 3 in any individual parameter	Low–medium	Urgent ward-based response*
Aggregate score 5–6	Medium	Key threshold for urgent response*
Aggregate score 7 or more	High	Urgent or emergency response**

* Response by a clinician or team with competence in the assessment and treatment of acutely ill patients and in recognising when the escalation of care to a critical care team is appropriate.

**The response team must also include staff with critical care skills, including airway management.

Fig. 3.2 Escalation. (Reproduced from: Royal College of Physicians, 2017. National Early Warning Score (NEWS) 2: Standardising the Assessment of Acute-illness Severity in the NHS. Updated report of a working party. RCP, London.)

preventive measures to be taken and identify those patients who might need a step up to higher levels of care (Mayo, 2017). In addition, trends in observations should also be noted because this provides a more detailed and accurate understanding of the patient's condition over time. Physiological observations and NEWS should form part of a comprehensive patient assessment (page 20).

A–E Assessment

USING ABCDE TO ASSESS PATIENTS

Although the NEWS (see p. 19) is a useful tool in identifying the effect of vital signs on the patient's physiological wellbeing, it does not give guidance regarding the details of assessment or how to prioritise patient need (Mayo, 2017). It is therefore recommended, that nurses use a systematic assessment framework when assessing ill adult patients, such as the ABCDE: Airway, Breathing, Circulation, Disability and Exposure (Resuscitation Council, 2021). Using this helps identification and appropriate management of critical illness (Mayo, 2017). This framework can be used in all clinical settings, and not only during emergency situations.

A: Airway

It is important to establish if the patient is responsive and therefore able to maintain his or her own airway. Talk to the patient, and note the ability to respond. Ask the patient specific questions such as 'Are you in pain?' or 'How are you feeling?' If the patient can talk, this indicates a patent airway. An unresponsive patient may not be able to protect their airway; therefore the following are signs of concern and warrant immediate reporting/intervention:

No response—the patient may be unconscious or unable to speak. If no air can be felt from the nose or mouth, this indicates an airway obstruction. Grunting, gurgling, snoring or 'barking'—noises other than talking may indicate a partial airway obstruction caused by swelling, spasm or inhalation of a foreign body.

Urgent help should be summoned and the patient's airway should be opened using head tilt/chin lift (see p. 331).

B: Breathing

When assessing the patient's breathing, it is important to 'Look, listen and report'.

Look—at the patient's chest

Are they struggling to breathe?

- Do they have an increased work of breathing (i.e. using accessory muscles in the neck, the abdomen and between the ribs)?
- Count the respiratory rate for 1 minute. The normal rate for adults is 12 to 20 breaths/min. Tachypnoea and bradypnoea should be reported (see p. 26).
- Is the chest rising equally (i.e. is the movement the same on both sides?)? Lack of symmetry may indicate an underlying lung or rib problem.
- Observe the depth of breathing—is it deep or shallow? Very deep slow breaths may indicate metabolic abnormalities or raised intracranial pressure. Shallow breaths may be due to pain or medication.
- Observe the peripheral oxygen saturation (SpO2) reading (normal 95% to 100%; see p. 36). A low SpO_2 could indicate hypoxia or respiratory distress (Elliott and Baird, 2019).

Listen—for any abnormal noises

Normal breathing is a relatively quiet activity. Noises such as wheezing (a high-pitched sound) may indicate narrowed airways, whereas gurgling or rattling may indicate fluid in the lungs. Coughing may be caused by infection or irritation within the lungs or airways.

Report any abnormalities found when assessing the patient's breathing must be reported immediately because they may indicate a serious problem. If the patient's condition allows, help the patient to sit in an upright comfortable position because this will help with lung expansion and breathing.

C: Circulation

The cardiovascular system can be affected by different problems such as haemorrhage, acute fluid loss or cardiac events such as myocardial infarction, sepsis or medication. The following should be assessed, and any abnormalities should be reported immediately because they may indicate a serious problem.

- Pulse (heart rate)—noting strength, rate and rhythm (see p. 78).
- Blood pressure (see p. 78).
- Capillary refill time, especially if haemorrhage is suspected.
- Urine output and fluid intake—poor urine output may indicate hypovolaemia.
- Temperature.
- Skin temperature—cool skin may indicate peripheral vasoconstriction; hot skin may indicate severe pyrexia.
- Does the patient need an electrocardiogram (ECG)? This is indicated if there is chest pain, collapse or difficulty in breathing.
- Has the patient undergone a surgical procedure? If so, check wound sites, drains, etc. for signs of bleeding.
- Central venous pressure (CVP)—if the patient has a central line, then a CVP measurement may be useful. Low CVP may suggest fluid loss; high CVP may suggest fluid overload or pulmonary oedema.

D: Disability (Including Diabetes and Drugs)

Disability in this context means the patient's neurological state, specifically their level of consciousness. Assess the patient's level of consciousness using the GCS or AVPU (p. 92). A patient with an altered level of consciousness is at risk of airway obstruction and should be observed closely or, if their condition allows, placed in the recovery position. Sudden-onset confusion or agitation must be reported.

Diabetes

   Low or high blood glucose levels can cause altered levels of consciousness; therefore the 'D' assessment should always include a blood glucose measurement if the patient is drowsy or unconscious for an unknown reason.

Drugs

   Certain medications (e.g. opiates, sedatives and anaesthetics) can cause an altered level of consciousness, therefore this needs to be taken into account. The patient's medication chart should be checked to see if this is the cause of the patient's deterioration.

Any abnormalities found when assessing 'Disability' must be reported immediately because they may indicate a serious problem.

E: Exposure (Plus Environment)

Maintain patient privacy and dignity, when the patient needs to be undressed to observe for other signs or causes of deterioration such as rashes, wounds, leg swelling or infected tissue. At this point the patient's overall skin integrity can be noted:

- Is it dry and flaky or warm and well perfused?
- Is the patient at risk of pressure ulcer formation? Is a further risk assessment needed (see p. 298?)
- Has the patient been incontinent when he or she is usually continent?

At this stage, consider 'Have I missed anything in my assessment?'

Any abnormalities found when assessing 'Exposure' must be reported immediately because they may indicate a serious problem.

Communicating Your Assessment Using Situation, Background, Assessment and Recommendation

Following assessment of the patient using ABCDE and/or EWS, it may be necessary to report your assessment to a doctor/senior nurse so that the patient can receive urgent care and treatment. Situation, Background, Assessment and Recommendation (SBAR) is an easily remembered mnemonic that provides a structure for such conversations. It is especially useful when trying to communicate in challenging or critical clinical situations where accuracy and time are critical. When used correctly, SBAR enhances patient safety and has been shown to improve outcomes for patients (Müller et al., 2018). When communicating with other healthcare professionals, a polite and professional approach is essential, no matter how stressed you may be feeling. Using a framework such as SBAR helps to achieve this and to obtain the optimal care and treatment for patients. The following example has been adapted from National Health Service (NHS) Improvement (2018) recommending the use of SBAR.

KEY POINTS

- Situation, Background, Assessment and Recommendation (SBAR) is an easy to use, structured form of communication that enables information to be transferred accurately between individuals.
- SBAR is used to share concise information often in an emergency setting.

SITUATION, BACKGROUND, ASSESSMENT AND RECOMMENDATION

All names and wards are fictitious. Each section of SBAR is broken down and used sequentially:

Situation
- Identify yourself by name and the ward/unit you are calling from
- Identify the patient by name and the reason for your call
- Describe your concern or the problem.

For example:

This is Elaine, staff nurse on Ward 16. I am calling about Mr Ahmed in bed 34. Mr Ahmed has suddenly become short of breath, and his respiration rate has increased to 24 breaths per minute. His oxygen saturations dropped to 88% on room air, so I started him on 24% oxygen, but there has been no improvement in the past 5 minutes (Fig. 3.3).

Background
- Give the patient's reason for admission and when he was admitted
- Explain any significant medical history (you may need the patient's notes for this).

He was admitted yesterday under the care of Dr Sharp, with an exacerbation of chronic obstructive pulmonary disease (COPD). After a chest x-ray this morning, he was started on intravenous (IV) antibiotics. He has been admitted a number of times with COPD, and he also has angina and prostate cancer.

Assessment
- Report any other important vital signs
- If you have found other clinical concerns or signs during your assessment, state them here.

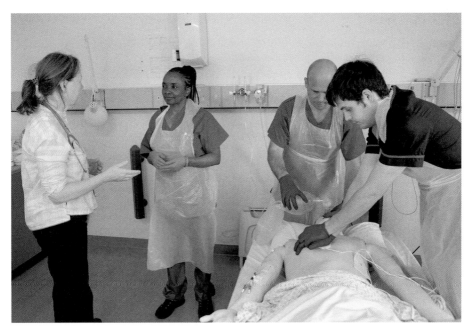

Fig. 3.3 Situation, Background, Assessment and Recommendation communication

When I assessed him just now, his heart rate is up to 110 and blood pressure is 85/50. He isn't pyrexial, but he looks flushed and unwell. He is really struggling to breathe and says that he has bilateral chest pain.

Recommendation

Explain what you need—be specific about your request and time frame, for example:

I am very concerned about Mr Ahmed and would like you to come to see him immediately. Should I keep him on 24% oxygen?

- Make suggestions (e.g. 'Shall I do an ECG?')
- Clarify your expectations (e.g. 'I will tell the family that you will be here within 30 minutes'.)
- If the person you call is unable to help, clarify who you should call next.

References

Ballantyne, N., 2016. Developing nursing care plans. Nurs. Stand. 30 (26), 51–57.

Barrett, D., Wilson, B., Woodlands, A., 2012. Care Planning: A Guide for Nurses, second ed. Routledge, Abingdon.

Carter C. Aedy H. Notter J. (2020). Covid-19 disease: assessment of a critically ill patient. Clinics in Integrated Care. 1. 100001. doi.org/10.1016/j.intcar.2020.100001

Elliott, M. and Baird, J., 2019. Pulse oximetry and the enduring neglect of respiratory rate assessment: a commentary on patient surveillance. British Journal of Nursing, 28(19), pp. 1256–1259.

Healthcare Improvement Scotland, 2020. SSKIN care bundle. https://www.healthcareimprovementscotland. org/our_work/patient_safety/tissue_viability/sskin_care_bundle.aspx.

NHS Improvement, 2018. SBAR Communication Tool-Situation, Background, Assessment, Recommendation. www.improvement.nhs.uk

NHS England, 2020. Rightcare: community rehabilitation tool kit. https://www.england.nhs.uk/rightcare/products/pathways/community-rehabilitation-toolkit/.

Nursing and Midwifery Council, (2018). The Code: professional standards of practice and behaviour for nurses, midwives and nursing associates. www.nmc.org.uk

Nursing & Midwifery Council, 2019. Future Nurse: Standards of Proficiency for Registered Nurses. London.

National Institute for Health and Care Excellence, 2020. National Early Warning Score systems that alert to deteriorating adult patients in hospital. Medtech innovation briefing. Published 18 February 2020.

Matthews, E., 2010. Nursing Care Planning Made Incredibly Easy! Lippincott Williams & Wilkins, Philadelphia, PA.

Mayo, P., 2017. Undertaking an accurate and comprehensive assessment of the acutely ill adult. Nurs. Stand. 32 (8), 53–61. September 2017. doi:10.7748/ns.2017.e10968.

Müller, M., Jürgens, J., Redaèlli, M., et al., 2018. Impact of the communication and patient hand-off tool SBAR on patient safety: a systematic review. BMJ Open. 8, e022202. doi:10.1136/bmjopen-2018-022202.

Peate, I., 2016. Health assessment. In: Peate, I. (Ed.), Medical-Surgical Nursing at a Glance. Wiley Blackwell.

Resuscitation Council (UK), 2021. Advanced Life Support, eighth edition RCUK, London.

Royal College of Physicians, 2017. National Early Warning Score (NEWS) 2: Standardising the Assessment of Acute-illness Severity in the NHS. Updated report of a working party. RCP, London.

Stonehouse, D., 2017. Understanding the nursing process. British Journal of Healthcare Assistants, 11(8), pp. 388–391.

Toney-Butler, T.J., Thayer, J.M., 2022. Nursing Process. In: StatPearls [Internet]. Treasure Island (FL). StatPearls Publishing. Available from: https://www.ncbi.nlm.nih.gov/books/NBK499937/.

CHAPTER 4

Respiratory Assessment

Respiratory Assessment

A well-functioning respiratory system is vital for the exchange of oxygen and carbon dioxide, which is an essential physiological function. A respiratory assessment is used as a key indicator of general health and forms a core element of the nursing assessment. A systematic approach using step-by-step methods are essential if a thorough assessment is to be completed. To carry out a comprehensive assessment, nurses need to have good communication, skills and the knowledge to observe and interpret key information. This involves analysing a range of data, including self-reports, history taking, observations, inspection, palpation, percussion and auscultation. Interpretation of objective data such as respiratory rate, depth, pattern, oxygen saturation levels and analysis of arterial blood gases (ABGs) is also essential to form a holistic assessment. This chapter will cover the key essential skills required to perform an in-depth respiratory assessment.

KEY POINTS

- Systematic approach to respiratory assessment is essential
- Detailed history taking is part of the respiratory assessment
- An accurate count of respiratory rate over 1 minute must be taken.
- Physical assessment involves three stages: auscultation, palpation and percussion
- Peripheral oxygen saturation (SpO_2) monitoring can be used in conjunction with other assessments but should not be used as a stand-alone method of respiratory assessment

History taking is an important element of assessment of respiratory function. Nurses need to ascertain information regarding general health and wellbeing as well as specific information. For any patient who is unable to give a an oral history, nurses must seek information from relatives/carers and medical notes (Simpson, 2015; Morgan, 2021). Information can include:

- History of presenting complaint e.g. coughing or breathlessness
- Social and lifestyle history (e.g. smoking, environmental factors and exercise tolerance)
- Relevant past medical history specifically checking for any chronic respiratory conditions
- Family health
- Travel history
- Employment history
- An assessment of any signs of confusion, agitation, anxiety or distress.
- Ask if any previous use of non-invasive ventilation (see p. 53).

Inspection

Ideally the patient should be sitting upright in a comfortable position, in a warm and well-lit environment.

Inspection includes:

1. Assessment of pattern of speech and any signs of shortness of breath, wheezing, stridor or gurgling
2. Assessment of whether patient has a cough (productive, dry or hacking)
3. Assessment of the use of accessory muscles, any nasal flaring and respiratory effort (work of breathing). Accessory muscles are the sternocleidomastoid and trapezius muscles in the neck and shoulders. If these are being used (noticed by contraction of these muscles), it indicates that the patient is unable to use their diaphragm and external intercostal muscles adequately (Massey and Meredith, 2010).
4. Observation of chest expansion and chest wall movement. The chest should rise and fall equally and symmetrically. If one side does not move as well as the other, this could indicate a pneumothorax (collapsed lung), bronchial obstruction or injury.
5. A full count a respiratory rate and rhythm over 1 minute (see p. 26). If breathing is very shallow and difficult to observe, lightly rest your hand on the patient's chest or abdomen to feel movement. The normal rate for an adult is 12 to 20 breaths per minute.
6. Identification of deformities, discolouration, scars, lesions or chest wall masses
7. Observation of sputum and type, amount, colour and consistency (see p. 27)
8. Evidence of clubbing or peripheral oedema
9. Observation of general health status and skin colour, including any signs of cyanosis (peripheral or central). Cyanosis is a blue discolouration of the skin and mucous membranes and is most noticeable around the lips, earlobes, mouth and fingertips. In darker-skinned patients, signs of poor perfusion or cyanosis may be more difficult to detected as changes in skin colour are less obvious.

Counting a Respiratory Rate

One of the key steps in a respiratory assessment is to count the number of respirations over 1 minute. The normal respiration rate for a patient at rest is 12 to 20 breaths per minute. Anything greater or less than this rate is abnormal and warrants further investigation (Simpson, 2015; Morgan, 2021). However, it has to be noted that normal respiratory rates vary between physiological textbooks and Early Warning Scores (Grant, 2018). Consequently, the respiratory rate should be applied within the context of the patient's condition and any increasing or decreasing trends noted.

It is important to count respirations over a full 1 minute because a shorter period may result in inaccurate results. A raised respiratory rate is one of the first signs of a rise in the work of breathing and critical illness (Resuscitation Council, 2021), and close attention must always be paid to this parameter. The respiratory rate should be regular and quiet. Normal breathing involves the diaphragm and the intercostal muscles, with both sides of the chest should showing equal expansion, with the trachea positioned in the middle. Any visible abnormalities such as tracheal deviation should be treated as a medical emergency. The normal inspiratory to expiratory (I:E) ratio is 1:2. Inspiration is active, and expiration is passive. This is an easy assessment can be performed in any clinical setting, however, it is often overlooked or incorrectly performed (Rolfe, 2019).

PROCEDURE

The patient should be relaxed and resting, or recent any activity must be taken into account.
If necessary, help the patient into as upright a posture as is possible and comfortable.

Do not inform the patient when you will be assessing breathing, because a more accurate observation is obtained if the patient is unaware that their respirations are being counted.

Using a watch with a second hand, count the respirations for 60 seconds.

Observe the movement of the chest wall for symmetry of chest movement—this is best observed in front of the patient rather than at the side.

Observe whether accessory muscles are being used.

Observe the rhythm and depth of respirations.

Observe for the following:

- difficulty in, or struggling with, breathing
- pain on breathing and its location
- Noisy respiration—whether there is any wheeze or stridor (high-pitched sounds).
- Cough—whether dry or productive.
- Sputum—amount, colour and consistency (see p. 27).

Observe the patient's colour for signs of cyanosis.

Document the respiratory observations according to local policy and report any deviation from the normal rate.

Adjust the frequency of observations as necessary.

Check the patient is comfortable. Breathless patients may be most comfortable sitting in a chair.

Observation of Sputum

Mucus is produced in the respiratory system and secreted by the goblet cells found in the epithelial surface lining the airways of the respiratory tract and from seromucous glands in the connective tissue beneath the mucosal epithelium (Shepherd, 2017). Mucus production is a normal function because it allows humidification of air passing through the respiratory tract, traps dust particles, bacteria, other inhaled debris and destroys bacterial. Smoking, infection (viral, bacterial or fungal), chronic lung diseases and cystic fibrosis may produce excess sputum which needs to be expectorated. Observation of sputum and the type, amount, colour and consistency is necessary to ascertain the requirement for obtaining a sputum specimen.

EQUIPMENT

Disposable sputum carton with lid
Tissues
Clinical waste bag
Personal protective equipment (PPE; see p. 5)

PROCEDURE

Explain the procedure, then gain consent and cooperation

Maintain privacy—the patient may be distressed or embarrassed at having to expectorate.

Decontaminate and wear gloves and aprons. Gloves and apron should be worn if the patient needs assistance with expectoration, use of tissues, etc.

Additional PPE may be necessary if indicated by the patient's condition e.g. Covid-19. (see Chapter 2).

Expectoration will be easier if the patient is sitting up, supported by pillows, or is sitting in an armchair.

Encourage the patient to expectorate into the sputum pot rather than swallowing the sputum. 'Huffing' may help the patient to expectorate. The assistance of a physiotherapist may be necessary to teach the patient how to breathe deeply and expectorate without strain rather than coughing ineffectively.

Observe the sputum for the following:

- Quantity
- Consistency: whether watery, frothy or tenacious (sticky)
- Colour: clear (normal mucous); white and frothy (pulmonary oedema); yellow/green (pus- infected); black flecks (smoke inhalation)
- Fresh blood (haemoptysis—trauma, tuberculosis or tumour)
- Odour: foul-smelling sputum may indicate a lung abscess.

A mouthwash or drink should be offered after expectoration.

Replace lid and remove used sputum pot after observation, and discard in clinical waste bin.

Provide the patient with clean sputum pot, and ensure they are comfortable. The patient may feel very tired after a bout of coughing.

Remove gloves and apron, and decontaminate hands.

Document findings and report any changes or abnormalities.

Obtaining a Sputum Specimen

A sputum specimen is the collection of a sample for laboratory analysis to identify the bacterial, viral of fungal causes of a suspected infection and its sensitivities to antibiotics. Ideally, sputum samples should be taken before antibiotics are started (Shepherd, 2017). Some tests require several samples for analysis; for example, three consecutive early-morning specimens may be requested for acid-fast bacilli (tuberculosis) or for cytology (malignant cells). Care must be taken when helping obtain a sputum specimen as droplets and aerosols may be generated during the procedure, PPE be used as per local policies (including gloves, apron and face masks).

EQUIPMENT

Universal specimen pot
Plastic specimen bag and label or laboratory request form
Drinking water and mouthwash
Tissues
Gloves and apron to be worn if the patient needs assistance with expectoration, use of tissues, etc.
Additional PPE if indicated by the patient's condition (see Chapter 2).

PROCEDURE

Explain the procedure and the number of specimens required.

Ask the patient to rinse their mouth thoroughly with water (not mouthwash) before expectoration, to reduce contamination of the specimen with food.

Ask/assist the patient to expectorate into the sterile pot. When obtaining the specimen, it is important to check that it is mucoid or mucopurulent, which indicates that it is sputum and not just saliva.

Seal the lid, and complete the label with the date, patient's full name, hospital number, ward and type of specimen (Fig. 4.1).

Place the pot and the laboratory request form in a plastic specimen bag, and dispatch it to the laboratory straight away. This is essential because respiratory pathogens do not survive for long periods. For example, if refrigerated for more than 12 hours, *Haemophilus*

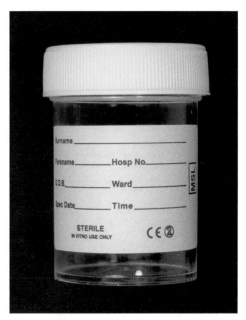

Fig. 4.1 Sputum specimen pot.

influenzae and *Streptococcus pneumoniae* may die and gram-negative organisms overgrow in the specimen.

Check that the patient is comfortable and offer a mouthwash and/or tissues as appropriate.

Dispose of any waste appropriately.

Remove gloves and apron. Decontaminate hands.

Document that the specimen has been obtained. Note colour, smell and consistency of specimen.

Auscultation

Auscultation is an important component of the respiratory assessment and is also used as part of cardiac and gastrointestinal examinations. This procedure should always form part of a holistic assessment (see p. 20) and must be considered with the patient's history (see p. 25) (Proctor and Rickards, 2020). Auscultation of the chest requires a stethoscope and a quiet environment, with the patient should ideally sitting in an upright position. Nurses need to recognise normal breath sounds and how they can be heard across the lung fields.

USING A STETHOSCOPE

If using a communal stethoscope, clean it, remember to use an alcohol-impregnated swab for the earpieces. Curving the ends of the stethoscope slightly forwards, place the ear pieces in your ears. This will help to create a seal and will reduce external noise.

If a stethoscope has two sides (Fig. 4.2), check that it is turned to the diaphragm side by tapping it with your fingers. In addition, if the stethoscope feels cold, it should be warmed between your hands before applying it to the chest to avoid discomfort for the patient.

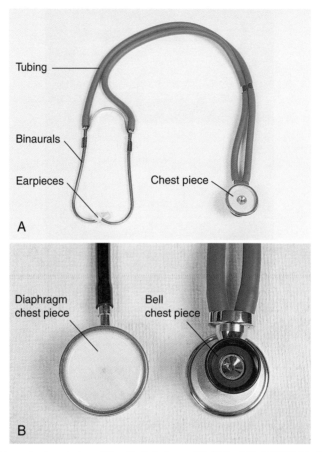

Fig. 4.2 Stethoscope showing earpieces [A] and ball diaphragm [B]. (Shiland, B. J. (2050). *Medical Assistant: Cardiopulmonary Systems, Vital Signs, Electrocardiography and CPR—Module D*, 2nd ed. Elsevier Inc.)

PROCEDURE

1. Discuss the procedure with the patient and gain informed consent.
2. Check that the patient is kept warm and the area is free from drafts.
3. Maintain privacy and dignity by screening the bed area.
4. Decontaminate hands, and wear personal protective equipment (PPE) as necessary (see chapter 2).
5. Position the patient comfortably so you can access the chest.
6. Remove or rearrange the patient's clothing as necessary to enable you to see the chest.
7. Gently place the chest piece of the stethoscope flat on the patient's chest, holding it between the index and middle fingers of your dominant hand.
8. Listen for breath sounds on the anterior chest first (Fig. 4.3). Each side should be compared in a systematic manner to detect any asymmetry. The stethoscope should be in contact with the chest for a full cycle of inspiration and expiration at each point on the chest. The scapula should be avoided as lung sounds cannot be heard through bone (Fig. 4.4).

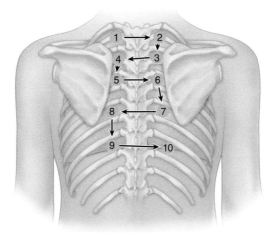

Fig. 4.3 Anterior landmarks for chest auscultation. (Silvestri, L., Kaushik, A., Silvestri, A. (2020). *Saunders Comprehensive Review for the NCLEX-RN® Examination*, 3rd South Asia ed. Elsevier Inc.)

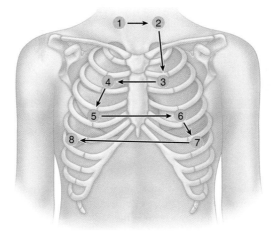

Fig. 4.4 Posterior landmarks for chest auscultation. (Silvestri, L., Kaushik, A., Silvestri, A. (2020). *Saunders Comprehensive Review for the NCLEX-RN® Examination*, 3rd South Asia ed. Elsevier Inc.)

9. Ask the patient to move their right arm to the side so the right lateral chest can be assessed. Starting with the upper lobe, move to the middle lobe and finally the lower lobe.
10. Repeat on the left side, where the lung is made up of an upper lobe and lower lobe.
11. Replace the patient's clothing and make them comfortable.
12. Explain your findings to the patient, and check whether they have any questions.
13. Decontaminate and clean your stethoscope.
14. Decontaminate hands and remove any PPE.
15. Document your findings.

Normal breath sounds include:
- Bronchial: A loud, high-pitched sound being blown through a hollow pipe, heard over the sternum. The expiratory phase is longer than the inspiratory phase.
- Bronchovesicular: Combination of bronchial and vesicular sounds that tends to be heard over the first and second intercostal spaces near the sternum. The inspiratory and expiratory phases are equal.
- Vesicular: A soft and low-pitched sound heard over the peripheries of the lungs. The inspiratory phase is longer than the expiratory phase, and there is no pause between the phases.

Other sounds include:
- Crackles: caused by the transmission of bronchial sounds through consolidated lung tissue, commonly associated with atelectasis and acute respiratory distress syndrome (ARDS). Described as a short, explosive, non-musical sound that can be either coarse or fine. Crackles are caused by sputum in the bronchi and trachea.
- Wheeze: Associated with musical noises, either monophonic (single) or polyphonic (multiple short and long noises) high or low pitch, and can be heard in either inspiration or expiration.
- Stridor is another type of wheeze but originates from an upper airway partial obstruction. Often heard without a stethoscope. May be heard following extubation due to laryngeal oedema.
- Pleural rubs: Heard in patients who have inflamed or thickened pleural membranes. They sound longer and lower pitched than a crackle and, depending on the size of the affected area, can be heard in different parts of the chest wall and may change between inspiration and expiration (Edwards and Williams, 2019).

Palpation

Palpation involves placing the palm of the hands lightly over the chest wall. The purpose of palpation is to provide information about underlying respiratory structures and to identify any abnormities. The procedure is carried out in the sequence is outlined in Figs 4.5 and 4.6.

PROCEDURE

1. Discuss the procedure with the patient, and gain informed consent.
2. Check that the patient is kept warm and the area is free from drafts.
3. Maintain privacy and dignity by screening the bed area.
4. Decontaminate hands, and wear PPE as necessary (chapter 2).
5. Position the patient comfortably so you can access the chest.
6. Remove or rearrange the patient's clothing as necessary to enable you to see the chest.
7. Confirm the central position of the trachea.
8. Place your hands on the chest, and feel for fremitus. Fremitus refers to vibrations which can be felt on palpation. These can be referred to as normal, increased or decreased.
9. Evaluate thoracic expansion for symmetry of movement. Normal palpation should reveal equal expansion on both sides of the chest. The degree of movement can also be considered.
10. Observe the chest to note any pain, scars, lumps or lesions. In addition, note any medication patches (e.g. glyceryl trinitrate (GTN) or slow-release analgesia).
11. Replace the patient's clothing and make them comfortable.
12. Explain your findings to the patient, and check whether they have any questions.

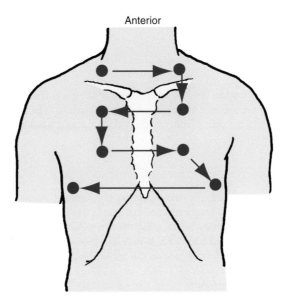

Fig. 4.5 Anterior landmarks for chest palpation. (Des Jardins, T., & Burton, G. G. (2019). *Clinical Manifestations & Assessment of Respiratory Disease*. Elsevier.)

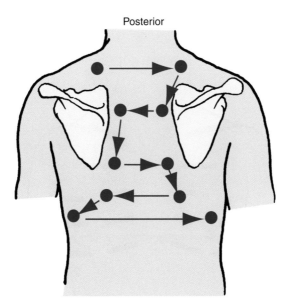

Fig. 4.6 Posterior landmarks for chest palpation. (Des Jardins, T., & Burton, G. G. (2019). *Clinical Manifestations & Assessment of Respiratory Disease*. Elsevier.)

13. Decontaminate and clean your stethoscope.
14. Decontaminate hands and remove any PPE.
15. Document your findings.

Percussion

Percussion of the chest provides further information about the underlying lung structure and assessing the lungs for the presence of air, liquid or solid material. The movement of the hands during percussion moves the tissue underneath, and as a result, audible sounds are produced (Simpson, 2015).

PROCEDURE

1. Discuss the procedure with the patient, and gain informed consent.
2. Check that the patient is kept warm and the area is free from drafts.
3. Maintain privacy and dignity by screening the bed area.
4. Decontaminate hands, and wear PPE as necessary (see chapter 2).
5. Position the patient comfortably so you can access the chest.
6. Remove or rearrange the patient's clothing as necessary to enable you to see the chest.
7. Percussion should be performed using two hands. One hand is placed on the chest with separated fingers. The middle finger of the other hand is used to strike the finger joint of the other hand. Loud sounds indicate air-filled spaces, whereas dull sounds indicate consolidation with either fluid or secretions. The procedure should be carried out as outlined in Figs 4.7 and 4.8.
8. Replace the patient's clothing and make them comfortable.

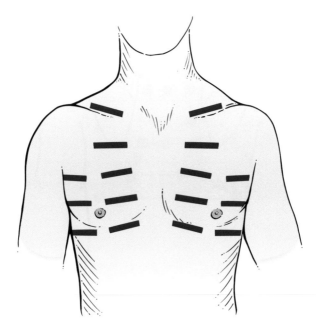

Fig. 4.7 Anterior landmarks for chest percussion. (Swartz, M. H. (2021). *Textbook of Physical Diagnosis: History and Examination*, 8th ed. Elsevier Inc.)

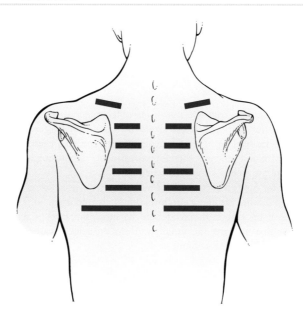

Fig. 4.8 Posterior landmarks for chest percussion. (Swartz, M. H. (2021). *Textbook of Physical Diagnosis: History and Examination*, 8th ed. Elsevier Inc.)

9. Explain your findings to the patient, and check whether they have any questions.
10. Decontaminate and clean your stethoscope.
11. Decontaminate hands and remove any PPE.
12. Document your findings.

Peak Expiratory Flow Rate

Peak expiratory flow rate monitoring is often used to evaluate patients who have respiratory failure. This test measures the speed of exhalation. Normal values are dependent on the individual height, gender, age and medical history. Lower than normal values are associated with exacerbation of some respiratory conditions. Normal readings for adults may vary between 400 and 700 L/min.

PROCEDURE

1. Peak expiratory flow rate measurement may be required before and after a nebuliser to monitor the patient's condition, or during patient assessment.
2. Attach a disposable mouthpiece to the peak flow meter and set the pointer to zero.
3. Instruct the patient to inhale deeply, place the lips around the mouthpiece to form a tight seal and, holding the meter horizontally, exhale forcibly. Make sure that the patient's fingers do not occlude the pointer.
4. Note the measurement.
5. Repeat steps 2 to 4 twice more.
6. Following the procedure, place the patient in comfortable position.
7. Document the highest of the three measurements. Record anything which could have impacted upon the peak flow reading should also be noted, such as nebuliser therapy or exercise.

8. Report any abnormality or significant variation from previous recordings.
9. The disposable mouthpiece may be reused for the same patient. Keep dry and protected from dust.

Using a Pulse Oximeter

Pulse oximetry monitoring is a common non-invasive technique used to detect pulsatile signals in an extremity, for example a finger. It calculates the amount of oxygenated haemoglobin and pulse rate. Pulse oximeter readings do not provide information about respiratory rate, tidal volume, cardiac output or blood pressure; therefore assessment, monitoring and recording of these observations in addition to pulse oximetry is essential.

The normal range for SpO_2 is 95% to 99%. Pulse oximetry is used extensively in acute settings in combination with all other respiratory information. It is important to point out that factors, such as temperature, light, carbon monoxide and haemoglobin level, may adversely influence readings. Also, that is does not give measurement of the presence of carbon dioxide, which may be higher than normal in respiratory failure.

KEY POINTS

- The SpO_2 probe should be attached to the patient according to the manufacturer's requirement.
- Common sites for SpO_2 monitoring include finger and earlobe.
- Care should be taken to ensure that the SpO_2 stays attached to patient, particularly during movements.
- In patients who are cool peripherally, consider alternative probe placement following manufacturer guidance.
- Alarms should be set according to target saturation levels

PROCEDURE

1. Assess the patient's peripheral circulation in order to choose an appropriate sensor and site. The most usual are those that clip onto the patient's finger, although sensors that clip onto the ears or adhesive nasal sensors are also available.
2. Before applying the sensor, check that the patient's skin is clean and dry.
3. If using a finger sensor, remove nail polish or false nails, as this could give an inaccurate reading. Avoid placing the finger probe on the same arm as a blood pressure cuff as the reading will be inaccurate during inflation of the cuff (Fig. 4.9).
4. Turn on the machine, and ensure the cable is plugged into the machine. Apply the sensor by clipping it on to the end of the finger (or earlobe etc).
5. Observe waveform fluctuations and check that the pulse waveform and oxygen saturation levels are registering, and document the reading.
6. Set alarm limits on the pulse oximeter if not preset by manufacturer.
7. If continuous oxygen saturation measurements are required, change the sensor site every 4 hours to prevent pressure damage or irritation from adhesive sensors.
8. If intermittent oxygen saturations are being measured, remove the sensor between readings and switch off the machine. Make the patient comfortable.

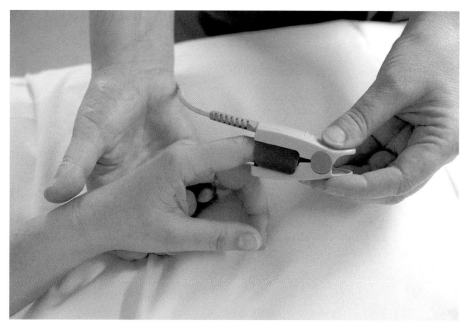

Fig. 4.9 Using a pulse oximeter finger probe.

9. Clean the machine and sensor according to local policy and manufacturers guidelines. Store the machine and cable as per manufacturer's instructions after use.
10. Remove PPE and decontaminate hands.
11. Document oxygen saturations, recording whether the patient is receiving oxygen therapy. Report any changes or abnormalities.

Arterial Blood Gases

ABGs are often measured in acute and critically ill patients to assess their acid–base status. ABGs can be measured from a peripheral sample or via an arterial line. In emergency departments and on wards, ABGs tend to be taken via a peripheral sample. As a student or newly qualified nurse, interpreting ABGs can be daunting, requiring time and experience. When learning how to interpret ABG results, you may find it helpful to think about how the results apply to the patient you are looking after. It also useful to have access to any previous ABGs to provide a comparison, especially when a patient has a chronic respiratory disease.

ABGs provide information regarding respiratory and metabolic status. Abnormal values are always indicative of an underlying disorder, which may be attributed to a respiratory, metabolic or mixed problem. You need to remember that respiratory and metabolic systems will try compensate for each other. For example, if the Partial pressure of carbon dioxide ($PaCO_2$) is high (referred as respiratory acidosis), the bicarbonate (HCO_3) will be increased to compensate as the body tries to restore homeostasis by moving the pH back into the normal range. If the HCO_3 is low (referred to as metabolic acidosis), the $PaCO_2$ will be decreased to reduce acid in the body, again trying to move the pH back into the normal range. When compensation fails, the pH will become abnormally high or low.

KEY POINTS

- ABG samples must be processed within 15 minutes (ideally as soon as taken)
- Sampling errors include: dilution (failure to remove solution from syringe), air bubbles in the sample (can affect the partial pressure of oxygen (PaO_2) level) and clotting, if samples are not mixed properly which (can affect the potassium result).
- The indications for an ABG include:
  - To assess oxygenation in deteriorating or high-risk patients
  - To assess effect of oxygen therapy and whether escalation of respiratory support is indicated
  - To assess or monitor acid–base balance
  - To assess the effect of therapeutic interventions
    - Cardiovascular stability
    - Changes in ventilation support
  - To measure lactate, haemoglobin and electrolytes (in particular potassium).
  - Ongoing monitoring for patients requiring invasive or non-invasive ventilation

NORMAL ABG VALUES

pH: 7.35 to 7.45
$PaCO_2$: 4.5 to 6.1 kPa
PO_2: 10 to 13 kPa
PaO_2: 95% to 100%
HCO_3^-: 22 to 26 mmol/L
Base excess (BE): -2 to $+2$

INTERPRETING AN ARTERIAL BLOOD GAS

There are several ways to interpret an ABG. The steps below follow the method suggested by the Resuscitation Council (UK) (2021):

Step 1: How is the patient?
Step 2: Assess oxygenation to determine if the patient is hypoxemic
Step 3: Determine the pH (or H+ concentration) to determine if the patient is acidaemic (pH low) or alkalaemic (pH high)
Step 4: Determine the respiratory component; is the $PaCO_2$ high or low?
Step 5: Determine the metabolic component; is the HCO_3 high or low?
Step 6: Match the pH with either the $PaCO_2$ or HCO_3
Step 7: Assess for compensation

Step 1: How is the Patient?

Using the A-E Assessment (page 20) identify the indications for taking an ABG. It is important to be aware that blood gas machines are able to provide range of results including supplementary values including haemoglobin, key electrolytes (potassium, sodium, chlorine), lactate levels and blood glucose (Resuscitation Council, UK, 2021). The results are used to determine how ill the patient is and if serial ABGs are taken, these can help determine if the patient is responding to treatment or deteriorating. This can indicate when escalation of care is needed.

Step 2: Assess Oxygenation

The concentration of oxygen in inspired air is 21% (partial pressure of 21 kPa). As the air passes through the respiratory system, it reduces, and at alveoli level the PaO_2 is approximately 13 kPa. The PaO_2 is always lower between the alveolar and arterial blood and affected by an underlying respiratory disease (acute or chronic). In a healthy individual this is normally approximately 10 kPa lower than the inspired partial pressure (Resuscitation Council (UK), 2021). For example, a patient breathing room air (21%) has a PaO_2 of 11 kPa. A low PaO_2 /SaO_2 indicates hypoxia but in this instance the pH is not significantly altered.

Step 3: Determine the pH

pH is the measure of hydrogen (H+) ion concentration in the blood. It is important to note, that H+ and pH have an inverse relationship; as one goes up the other comes down, indicating the level of acid or alkaline in the blood. A low pH (less than 7.35) indicates it is acidic and a high pH (more than 7.45) indicates alkalosis.

7.35   to 7.45
acidosis   alkalosis

Step 4: Assessing $PaCO_2$

Carbon dioxide is a waste product of metabolism and is normally transported by blood to the lungs, where is it excreted during expiration. $PaCO_2$ refers to the pressure or tension exerted by dissolved CO_2 gas in arterial blood. CO_2 levels are primarily regulated by the ventilatory function of the lungs and a potential acid. If the $PaCO_2$ is less than 4.5kPa it indicates alkalosis and if it is more than 6.0kPa it indicates acidosis.

KEY POINT

If the $PaCO_2$ goes in the opposite direction to the pH, **this** is the primary disorder.

Step 5: Assessment Metabolic Element

Bicarbonate (HCO_3^-) is the main buffer found in the blood and regulated by the kidneys. The normal HCO_3^- range is 22–26mmol/L. Acids that cannot be eliminated by the respiratory system can be 'mopped up' by HCO_3^-. The metabolic response of the kidneys is slower than the respiratory response, therefore, changes may take a few days to become effective. Alternatively, base excess (BE) can also be used to measure the metabolic acid-base. The normal BE range is −2 to +2.

> −2   to   > +2
> 22 mml/L   > 26 mmol/L
acidosis   alkalosis

KEY POINT

If the bicarbonate follows the same direction as the pH, **this is** the primary disorder.
  Base excess (BE)/deficit is the amount of acid required to restore 1 L of blood to a normal pH of 7.4.

−2   to   +2
Acidosis   Alkalosis

  A BE of greater than −2 indicates a metabolic acidosis, and a BE greater than +2 indicates a metabolic alkalosis.

Step 6: Match the pH with Either the $PaCO_2$ or HCO_3

Types of acid–base abnormalities include respiratory acidosis or alkalosis, metabolic acidosis or alkalosis and respiratory and compensation.

Respiratory Acidosis

Respiratory acidosis occurs when gaseous exchange or lung ventilation is affected (e.g. due to pulmonary oedema, opioid overdose, airway obstruction or chest wall injury). For example, if the pH less than 7.35, and the $PaCO_2$ greater than 6.0 kPa (45 mmHg), this is a respiratory acidosis. A lower than normal pH represents an acidosis, and a higher than normal pH represents an alkalosis.

Metabolic Acidosis

Metabolic acidosis occurs when there is severe loss of bicarbonate (e.g. diarrhoea, circulatory failure/ hypovolaemia, renal failure, untreated diabetes or high extracellular potassium concentrations). For example, if the pH is less than 7.35, and the HCO_3- less than 22 mmol/L (base excess < -2 mmol/L), this indicates a metabolic acidosis.

Respiratory Alkalosis

Respiratory alkalosis occurs due to hyperventilation (e.g. overventilation [large tidal volumes and/ or fast respiratory rate], acute anxiety, traumatic brain injury, early stages of chronic obstructive pulmonary disease, asthma). For example, if the pH greater than 7.45, and the $PaCO_2$ less than 4.7 kPa (35 mm Hg) indicates a respiratory alkalosis.

Metabolic Alkalosis

Metabolic alkalosis is caused by excessive loss of acids (e.g. vomiting or gastric suctioning, selected diuretics, ingestion of sodium bicarbonate, constipation, excessive aldosterone [tumours]). For example, if the pH greater than 7.45, and the HCO_3- greater than 26 mmol/L (base excess $> +2$ mmol/L), indicates a metabolic alkalosis.

Step 7: Compensation

In addition to the acid–base abnormalities listed earlier, both respiratory and metabolic changes may occur, whereby the respiratory and metabolic components change in the opposite directions, with minimal disturbances of the pH. This is a compensatory mechanism to prevent long-term changes to pH. A raised $PaCO_2$ (acidosis) and BE greater than $+2$ or bicarbonate greater than 26 mmol/L (alkalosis) indicates a primary respiratory acidosis, with the aim of a metabolic alkalosis trying to bring the pH back to normality.

Condition	pH	$PaCO_2$	HCO_3
Respiratory acidosis	Low	High	Normal
Respiratory alkalosis	High	Low	Normal
Metabolic acidosis	Low	Normal or low	Low
Metabolic alkalosis	High	Normal	High

References

Carter, C., Aedy, H., Notter, J., 2020. COVID-19 Disease: Assessment of a Critically Ill Patient. Clinics in Integrated Care https://doi.org/10.1016/j.intcar.2020.100001.

Chung, F., Adbullah, H.R., Liao, P., 2016. STOP-BANG questionnaire. A practical approach to screen for obstructive sleep apnoea. Chest. 149 (3), 631–638.

Edwards S. Williams J. (Edt). (2019). A nurse's survival guide to critical care. Elsevier

Grant, S., 2018. Limitations of track and trigger systems and the National Early Warning Score. Part 1: areas of contention. Br. J. Nurs. 27 (11), 624.

Khanna, A.K., Sessler, D.I., Sun, Z., et al., 2016. Using the STOP-BANG questionnaire to predict hypoxaemia in patients recovering from non-cardiac surgery: a prospective cohort analysis. Br. J. Anaesth. 116 (5), 632–640.

Massey, D., Meredith, T., 2010. Respiratory assessment 1: why do it and how to do it. Br. J. Card. Nurs. 5 (11), 537–541.

Morgan, S., 2021. Respiratory assessment: undertaking a physical examination of the chest in adults. Nursing Standard (Royal College of Nursing (Great Britain): 1987).

Proctor, J., Rickards, E., 2020. How to perform chest auscultation and interpret the findings. Nurs. Times [online] 116 (1), 23–26.

Resuscitation Council (UK), 2021. Advanced Life Support Manual. 8th ed. London.

Rolfe, S., 2019. The importance of respiratory rate monitoring. British Journal of Nursing, 28(8), pp.504–508.

Shepherd, E., 2017. Specimen collection 4: procedure for obtaining a sputum specimen. Nurs. Times [online 113] (10), 49–51.

Simpson, H., 2015. Respiratory assessment. Br. J. Nurs. 15 (9), 484–488.

STOP-BANG, 2012. STOP-BANG Questionnaire. http://www.stopbang.ca/osa/screening.php#.

Williams, J. and Edwards, S., 2019. A Nurse's Survival Guide to Critical Care-Updated Edition. Elsevier.

CHAPTER 5

Respiratory Support

Oxygen Delivery Devices

Oxygen therapy is a treatment used for patients who are hypoxaemic, which means they have an abnormally low level of oxygen in the blood. This can be caused by several conditions, such as chest infections and pneumonia. In medical terms, oxygen is a drug and as with other drugs must be prescribed (unless in a medical emergency) and closely monitored. Oxygen administration must be titrated (increase/decrease) according to the patients condition. Monitoring is usually through measuring respiratory rate, pulse oximetry monitoring (see p. 36) in acute areas and as arterial blood gas (ABG) analysis (see p. 37) in critical care/emergency areas for more precise measurements. All patients requiring oxygen therapy need regular medical reviews and close observation. With the increasing patient acuity and complexity, conditions that previously were solely nurses in specialist areas can now be found in a range of clinical settings, therefore, this chapter also includes an overview of the use of High Flow Nasal Oxygen and Non Invasive Ventilation. You would not be expected to care for these patients unsupervised, but it is important that you understand the principles of these additional respiratory interventions.

KEY POINTS

- Oxygen is a drug and, unless in an emergency situation, must be prescribed.
- Target oxygen saturations are 94%–98% in adults and 88%–92% in patients with chronic obstructive pulmonary disease (COPD) or risk factors for developing hypercapnia (British Thoracic Society [BTS], 2019).
- Oxygen delivery devices can be either fixed or variable performance (Carter et al., 2020).
  - In variable performance the amount of oxygen delivered is unknown as it is dependent upon the patient's ventilator pattern.
  - Fixed performance is independent of the patient's ventilator pattern.

ADMINISTERING OXYGEN

Oxygen is highly flammable and can be provided via a wall supply, oxygen cylinder and in some settings via an oxygen concentrator. Oxygen cylinders come in different sizes and must be clearly labelled oxygen (Fig. 5.1). Oxygen tubing may come in prepacked lengths or as a continuous roll, with a 'bubble' (widened portion) at regular intervals. Cut through the centre of the bubble, and then further trim as necessary to make a secure fit onto the flow meter and mask. The length should allow freedom of movement for the patient but not be so long that it may become kinked or touch the floor.

If using a flow meter, the centre of the ball in the flow meter must sit at the level of the flow rate prescribed (Fig. 5.2). When using an oxygen cylinder (Fig. 5.3), it is important to check the amount of oxygen in the cylinder to allow for time for change of cylinder, particularly when using cylinders during patient transfer.

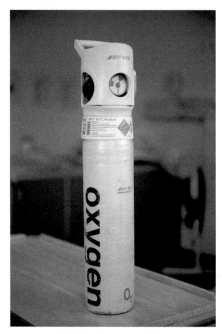

Fig. 5.1 Oxygen cylinder.

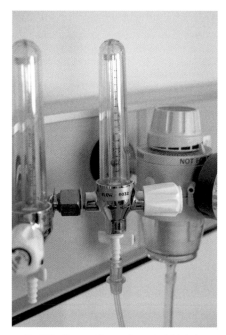

Fig. 5.2 Oxygen flow meter set at 2 L/min.

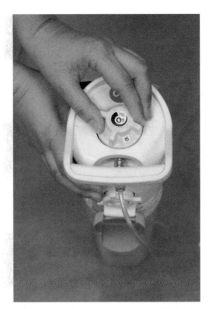

Fig. 5.3 Cylinder oxygen set at 15 L/min.

TYPES OF OXYGEN DELIVERY DEVICES

Oxygen delivery devices are classified as either variable or fixed rate (Table 5.1). Variable delivery devices (e.g. nasal cannulae) use oxygen prescribed and delivered using litres per minute (L/min) rather than fixed percentages. Other examples, including a non-rebreath mask with reservoir bag, which is used to deliver very high concentrations of oxygen and 10 to 15 L/min. In consequence,

TABLE 5.1 ■ **Examples of Variable and Fixed Rate**

Device	Use	Oxygen Delivery
Reservoir mask	Critical illness such as sepsis or acute deterioration. Variable performance mask (Fig. 5.4).	15 L/min
Venturi mask	Able to deliver a range of oxygen percentage according to patient need. Fixed performance oxygen device (Figs 5.5 and 5.6).	These are colour-coded and specify the flow of oxygen required to deliver 24%, 28%, 35%, 40% and 60% oxygen 24%, 28%, 35%, 40% and 60%
Nasal cannula	Allows low flow oxygen. Useful for patients requiring low levels of oxygen. Variable performance mask (Fig. 5.7).	1–4 L/min (24%–40%)
Simple face mask	Allows low flow oxygen. The side ports allow carbon dioxide to escape. Variable performance mask (Fig. 5.8).	6–10 L/min

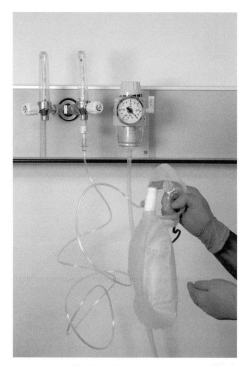

Fig. 5.4 Reservoir mask.

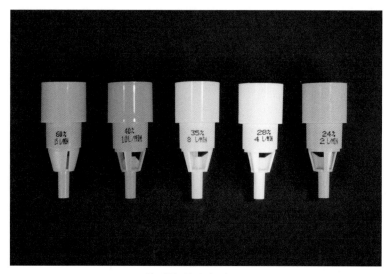

Fig. 5.5 Venturi valves.

the amount of oxygen delivered (FiO2) is unknown, as it is dependent upon the patient's ventilatory pattern. Conversely, fixed delivery devices are independent of the patient's ventilatory pattern (e.g. using the Venturi system).

Humidified Oxygen

As oxygen therapy dries the mucous membranes of the mouth, frequent drinks should be offered mouth care provided. Therefore, humidifications should always be considered when oxygen therapy is required for prolonged periods and for patients with respiratory infections who have difficulty expectorating sputum. The use of oil-based preparations such as Vaseline or petroleum jelly should be avoided (Olive, 2016).

Humidification is not normally required for patients who are receiving low-flow oxygen or high levels of oxygen for a very short period of time. However, in those patients who may have thick or difficult to expectorate respiratory secretions, humidification will help to loosen and moisten respiratory secretions. The decision to use humidified oxygen is based on individual clinical assessment/need. Humidification may also improve patient comfort by reducing nasal and oral dryness.

KEY POINTS

- It is important that the flow is set at the rate indicated to achieve the prescribed percentage of oxygen. This is usually indicated on the top of the humidifier where it attaches to the flow meter. There may also be a valve adjustment, which should be turned to the correct setting.
- Water that collects in the wide-bore tubing should be emptied or the tubing changed according to local policy.

PROCEDURE

1. Check the prescription regarding the percentage of oxygen to be administered.
2. Connect the humidifier to the oxygen flow meter according to the manufacturer's instructions.
3. Connect the wide-bore tubing to the mask and set the flow meter to the flow required to achieve the prescribed percentage of oxygen.
4. A fine mist should appear in the mask. Ask/assist the patient to put on the mask and adjust the retaining strap to prevent pressure on the ears. The nose part of the mask may need to be adjusted to prevent mist going into the eyes.
5. Check the patient is comfortable. The humidified oxygen may encourage the patient to cough, so a sputum pot and tissues should be provided.
6. Document humidified oxygen therapy.
7. If using an oxygen cylinder, monitor the amount remaining and order a replacement when it is down to a quarter full.
8. Check regularly to see if water is collecting in the tubing. The water reservoir should be replaced when empty. The tubing and mask should be changed every 24 hours.
9. Connect humidifier according to manufacturer's instructions (Fig. 5.9).
10. In this case the water bottle is connected to the oxygen flow meter via the screw top.
11. Prescribed oxygen level is set on oxygen flow meter.
12. Elephant tubing is then attached to the oxygen mask and fed back to the water pack.
13. Tubing should be observed regularly to ensure water is not collecting.
14. Any water found in the tubing should be removed according to local policy.

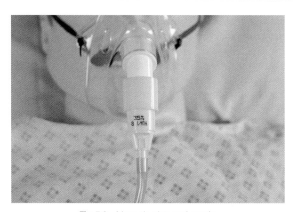

Fig. 5.6 Venturi valve and mask.

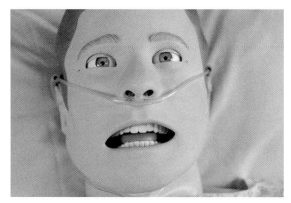

Fig. 5.7 Nasal cannula.

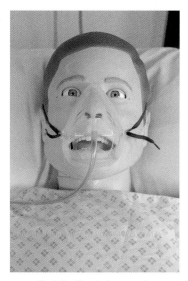

Fig. 5.8 Simple face mask.

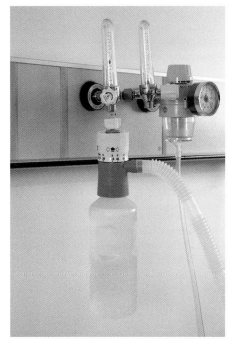

Fig. 5.9   Assembled humidified oxygen.

Use of a Nebuliser

A nebuliser converts liquid medication into an aerosol for the patient to inhale. The use of air or oxygen to drive the nebuliser will depend on the underlying disease process. Most patients with asthma will be prescribed oxygen, whereas those with chronic obstructive pulmonary disease (COPD) are usually prescribed nebulisers with air. In some instances, compressed air boxes are used to 'drive' the nebuliser, operated with a simple on/off switch. When using a wall supply or oxygen the flow rate is critical to the delivery of the drug and although manufacturer's guidance should be followed, generally the flow needs to be greater than 6 L/min to produce the small aerosol particles (BTS and SIGN, 2019). Flow rates greater than 8 L/min are generally too forceful and may cause the oxygen tubing to disconnect from the nebuliser pot.

Either a mouthpiece or mask can be used; if the patient is having nebuliser therapy regularly, the mask or mouthpiece may be kept at the bedside between uses. Nebuliser therapy is usually administered 2 to 4 times per day. Drugs to be nebulised (e.g. a bronchodilator) must be prescribed, and checked according to local policy (see p. 195).

PROCEDURE

1. Check the prescription regarding the percentage of oxygen to be administered.
2. Connect the humidifier to the oxygen flow meter according to the manufacturer's instruction. Oxygen may be delivered via a flow meter connected to a walled supply, cylinder or oxygen concentrator. The centre of the ball in the flow meter must sit at the level of the flow rate prescribed.

3. Connect the tubing to the nebuliser pot and mask. Set the flow meter to the flow required to achieve the prescribed percentage of oxygen or turn on the nebuliser box.
4. A fine mist should appear in the mask. Ask/assist the patient to put on the mask and adjust the retaining strap to prevent pressure on the ears. The nose part of the mask may need to be adjusted to prevent mist going into the eyes (Fig. 5.10).
5. Check the patient is comfortable.
6. Remember if using an oxygen cylinder, monitor the amount remaining and order a replacement when it is down to a quarter full.
7. Observe the patient's respiratory pattern and oxygen saturation to check that the therapy is working. Vital signs, and an National Early Warning Scoring Early Warning Score, should be assessed regularly.

Positioning the Breathless Patient

Patients with respiratory conditions who are breathless may need to be positioned sitting upright, to maximise respiratory functioning while reducing physical effort and maintaining comfort. Pillows should be used to support the small of the back so that the patient does not sag into the bed and thus restrict chest movement. In the patient with poor or restricted mobility, regular repositioning is necessary to prevent pressure ulcers (see Chapter 17).

EQUIPMENT

1. Bed with adjustable backrest or electric raising mechanism
2. Four or five pillows
3. Bed table with brakes

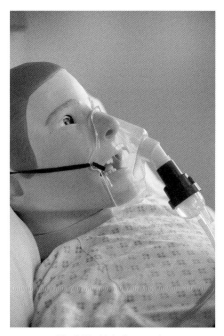

Fig. 5.10 Nebuliser mask.

4. Firm, supporting armchair
5. Additional staff and use a hoist or sliding aid may be needed if the patient is unable to move up the bed unaided.

PROCEDURE

1. Explain the procedure, then gain consent and cooperation.
2. Provide reassurance if the patient is anxious because of the difficulty in breathing.
3. Explain to the patient exactly what is planned so that movement is reduced to a minimum.
4. Ask/assist the patient to sit forward. A second nurse may be needed to support the patient while the backrest is adjusted and the pillows are arranged.
5. Adjust the backrest or raise the head of the bed.
6. Arrange the pillows so that the patient feels supported. This will vary according to patient preference, but you should check that the lumbar region is supported.
7. If the foot of the bed can be raised slightly, this may help to prevent the patient from slipping down.
8. For a short periods, the patient may find they can breathe more easily by leaning forwards with the forearms resting on a pillow on a bed table.
9. If able to get out of bed, the breathless patient maybe most comfortable sitting in an armchair, and many prefer to sleep in this position.
10. As you help the patient to reposition, observe for changes in respiratory pattern, cough, colour, etc.
11. When completed, check if the patient needs a drink and that call bell, etc. are close to hand.
12. If sitting for long periods, a pressure-relieving mattress or cushion may be needed to prevent pressure ulcers.
13. Document the care given and report any change(s) in condition.

High-Flow Nasal Oxygen

RATIONALE

High-flow nasal oxygen (HFNO) combines active humidification, air/oxygen blender, a heated circuit and a nasal cannula (Nishimura, 2015). This therapy can deliver high flow rates of oxygen (up to 60 L/min). The aim of this therapy is to treat hypoxaemic respiratory failure as well as a wide range of conditions.

Indications for HFNO include:

- Increased respiratory effort (e.g. tachypnoea, shortness of breath, increased work of breathing in the presence of hypoxia)
- Evidence of type I respiratory failure (PaO_2 <10 kPa)
- Desaturation despite increasing oxygen requirements

Contraindications include:

- Severe respiratory distress, severe cardiovascular instability
- Unconscious patient
- Upper airway obstruction
- Basal skull fractures
- Epistaxis
- Impaired ability to cough or clear secretions

Prior to commencing HFNO, a clear plan of care must be agreed on and documented in the medical notes. This includes treatment escalation plans and end-of-life care pathway if the treatment is unsuccessful.

KEY POINTS

- HFNO tends to initially be commenced at a flow rate of 60 L/min and oxygen at a percentage to achieve the target oxygen saturation (SpO_2). The temperature of the humidification circuit should be set at 37°C.
- Patients must be continuously monitored (to ensure the target oxygen saturation is maintained) and vital signs assessed.
- The patient should be assessed to determine if there is any improvement in vital signs. The therapy can then be titrated. The patient should be observed for signs of improvement or deterioration (Box 5.1). If the patient does not initially improve, the oxygen percentage should be increased until target saturations are achieved. If the oxygen is greater than 50%, the patient should be urgently reassessed as intubation may be an appropriate next step.
- Patients receiving HFNO should be nursed in an area where they can be continuously observed by appropriately trained nursing staff. Signs of deterioration include changes in respiratory observations, vital signs and neurological observations (Box 5.2).

PROCEDURE

1. When setting up HFNO, a double oxygen connector (one to connect HFNO, the other oxygen flow meter) must be used. This allows for supplementary oxygen, and emergency equipment to be used quickly.

BOX 5.1 ■ Criteria for High-Flow Nasal Oxygen Success and Failure

Success

- Able to maintain target saturation
- Improved respiratory rate and breathing effort
- Improved partial pressure of oxygen (PaO_2)
- Improved patient comfort

Failure

- Unable to maintain target saturation
- Increased or worsening respiratory rate and effort
- Worsening PaO_2 and increasing $PaCO_2$

BOX 5.2 ■ Signs of Deterioration

Respiratory Observations

- Increased work of breathing or worsening breathing pattern
- Use of accessory muscles and mouth breathing
- Tachypnoea and bradypnoea
- Decreasing saturations or continuously increasing oxygen requirements to maintain oxygen saturations.
- Sudden increase or gradual increase in oxygen greater than 50%

Vital Signs

- Deteriorating vital signs/rising early warning score (EWS) (e.g., national early warning score (NEWS))

Neurological Observations

- Anxiety
- Agitation
- Confusion/disorientation
- Reduced consciousness

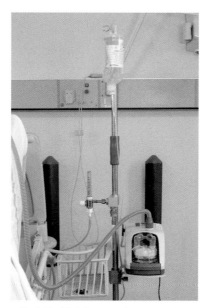

Fig. 5.11 High-flow nasal oxygen setup.

2. HFNO is usually provided as a complete circuit including tubing and nasal cannula (Fig. 5.11).
3. The oxygen/air blender should be attached to piped oxygen and air.
4. Sterile water is provided as part of the circuit. This should be attached via the tubing provided.
5. Depending on the machine used, specialised oxygen tubing will need to be used. One tube (usually the shorter tube) should be attached to the oxygen and air blender. The other tube must also be attached to the humidifier.
6. The longer tube contains the nasal cannula, which need to be fitted and adjusted to the patient's requirements.
7. The flow rate and oxygen level must be selected according to prescription.
8. The humidifier must be switched on and an appropriate temperature selected. This is usually set at 37°C.
9. The nasal cannula should be fitted to the patient and the tape adjusted for comfort.
10. Continuous SpO2 monitoring should be utilised.
11. Oxygen level and flow should be titrated according to individual parameters. When weaning, the flow should be reduced by 5L at a time, as tolerated by the patient, and should not be less than 30 L/min (Fig. 5.12).
12. The humidification water chamber and fluid bag must be checked regularly to ensure sufficient water levels.

Nursing a Patient on Non-Invasive Ventilation

RATIONALE

Non-invasive ventilation (NIV) is often used in short-term life-threatening conditions (e.g. pulmonary oedema) or when intubation carries a greater risk than other benefits (e.g. patients with chronic type II respiratory failure from COPD) (Intensive Care Foundation, 2015). NIV refers to the provision of ventilatory support through the patient's upper airway using a mask or

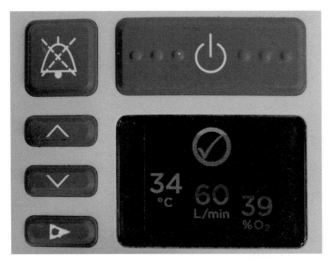

Fig. 5.12 High-flow nasal oxygen settings.

similar device. Other forms of ventilation delivered by an endotracheal tube, tracheostomy tube or laryngeal mask are described as invasive ventilation.

NIV encompasses the use of continuous positive airway pressure (CPAP) and bilevel positive airway pressure (BiPAP) (see below). NIV is used for a range of respiratory conditions and may be used to assist early extubation (Intensive Care Foundation, 2015; Davies et al., 2018). NIV and CPAP are common terms which are often used interchangeably but are distinct from each other. It is vital that nurses understand the difference between the two as they are indicated for different respiratory conditions.

Nurses caring for patients receiving NIV need to be experienced in the use of the equipment and local policies and guidelines. This is a specialist area of care that requires in-depth knowledge of respiratory physiology, pulse oximetry and ABG analysis.

NIV assists breathing by giving the patient a mixture of air and oxygen through a tightly fitting facial or nasal mask. This helps the patient to take a full breath, thus providing adequate oxygen supply to the body. NIV is usually prescribed as either CPAP or BiPAP (National Confidential Enquiry Into Patient Outcome and Death Acute Non-Invasive Ventilation: Inspiring Change (NCEPOD), 2017). Complications of NIV are outlined in Box 5.3.

NURSING CONSIDERATIONS

Nurse the patient in an area enabling increased observation and access to specialist-trained and experienced nurses in managing a patient on NIV.

Provide reassurance, particularly when starting treatment, as patients may find the mask and tight-fitting straps cause anxiety and fear.

Before commencing treatment, measure the mask to check it is the correct size.

During acute episodes, a full face mask is advised.

The mask needs to be fitted securely but not excessively tight. Many NIV machines measure 'leak' to determine if the mask is fitted too loosely.

Observe the pressure points on the face and apply a protective dressing if necessary, particularly if the patient has a nasogastric tube in situ.

Mucous membrane may become dry, and regular mouth care is required.

Patients will need to maintain hydration and nutrition; consequently, planned breaks will be required to allow patients to drink and/or eat.

Ensure the patient can access the nurse call bell.

Input from a chest physiotherapist will be required.

Undertake continuous cardiac monitoring and oxygen saturations.

Assess vital signs and National Early Warning Score (NEWS) monitoring at least hourly.

Observe for potential complications (Box 5.3).

Continuous Positive Airway Pressure

CPAP is a therapy used to increase functional residual capacity and therefore to improve oxygenation. It can be described as a positive pressure applied to the airway continuously to keep alveoli expanded at the end of expiration. This is delivered through a specialised facial or nasal mask. CPAP delivers a constant flow of oxygen at a prescribed pressure which remains constant during inspiration and expiration. The continuous pressure increases lung volume and keeps the alveoli open at the end of each breath to allow more time for gaseous exchange (Olive, 2016; Intensive Care Foundation, 2015; Carter et al., 2021). For CPAP to work, a sealed system is required, using a tight-fitting mask or a hood.

(Intensive Care Foundation, 2015; Davies et al., 2018).

Indications for CPAP include

- Type I respiratory failure (hypoxaemia)
- Some types of sleep apnoea
- Post-operatively for mild alveolar collapse
- To manage pulmonary oedema while awaiting other treatments effects.

Patients receiving CPAP therapy, particularly in acute hospital settings, require close observation including continuous pulse oximetry monitoring.

EQUIPMENT REQUIRED

CPAP mask

CPAP flow generator (NB most mechanical ventilators can also deliver CPAP)

BOX 5.3 ■ Potential Complications of Non-Invasive Ventilation and Contraindications

Potential Complications

- Continuous positive airway pressure (CPAP):
    - Pressure damage to the nasal bridge
    - Under pressure, air can be swallowed, leading to gastric distention.
    - Air leaks from the mask may lead to corneal/conjunctival irritation.
    - Pneumothorax

Contraindications to Non-Invasive Ventilation (NIV)

- The patient cannot maintain/protect an airway
- Compliance is a problem (e.g. agitation)
- Risk of apnoea
- Head or facial injuries
- Factors making it difficult to create a seal (e.g. facial deformity or recent surgery)
- Consolidation on the chest x-ray

(Intensive Care Foundation, 2015).

'Elephant' (wide bore) oxygen tubing
SpO_2 monitor

PROCEDURE

1. Ensure an adequate-fitting mask to suit patient comfort. Many different types exist, and every effort must be made to effectively fit the mask.
2. The level of CPAP should be set via the CPAP machine. This will be directed by patient condition and usually starts at 5 cm H_2O.
3. The mask should be attached to tubing.
4. An expiratory valve should always be present.
5. Check that the pressure is present by putting hand over mask.
6. The mask can then be adjusted to fit the patient's face.
7. Close attention should be paid to patient comfort, as ill-fitting or extremely tight masks can cause patient intolerance and pressure damage.
8. SpO_2 monitoring and ABGs should be used to check for treatment effectiveness.
9. Alarms should be set according to patient condition.
10. Pressure areas should be inspected regularly. Consider alternative masks if pressure damage is apparent.
11. Eye and mouth care should be performed regularly to prevent dryness and discomfort.

Bilevel Positive Airway Pressure

BiPAP refers to ventilatory support provided via a mask. It can help facilitate gas exchange by providing positive pressure in varying levels throughout the respiratory cycle. NIV in indicated in those patients who have

- Acute type II respiratory failure (hypercapnia),
- Chronic hypercapnic respiratory failure
- Acute or chronic type II respiratory failure (e.g. exacerbation of COPD by a community-acquired

BiPAP is an essential component of the care of patients with chronic obstructive airways disease (COPD) when there is persistent acidotic hypercapnic ventilator failure that has not improved after 1 hour following conventional therapy of bronchodilators, oxygen, steroids and antibiotics (National Institute for Health and Care Excellence (NICE), 2016).

BiPAP works through setting the following parameters:

- Inspiratory positive airway pressure (IPAP): When the patient initiates a breath, the ventilator supports the breath to a preset inspiratory pressure.
- Expiratory positive airway pressure (EPAP): Prevents the alveolar collapsing on expiration.
- Pressure support (PS): Breathing on a ventilator is difficult, due to the valves, tubing etc.; therefore PS makes respiration easier for the patient. PS is calculated by
  IPAP − EPAP = PS
- Supplementary oxygen (FiO2)

KEY POINTS

Patients requiring NIV must be involved in their own care.
A multidisciplinary team approach to care is necessary to agree on appropriate parameters for treatment.

Treatment (including NIV) should be started within 1 hour of blood gas measurement regardless of location.

NIV is not suitable for patients who

- Have a reduced level of consciousness or are unable to protect their own airway
- Patients who have had facial surgery
- Patients with known poor tolerance levels

NIV can be used to prevent tracheal intubation and invasive mechanical ventilation in patients who are not suitable for a critical care admission. ABG analysis is essential for patients receiving NIV, to monitor $PaCO_2$ and PaO_2 levels and monitoring its effectiveness. An appropriate prescription and care plan should be in place.

Equipment Required

The most commonly used manufacturers in UK hospitals include BIPAP machines (biphasic or bilevel IPAP) and NIPPY machines (non-invasive positive pressure ventilation) (Fig. 5.13). It is essential that all nurses who are required to use these machines have ongoing training and regular updates.

On the machine shown in Fig. 5.14, two pressure levels are set. This is referred to as the IPAP and the EPAP. IPAP is commonly set at 10 to 15 cm H2O, and EPAP is commonly set at 5 to 10 cm H2O (see Fig. 5.14). The setting of these levels is directed by the medical team and patient condition. Many NIV machines also have an apnoea backup mode which will start if no patient breaths are detected. This should always be checked and active before starting NIV. If this mode is activated, then this is a medical emergency and help should be summoned immediately. Supplementary oxygen can also be provided via NIV if necessary (See Table 5.2). The setup of NIV

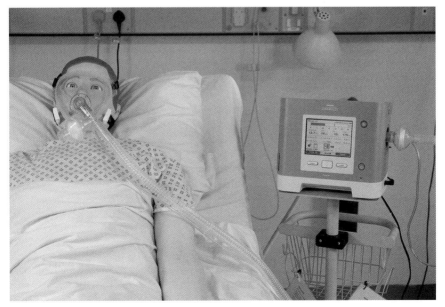

Fig. 5.13 Bilevel positive airway pressure machine.

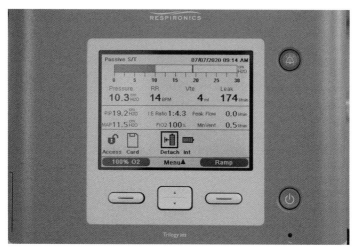

Fig. 5.14   Bilevel positive airway pressure settings.

TABLE 5.2 ■ Inclusion/Exclusion Criteria for Non-Invasive Ventilation

Inclusion Criteria

- Primary diagnosis of COPD
- Able to protect the airway
- Conscious and cooperative
- Potential for recovery
- Patient consent

Exclusion Criteria

- Facial trauma, burns, recent faction or upper airway surgery
- Upper gastrointestinal surgery
- Fixed obstruction of the upper airway
- Inability to protect the airway
- Life-threatening hypoxaemia
- Haemodynamic instability requiring vasopressors or inotropes
- Severe comorbidity
- Patient moribund
- Confusion, agitation or severe cognitive impairment
- Vomiting
- Bowel obstruction
- Copious respiratory secretions
- Undrained pneumothorax

COPD, Chronic obstructive pulmonary disease.
Fraser, J., 2016. Non-invasive ventilation in type 2 respiratory failure. In: Price, A.M., Smith, S.A., Challiner, A.
   (Eds.), Ward-Based Critical Care, a Guide for Health Professionals. Second ed. M&K Publishing.

is very similar to that of CPAP. However, extra monitoring is required in the form of regular ABGs to ensure NIV is effective. Humidification is not usually routinely required but may be used for patient comfort when using NIV (BTS, 2018). Alarms should be set according to patient condition and aims of treatment. When nursing a patient on NIV, if you have concerns at all or note any deterioration of the patient, you must immediately call for help. While you are waiting for help assess the patient using the ABCDE approach, document and act on what you find. Potential problems may include there is an excessive leak from the mask and straps need to be adjusted (this requires two people), connections have become loose, the development of a pneumothorax, not synchronising with with ventilator, respiratory fatigue or the settings need to be adjusted to improve oxygenation and / or carbon dioxide levels (Fraser, 2016).

Chest Drain Care

Chest drains are inserted to drain air, fluid, blood or pus from the pleural space. The pleural space contains a small volume of serous fluid for lubrication of the pleural membranes. Any other substances present in the pleural space may cause problems with ventilation, and therefore it may be necessary to remove these via a chest drain. An underwater seal chest drain provides a one-way valve for drainage of substances such as fluid or air. Chest drain insertion is a sterile procedure performed by trained medical staff. Nurses should be able to assist in gathering equipment, setting it up and monitoring the patient during the procedure.

EQUIPMENT REQUIRED

- Sterile chest drain insertion pack
- Ultrasonography equipment
- Sterile gown, gloves and goggles for medical staff
- Apron, gloves and goggles for nursing staff
- Dressing trolley or another clean surface
- Local anaesthetic
- Suture pack
- Clamps for initial insertion
- Scalpel
- Chest drain bottle and tubing
- One bottle of sterile water
- Tubing
- Sharps bin

PROCEDURE

Medical staff direct the procedure; however, nurses must be familiar with the equipment required and be able to anticipate procedural steps, to maximise the efficiency of the procedure and minimise discomfor for the patient.

1. The patient should be sitting in an upright position.
2. SpO2 monitoring should be applied. Respiratory observation should be carried out during the procedure.
3. The chest drain bottle should be assembled and sterile water added up to the desired prime level (Fig. 5.15). This should be clearly marked on the chest drain bottle.
4. When directed, the sterile chest drain pack should be opened.
5. Local anaesthetic should be prepared and checked with medical staff prior to administration. Medical staff should administer this along with any other required pain relief.
6. Ultrasonography can be used to ascertain correct chest drain position on insertion.
7. When the chest drain is inserted, there is a brief period where tubing may be clamped until the drainage bottle is connected.
8. The chest drain will be sutured in place and a clean sterile dressing applied over the site.
9. Once the drainage bottle is connected, all clamps should be removed.

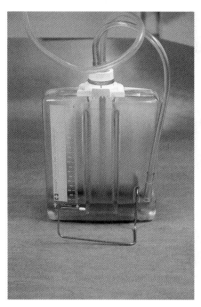

Fig. 5.15 Chest drain with an underwater seal.

10. The bottle should always be kept below the level of the thorax; this should be explained to the patient.
11. A chest x-ray will be required to confirm position.
12. A care plan should be in place.

NURSING CARE

Nurses should observe the drain for:

- **Swinging/oscillating.** This refers to water being pulled back up into the tube by negative intrathoracic pressure (Millar and Hillman, 2018). This is an indication that the chest drain is patent (i.e. not blocked and working correctly).
- **Bubbling.** A bubbling chest drain occurs when air is drained from the pleural space (pneumothorax) and may be indicative of an ongoing air leak. Bubbling should gradually reduce and then resolve completely as air is drained. A chest drain which suddenly stops bubbling is a cause for concern. A respiratory assessment should be carried out immediately, and chest drain tubing should be observed closely for any kinks or disconnection.
- **Draining.** Any fluid above the level of the priming fluid should be carefully recorded. Colour and consistency of any drainage should also be noted.
- Vital signs should be checked at least once every 4 hours unless otherwise indicated.

Other points to note

- Low pressure suction may be applied to chest drains to aid lung re-expansion. This must be prescribed, and low-pressure thoracic suction unit should always be used (usually −5 kPa) (Fig. 5.16).
- Chest drains rarely require clamping; however, if it becomes necessary, it should be done under medical supervision and only for a short period of time

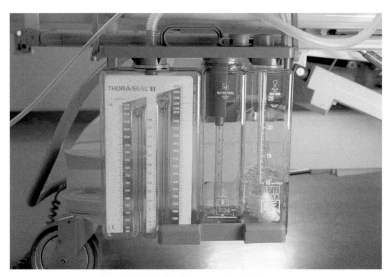

Fig. 5.16 Underwater chest drain.

- Chest drain bottles should be changed before the drainage reaches three-quarters full. A full chest drain bottle will result in ineffective drainage as the pressure generated may be too high to allow further drainage
- Flushing of chest drains should be carried out rarely and only under direct medical supervision
- Milking' and 'stripping' of chest drain should be avoided as this can create high intrathoracic pressures and cause difficulty in breathing

REMOVAL OF CHEST DRAINS

Chest drains should be removed when the original reason for insertion has resolved or the chest drain has become blocked.

Chest drain removal can be very painful, therefore analgesia must be offered.

Chest drains should be always be removed on expiration and an airtight dressing applied immediately.

An aseptic technique should be used.

A chest x-ray should be carried out after removal along with a repeat respiratory assessment.

References

British Thoracic Society (BTS), 2018. Quality Standards for Acute NIV in Adults. https://www.brit-thoracic. org.uk/quality-improvement/quality-standards/niv/.

British Thoracic Society (BTS), 2019. BTS Guideline for Oxygen Use in Healthcare and Emergency Settings. https://www.brit-thoracic.org.uk/quality-improvement/guidelines/emergency-oxygen/.

British Thoracic Society, SIGN, 2019. British guideline on the management of asthma. SIGN 158. www. sign.ac.uk.

Carter, C., Aedy, H., Notter, J., 2020. COVID-19 disease: assessment of a critically ill patient. Clinics in Integrated Care.

Carter, C. and Notter, J., 2021. Covid-19: An Open Access Critical Care Textbook. Elsevier Health Sciences.

Davies, M., Allen, M., Bentley, A., Bourke, S.C., Creagh-Brown, B., D'Oliveiro, R., Glossop, A., Gray, A., Jacobs, P., Mahadeva, R. and Moses, R., 2018. British Thoracic Society Quality Standards for acute non-invasive ventilation in adults. BMJ open respiratory research, 5(1), p.e000283.

Fraser, J., 2016. Non-invasive ventilation in type 2 respiratory failure. In: Price, A.M., Smith, S.A., Challiner, A. (Eds.), Ward-Based Critical Care, a Guide for Health Professionals. Second ed. M&K Publishing.

Intensive Care Foundation, 2015. Handbook of Mechanical Ventilation – A Users Guide. London.

Millar, F.R., Hillman, T., 2018.. Managing chest drains on medical wards. BMJ. 363, k4639. doi:10.1136/bmj.k4639.

National Confidential Enquiry Into Patient Outcome and Death Acute Non-Invasive Ventilation: Inspiring Change (NCEPOD), 2017. tinyurl.com/NCEPOD-NIV.

National Institute for Health and Care Excellence, 2016. Chronic obstructive pulmonary disease in adults. Quality Standard 10. Quality statement 7: Non-invasive ventilation I Chronic obstructive pulmonary disease in adults I Quality standards I NICE.

Nishimura, M., 2015. High-flow nasal cannula oxygen therapy in adults. J Inten. Care. 3 (1), 15.

Olive, S., 2016. Practical procedures: oxygen therapy. Nurs. Times. 112 (1/2), 12–14.

CHAPTER 6

Tracheostomy Care

Tracheostomy

RATIONALE

A tracheostomy is a surgical opening in the anterior wall of the trachea to enable insertion of a tube to facilitate ventilation. With the advances in medical care and treatment, Tracheostomy insertion and management are becoming increasingly common in critical care units and general wards. Indications for a tracheostomy include weaning from prolonged mechanical ventilation, upper airway obstruction (for example, a tumour), prolonged absence of laryngeal reflex or inability to swallow, and those with head and neck injuries/cancers. An estimated 10% to 15% of critical care patients in the UK require a tracheostomy as part of their care (Billington and Luckett, 2019) and a percentage of these patients maybe transferred to ward areas with a tracheostomy still insitu. Therefore, nurses need to have the knowledge and skills necessary to care for these patients (Mc Grath et al., 2020).

KEY POINTS

- The placement of a tracheostomy tube changes airway anatomy and physiology (National Tracheostomy Safety Project [NTSP], 2022). The warming, filtering and humidification functions performed by the upper airway are lost when a tracheostomy is placed, and, therefore, all tracheostomies require some form of artificial humidification.
- The patient's ability to speak is also removed, and it makes it much more difficult for the patient to communicate and swallow. This means that patients with tracheostomies always require close attention to minimise the risk of complications.

TYPES OF TRACHEOSTOMY TUBES

Hospitals use tracheostomy tubes from a variety of manufacturers, so it is important that you are familiar with the types and sizes of tubes used in your clinical setting.

A cuffed tracheostomy tube is used with positive pressure ventilation. This protects the airway from aspiration, and is usually inserted when a new tracheostomy is formed.

An uncuffed tracheostomy tube allows airflow through the nose and mouth. It can be used as a weaning tool when planning the complete removal of tracheostomy. It cannot be used in positive pressure ventilation.

A tracheostomy tube with an opening in the outer cannual which allows air to circulate through the oral/nasal pharynx is referred as an fenestrated tube. It can be useful as it allows a patient to speak. However, it may increase the risk of aspiration. Therefore, a non-fenestrated inner cannula should be used when suctioning is required.

Traditionally, single lumen trachesotomies were inserted in critical care as the first tube to be sited, as it allowed for lower inflation pressures to be used when a patient is ventilated. However, over a decade ago it was no longer recommended to use these tubes due to the high risk of the tube becoming blocked. In consequence, today double lumen tracheostomy

tubes tend to be used (NTSP, 2022). For example, a reinforced tracheostomy tube with an adjustable flange are usually single lumen and used in patients with unusual anatomy.
Double lumen tracheostomies have an inner and outer tube, which allows the inner tube to be removed regularly for inspection and cleaning, which reduces the risk of blockage (Fig. 6.1). These types of tracheostomies are usually safer as there is the option to replace the inner tube should this happen. Some tracheostomy tubes also have a supraglottic port which allows for aspiration of secretions above the cuff (Fig. 6.2).

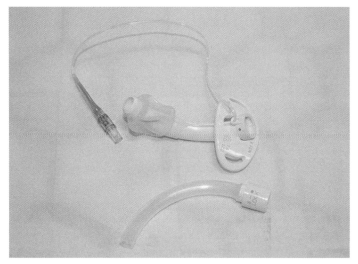

Fig. 6.1   A cuffed double lumen tracheostomy tube with inner tube.

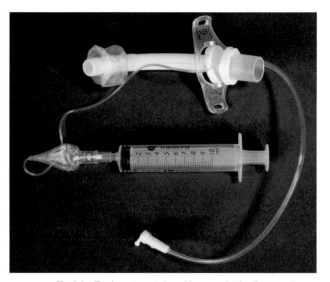

Fig. 6.2   Tracheostomy tube with supraglottic port.

TRACHEOSTOMY HUMIDIFICATION

All patients with a tracheostomy require humidification. Types of humidification include heat or cold humidification (Fig. 6.3), heat moisture exchangers (HMEs), saline nebulisation and stoma filters or bibs (NTSP, 2022). The method of humidification must:

- Provide adequate humidification for chest secretions.
- Help maintain body temperature
- Be appropriate for the patient
- Be readily available, simple to use and cost effective.

This can be either active or passive (Fig. 6.4). The type of humidification required will be dependent upon how new the tracheostomy is and whether supplemental oxygen therapy is required. Patients who have a high sputum load may need more humidification to prevent blockage of the tracheostomy.

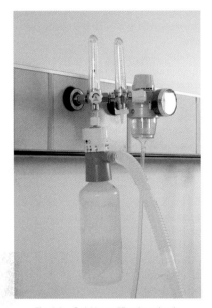

Fig. 6.3 Cold humdification circuit.

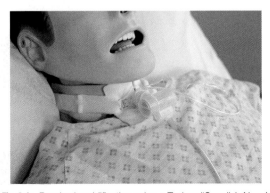

Fig. 6.4 Passive humidification using a T-piece/'Swedish Nose'.

Humidified moisture exchangers (HMEs) contain materials that conserve heat and moisture on expiration. These are good for patients who have a low secretion load; however, they need to be checked and replaced at least once every 24 hours as they can easily become blocked.

Tracheostomy Assessment

The National Confidential Enquiry into Patient Outcome and Death (NCEPOD) (2014) found that there was potential for improvement in tracheostomy care in relation to cuff management, the monitoring and frequency of clinical observations, tube selection, and the weaning process. Consequently, nurses caring for a patient with a tracheostomy must be able to perform a full respiratory assessment (see Chapter 4). Nurses should use the ABCDE framework to assess, clinical areas may also use a tracheostomy care bundle to guide care. Key elements specifically related to the assessment of a patient with a tracheostomy are given below:

Handover:

- Reason for tracheostomy tube insertion (e.g. an emergency due to airway obstruction, long-term intubation, improved respiratory function, neurological compromise, secretion management)
- Date of tracheostomy insertion
- Type of procedure (percutaneous or surgical)
- Any reported complications arising from the tracheostomy
- Bedside safety/emergency equipment availability

Patient Assessment:

- Tracheostomy type (e.g., fenestrated, cuffed, single or double lumen)
- Size of tube
- Tracheostomy tube ties secure (see page 67)
- Cuff status, e.g., inflated or deflated, any concerns with cuff leak
- Suctioning needs
- Inner tube check and confirmation of when last changed/cleaned.
- Stoma site checked and dressing intact and clean
- Assessment of cough reflex
- Assessment of patient's sputum load
- Tracheostomy tube cuff pressure (see page 66)
- Oxygen requirement and amount
- Type of humidification in use (e.g. Heat Moisture Exchange filter, Buchanan Bib
- Patient position (e.g., upright)
- Assessment of vital signs and national early warning score (NEWS)
- Nutrition assessment including: Nasogastric or percutaneous endoscopic gastrostomy (PEG) feeding, oral intake or oral trials
- Mobility assessment
- Communication methods, e.g., figure boards or letter boards that contain common phrases and messages to aid communication
- Documentation of all elements of assessment

Measuring a Tracheostomy Cuff Pressure

A tracheostomy with a cuff near the end of the tube provides a closed circuit for mechanical ventilation. Cuffed tubes are usually used in patients at the initial tracheostomy insertion as the risk of aspiration is high. Tracheostomy cuffs should neither be over- nor under-inflated, and the cuff pressure must be checked regularly to prevent complications (Credland, 2015). For example, occlusion of the tracheal mucosa blood supply can occur if the tracheostomy cuff pressures of 30

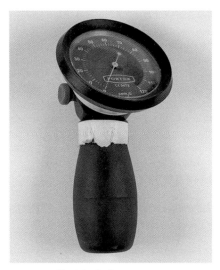

Fig. 6.5   Cuff manometer.

to 32 mmHg; therefore, the maximum cuff pressure of 25mmHg is deemed the safer upper limit for patients (Credland, 2015). This can be measured by using a cuff manometer (Fig. 6.5). Fingertip estimation of cuff pressure is inaccurate and must never be used.

KEY POINTS

- Nurses should aim for a tracheal capillary pressure to be within the safe range using a cuff manometer. High pressure represent over-inflation, and low pressures represent under-inflation.
- Over-inflated cuffs may result in tracheal mucosal damage and could result in long term problems such as tracheal stenosis. Over-inflated cuffs may also result in a reduced cough reflex and reduced sound production.
- Conversely, under-inflated tracheostomy cuffs should also be avoided as a deflated cuff may increase the risk of aspiration. If the cuff is constantly leaking and requires frequent 'top-ups' with air, then it is possible that the tracheostomy tube is damaged. This should be treated as a medical emergency and in this situation…. In this situation, the tracheostomy tube should be replaced by a suitably qualified person.
- For Patients who have had a laryngectomy, the cuff pressure may be considerably higher than for a patient with a temporary tracheostomy.

PROCEDURE

1. Explain the procedure to the patient to gain informed consent and reduce anxiety.
2. Decontaminate hands and put on a clean pair of gloves and an apron to reduce the risk of cross-infection.
3. Connect the balloon to the gauge and note current pressure. If this is between 20 to 25 cmH20, no further action is required.
4. If more pressure is required, use a 10 mL syringe to inflate the cuff (with air) to desired target pressure.

5. If the pressure reading is higher than 25 cm H_2O, allow some of the air to escape by pressing the red deflate button on the manometer or, alternatively, use the 10 mL syringe to deflate the cuff to the required level.

6. Recheck the pressure on the gauge and disconnect from the balloon.

7. Also, check for air escaping, place a stethoscope at the suprasternal notch and listen for any air escaping. If noise can be heard, the seal between the tracheal mucosa and the tracheostomy cuff may not be adequate, more air needs to be added via the pilot balloon until the leak can no longer be heard. The tracheostomy cuff pressure should then be rechecked and documented.

8. If there is still an air leak occurring, report this to the medical team immediately as the tube may need to be changed.

9. Each patient should have a dedicated manometer.

Securing a Tracheostomy Tube and Changing a Tracheostomy Dressing

Tracheostomy tubes need to be secure to prevent accidental decannulation (Credland, 2015). The tracheostomy ties should be checked regularly so that they remain secure and changed if they become soiled, wet or too tight/loose. As a guide, it should be possible to insert two fingers under the ties.

A tracheostomy stoma can easily become infected, particularly if a patient has a high sputum load and lots of moisture is present around the wound site. The areas should be inspected as per local policy, however, it is recommended, at least once in each twenty-four hour. For any signs of redness, swelling, bleeding or pressure damage. Tracheostomy dressings can be a source of infection, therefore, an aseptic, non-touch dressing technique is essential (see p. 5). Dressings must be changed as soon as soiled, and skin can be protected by using a barrier cream or film (Mallett et al., 2013; Credland, 2015).

KEY POINTS

- Tracheostomy dressings should be changed if visibly soiled or wet or as a minimum once every 24 hour at a period.
- Tracheostomy ties should be assessed and adjusted as indicated.
- Two nurses are needed to safely change a tracheostomy dressing.
- Often the tracheostomy dressing and ties are changed at the same time, as two nurses are needed for each procedure.

EQUIPMENT

- Sterile gloves, eye protection and protective apron
- 1 dressing pack and 1 sachet of 0.9% saline
- 1 pre-cut keyhole dressing for low exudate site or foam dressing for high exudate site
- 1 pair of scissors and 1 pair of Spencer Wells forceps
- Clinical waste bag
- Emergency tracheostomy box

PROCEDURE

1. It is a good idea to perform tracheal suction (see p. 73) prior to the dressing change, to minimise the risk of coughing and possible dislodgement of the tube during the procedure.

2. Prepare the trolley and equipment as for an aseptic dressing.
3. Raise the bed to a safe working height.
4. Decontaminate hands and put on PPE.
5. Remove any humidification/oxygen apparatus from the tracheostomy site, but leave the ties in place. If possible, hold/position the oxygen mask close to the tracheostomy throughout the dressing change.
6. Remove gloves and decontaminate hands.
7. Open the dressing pack, keyhole dressing and cleansing solution, and use the yellow waste bag as a 'glove' to remove the old dressing (see p. 226).
8. Attach the waste bag to the side of the trolley nearest the patient. Re-wash your hands or clean them using an alcohol hand-rub. Put on the sterile gloves.
9. Use gauze swabs and cleansing solution to clean around the tracheostomy as necessary. Use gauze swabs to gently dry the site.
10. Apply the keyhole dressing (Fig. 6.6).
11. With a second nurse holding the tube in position, undo one Velcro fastener, and pass the tie behind the patient's neck to the other nurse. Remove the other Velcro fastener and remove the tie.
12. Use the old tie to measure and cut the new tie to size (Fig. 6.7). Thread the Velcro fastener of the long length of padded tape through one side of the tracheostomy tube and secure. Pass the tape behind the patient's neck (Fig. 6.8). Attach the Velcro fastener of the short tape to the other side of the tracheostomy tube and then attach it securely to the long tape using the Velcro provided (Fig. 6.9).
13. Check that the fit is snug but it is not too tight. It should just be possible to slip two fingers between the tie and the patient's neck (Fig. 6.10).
14. Replace any humidification/oxygen equipment.
15. Check the patient is comfortable, and there is no respiratory distress.
16. Discard all clinical waste appropriately.
17. Remove apron and decontaminate hands.
18. Document the dressing change, describing the appearance of the tracheostomy site.

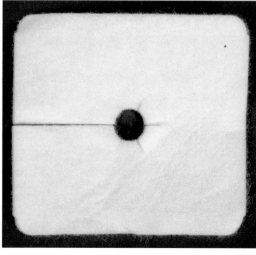

Fig. 6.6 Tracheostomy dressing.

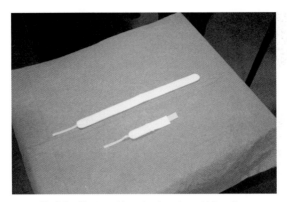

Fig. 6.7   Short and long tracheostomy Velcro ties.

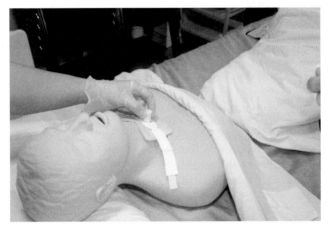

Fig. 6.8   Passing the short part of the Velcro tie through the tracheostomy flange.

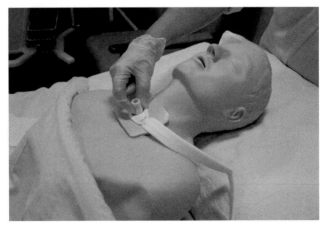

Fig. 6.9   Passing the long part of the Velcro tie through the second hole of the tracheostomy flange.

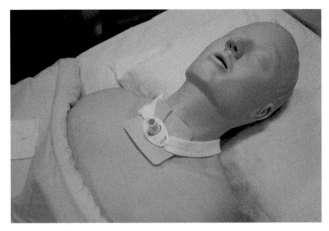

Fig. 6.10 Tracheostomy tube secured using Velcro ties.

Changing an Inner Tube

As mentioned previously, double lumen tubes are preferred as a safety measure to prevent occlusion by secretions. Types of inner cannula/tube include:

- Non-fenestrated: for use in both fenestrated and non-fenestrated tracheostomy tubes; in the latter, it is used during suction and when respiratory support is required.
- Fenestrated: For example, the Tracoe Twist has one large hole which allows air to be exhaled up through the upper respiratory tract.

Secretions can adhere to the internal lumen of the tracheostomy tube and significantly reduce the inner lumen diameter, increasing the effort involved in breathing and or obstructing the patient's airway. The removable inner cannula/tube can be changed and cleaned every 2 to 4 hours, thereby reducing the risk of occlusion (NTSP, 2022). If the sputum is particularly thick or sticky, it may need to be carried out more frequently, and if the patient is in respiratory distress, the inner cannula/tube should be removed and checked (Credland, 2016).

KEY POINTS

- Double lumen tracheostomies should be checked at least once every 2 to 4 hours and more if the patient has a high respiratory secretion load.
- Patients who have a double lumen tracheostomy should have at least one spare inner cannula/tube at the bedside with the emergency equipment. Depending on the manufacturer, inner tubes may be single use, i.e., disposable, or reusable.

EQUIPMENT

- Spare inner cannula/tube of the same size and type
- Clean gloves and apron
- Suction equipment
- Sterile water
- Disposable bowl
- Tracheostomy cleaning swab.

PROCEDURE

1. Hand hygiene must be performed before and after the procedure and when gloves are changed. Wear gloves, apron and eye protection (offer patient eye protection if required).
2. Inform the patient of the procedure.
3. Assess the patient and consider if supplemental oxygen is required prior to the procedure.
4. Open the clean inner cannula tube packaging or container. To remove the inner tube safely, use standard precautions and stabilise the outer tracheostomy tube prior to the removal of the inner cannula. The mode of removal of the inner tube/cannula will vary depending on the make and model used. Always check the manufacturer's guidelines prior to commencing the procedure. Remove the used inner tube and immediately replace it with the clean tube (Fig. 6.11).
5. If the inner tube cannula is reusable and appears clear when changing it, flush with sterile water (depending on local policy) (Figs. 6.12 and 6.13), make sure the neck of the bottle does not touch the inner tube, collect the 'flushed' water in a disposable container and disposing of it in the macerator in the sluice; then leave it in a drainage position on a piece

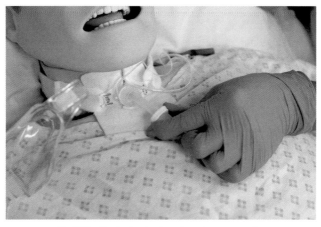

Fig. 6.11   Replacing tracheostomy inner cannula.

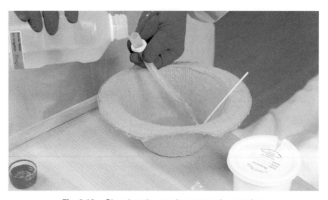

Fig. 6.12   Cleaning the tracheostomy inner tube.

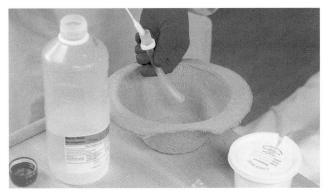

Fig. 6.13 Using a tracheostomy cleaning swab to clean the tracheostomy inner tube.

of gauze in a closed container. Inner tubes should never be cleaned using tap water, as increases the risk of microbe invasion.

6. If soiled, repeat this again, but flush longer, holding the cannula under the sterile water and turning it so that the water flows through one end then the other; this is to clean and remove any encrustation. If clean, store as before.

7. If the tube cannula remains soiled, to soften stubborn encrustation, it may be soaked in sterile water for 10 minutes, then clean as outlined above. Or gently clean the tube with the appropriate swab as advised by the manufacturer while flushing with sterile water, moving only halfway into the tube to minimise the risk of kinks and fractures. The swab should only be used as a last resort, as it may damage the smooth lining of the cannula and create grooves, which may harbour microorganisms.

8. If the secretions cannot be removed easily, replace the soiled tube with a new one, this is to minimise the risk of obstruction and infection. Soiled tubes must be disposed of as clinical waste.

9. Assess the type and quantity of secretions to check appropriate humidification is being used, as this will keep the airways warm and humidified.

10. If the patient is producing large amounts of thick or sticky secretions, nebulisers or mucolytic agents may be indicated. This is to prevent encrustation and minimise the risk of obstruction.

11. The patency of inner cannulas should be closely monitored at all times because the presence of secretions may increase resistance to airflow by decreasing the lumen size and leading to blockage.

Tracheal Suctioning

Tracheal suctioning should be carried out regularly to clear secretions from the tracheostomy tube (Billington and Luckett, 2019), and should be performed when clinically indicated. The frequency will depend on the patient's condition. Indications for tracheal suctioning include:

- Patients who are unable to maintain a patent airway, by clearing their secretions effectively and/or have an ineffective cough
- Abnormal breath sounds e.g., coarse breath sounds or crackles on auscultation
- Audible secretions
- Increasing respiratory effort in a self-ventilating patient
- Deteriorating oxygen saturation or arterial blood gas readings

- Suspected aspiration of food, fluids, saliva and/or stomach contents
- Changes in quantity, tenacity and colour of secretions
- Irregular respiratory pattern
- Changes in skin colour
- Patient anxiety, for example, patient distress due to breathing difficulties
- To obtain a sputum sample

KEY POINTS

- The suction catheter diameter should be no more than half the size of the diameter of the tube to allow for adequate flow of oxygen around the catheter during suction
- Sterile distilled water is used to clean the suction tubing after use and must be kept closed to discourage bacterial growth. The bottle must be changed every 24 hours.
- Suction pressure should be 80 to 120 mm Hg/12 to 16 kPa
- Suction should take no more than 15 seconds, to prevent hypoxia. A guide is to hold your own breath as you insert the catheter and aim to complete suctioning by the time you need to breathe again.
- Non-fenestrated inner cannula/tube must always be used for suctioning.

The use of sterile versus non-sterile gloves remains controversial, with local guidelines and policies varying. Therefore, it is important to check and follow local policies. The procedure outlined below details tracheal suctioning using sterile gloves, however, if non-sterile gloves are used, a clean glove is used instead.

EQUIPMENT

- Stethoscope
- Functional wall or portable suction unit.
- Sterile suction catheters
- Disposable non-sterile gloves and apron
- Sterile gloves
- Protective eyewear/facemask
- Oxygen therapy
- Sterile water for cleaning suction tubing post-treatment (labelled and dated)
- Disposable bowl
- Yankauer suction catheter
- Continuous pulse oximetry

PROCEDURE

1. Turn on the suction machine and test the suction pressure.
2. Open the suction-control end of a suction catheter, but leave it in its packet. Attach the end to the suction tubing, ensuring a good fit so that suction pressure is not lost.
3. Place the tubing and suction catheter (still in its packet) in a convenient position, ready for use. If a sputum specimen is needed, use a sputum trap (Fig. 6.14).
4. Open a sterile glove and put it on your dominant hand.
5. With your non-dominant hand (non-sterile gloved hand), remove any humidifying/oxygen apparatus from the endotracheal/tracheostomy tube/tracheostomy.

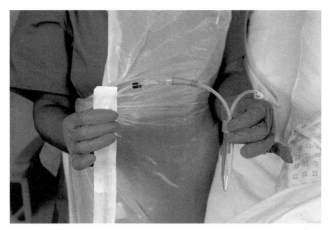

Fig. 6.14 Sputum trap attached to suction catheter.

6. With the same hand, pick up the suction tubing and carefully pull the suction catheter out of its packet. As the suction catheter emerges, take hold of it in your sterile-gloved hand 10 to 15 cm from the end of the catheter. Do not allow the catheter to touch anything.
7. Insert the suction catheter into the tracheostomy tube and, after warning the patient, advance it until it reaches the bifurcation of the right and left main bronchi (Fig. 6.15). This will make the patient cough.
8. When the patient coughs, withdraw the suction catheter 1 to 2 cm and then apply suction by occluding the suction-control apparatus with the thumb of your non-dominant hand.
9. Continue to apply suction and gradually withdraw the catheter. The patient cannot breathe during suction; therefore, it should be performed for no more than 10 to 15 seconds each time.
10. Remove the catheter from the ET tube/tracheostomy and wrap it around the fingers of your sterile-gloved hand. Remove the glove, turning it inside out with the catheter contained within it.
11. Disconnect the catheter from the suction tubing and discard.

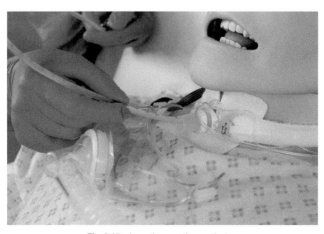

Fig. 6.15 Inserting suction catheter.

12. Repeat as necessary using a new catheter and sterile glove each time, allowing the patient time to recover before it is repeated.
13. Replace any humidification/oxygen equipment.
14. If the tracheostomy tube has a supraglottic port, aspirate the port (Fig. 6.16).
15. Check the patient is comfortable and breathing has returned to its usual rate.
16. Clean the suction tubing by suctioning sterile water through it until all traces of sputum have gone. The tubing should be replaced every 24 hours.
17. Check that there are more suction catheters available close by to the patient, ready for the next tracheal suction.
18. Replace the cap on the bottle of sterile water.
19. Remove gloves and apron and decontaminate hands.
22. Document suctioning, including the amount and appearance of the secretions.
21. Monitor the amount in the suction container. If the suction machine has a disposable sealed container, this does not need to be emptied but sealed and discarded when full or when the patient no longer requires suctioning. Eye protection should be worn when emptying it as there is a high risk of splashing.

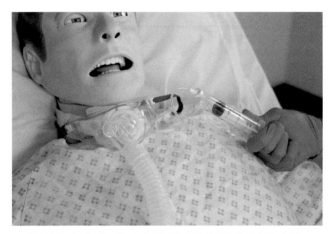

Fig. 6.16 Aspirating the supraglottic port of a tracheostomy tube.

References

Billington, J., Luckett, A., 2019. Care of the critically ill patient with a tracheostomy. Nurs. Stand. doi:10.7748/ns.2019.e11297.

Credland, N., 2015. How to measure tracheostomy tube cuff pressure. Nurs. Stand. 30 (5), 36–38.

Credland, N., 2016. How to perform a tracheostomy dressing and inner cannula change. Nurs. Stand. 30 (30), 34–36.

Mallett, J., Albarran, J.W., Richardson, A. (Eds.), 2013. Critical Care Manual of Clinical Procedures and Competencies. Wiley-Blackwell, Oxford.

McGrath, B.A., Wallace, S., Lynch, J., Bonvento, B., Coe, B., Owen, A., Firn, M., Brenner, M.J., Edwards, E., Finch, T.L. and Cameron, T., 2020. Improving tracheostomy care in the United Kingdom: results of a guided quality improvement programme in 20 diverse hospitals. British journal of anaesthesia, 125(1), pp.e119–e129.

National Confidential Enquiry into Patient Outcome and Death, 2014. On the Right Trach? A Review of the Care Received by Patients who Underwent a Tracheostomy. www.ncepod.org.uk/2014report1/downloads/OnTheRightTrach_FullReport.pdf.

National Tracheostomy Safety Project (NTSP), 2022. https://www.tracheostomy.org.uk/.

CHAPTER 7

Cardiovascular Assessment

Recording a Pulse Rate

A crucial element of patient assessment is the taking and recording of vital signs, which includes the pulse. The usual site for recording the pulse rate is at the wrist, where the radial pulse is easily felt. Pulses may also be felt at other sites (see p. 78) including the carotid, femoral, brachial, aortic, popliteal and dorsalis pedis (Fig. 7.1), and these may be used to check tissue perfusion (e.g., following surgery to a limb) or in an emergency (Williams and Edwards, 2019).

A patient's pulse should be felt even if it is shown on a pulse oximeter, automatic blood pressure machine or cardiac monitor. Assessment includes measuring the rate, rhythm, pressure (volume) and, if appropriate, deficits with the apex beat (Williams & Edwards, 2019). If an abnormality is detected, for example, an irregularity, a 12 lead electrocardiography (ECG) should be performed and investigated further.

KEY POINTS

- Use light pressure only; pressing too hard can occlude the artery, and you will be unable to feel the pulse. Do not use your thumb as the pulse in your thumb may result in you feeling your own pulse rather than the patient's.
- It is important to feel the patient's pulse even if the pulse rate is shown on the pulse oximeter or automatic blood pressure machine.

PROCEDURE

1. Choose a site to record the pulse. For most routine recordings, the radial pulse is used (Fig. 7.2).
2. Using your first and second fingers to feel the pulse, lightly compress the artery. Do not use your thumb.
3. Ideally, count the number of beats for 1 full minute. However, if the pulse is regular, it is sufficient to count for 30 seconds and double the result. If the pulse is irregular, you must count for the full minute.
4. Also, note the rate, rhythm, and the volume/strength of the pulse felt.
5. Check and record the colour of the patient's skin and mucous membranes (inside the lower eyelid). Pallor may indicate anaemia, while a bluish colour (cyanosis) indicates a lack of oxygen. In darker-skinned patients, it may be easier to detect this in the nail beds.
6. Document the findings according to local policy and report any abnormalities or changes from previous recordings of more than 20 beats per minute. The normal range in adults is 60 to 80 bpm.
7. Use an alcohol rub or wash and dry your hands.

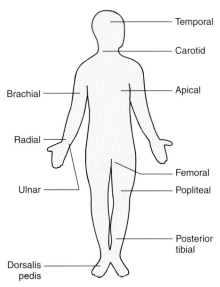

Fig. 7.1 Location of peripheral pulses. (Sharma, S.K., Stockert, P.A., Perry, A.G., Hall, A.M., Potter, P.A. (2021). *Potter & Perry's Essentials of Nursing Foundation*, South Asia Edition. Elsevier Inc.)

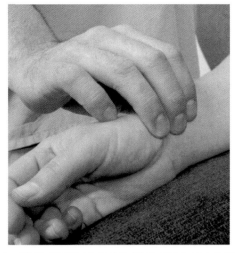

Fig. 7.2 Taking a radial pulse. (Zenith (2050). *Medical Assistant: Introduction to Medical Assisting—MAIntro*, 2nd ed. Elsevier Inc.)

Blood Pressure

Blood pressure (BP) is the force or pressure exerted by the blood on the walls of the blood vessels. The pressure is higher in arteries than in veins. When the ventricles contract, blood is forced into the aorta; the pressure created is called systolic pressure. When the heart relaxes following contraction, the arteries, such as the aorta, recoil and will still maintain some constriction; the pressure created in the walls is known as the diastolic pressure. The difference between the systolic and diastolic is known as the pulse pressure. The normal value is <40 mmHg (Williams and Edwards, 2019). BP varies throughout the heart and vascular system, with the highest in the aorta and gradually reducing with the lowest pressure in the arterioles and capillaries.

Blood pressure can be measured using either a non-invasive sphygmomanometer and stethoscope or automated device, or invasively via an arterial line. In emergencies, when a sphygmomanometer or automated device is not available, e.g. in a pre-hospital setting, it is possible to estimate the systolic blood pressure (SBP) by palpating a pulse. A radial pulse is equivalent to an SBP >90 mmHg, a femoral pulse 70 to 90 mmHg and a carotid pulse >60 mmHg.

Mean arterial pressure (MAP) is the average pressure reading within the arterial system. A MAP of 70 mmHg is required to maintain adequate perfusion. On automated BP machines and transduced BP MAP shows continuously. MAP is calculated by:

$$MAP = \frac{SBP + 2\ DBP}{3}$$

KEY POINTS

- Non-Invasive BP is the most common method of recording blood pressure.
- The sphygmomanometer may be an aneroid or a mercury type. The bladder part of the cuff must cover at least 80% of the circumference of the upper arm; a sizing guide is normally indicated on the cuff.
- Electronic BP machines are now commonly used. The cuff is positioned in the same way as described in step 4, but no stethoscope is required because the machine provides a digital display of the systolic and diastolic pressures. These machines must be plugged into the main electricity after use to re-charge the battery.
- Cuff width is an essential determinant of the accuracy of the pressure reading. The cuff should be 40% of the mid-circumference of the limb (the length should be twice the width). Cuffs that are too narrow tend to overestimate BP, while those who are too wide tend to underestimate.
- Potential complications include ulnar nerve injury (usually associated with the cuff being placed too low on the upper arm), oedema of the limb, petechiae and bruising, friction blisters and intravenous fluid failure.

PROCEDURE

1. Check the patient is resting in a comfortable position and discourage them from talking during the procedure. If a comparison between lying and standing blood pressure is required, the 'lying' recording should be done first. The patient should be rested and lying or seated comfortably with the legs uncrossed and should have rested for the previous 5 minutes. If there is a difference between the BP in each arm, use the arm with the higher BP for measurements (BIHS, 2021).
2. When applying the cuff, no clothing should be underneath it. If clothing constricts the arm, remove the arm from the sleeve.
3. Apply the cuff such that the centre of the inflatable 'bladder' is over the brachial artery (located on the medial aspect of the antecubital fossa) and 2 to 3 cm above the antecubital fossa. If the patient is receiving intravenous therapy, avoid using the arm that has the intravenous cannula or infusion in progress. Also, avoid using the same arm as the pulse oximeter.

4. The arm should be horizontal and supported at the level of the heart; it may be more comfortable resting on a pillow. If the arm is too low, it could lead to overestimation of the systolic BP by up to 10 mmHg. If the arm is raised above the heart, this may lead to underestimation (BIHS, 2021).
5. The sphygmomanometer should be placed on a firm surface, with the dial clearly visible and the needle at zero.
6. Estimate systolic BP by locating the radial or brachial pulse (Figs 7.3 and 7.4). Squeeze the bulb slowly to inflate the cuff while still feeling the pulse. Observe the dial and note the level when the pulse can no longer be felt. Open the valve fully to quickly release the pressure in the cuff. By estimating the systolic blood pressure in this way, you avoid having to inflate the cuff unnecessarily high during step 11.

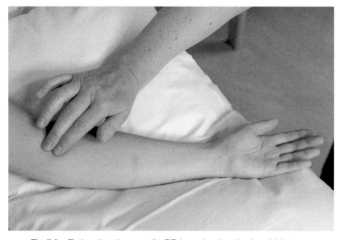

Fig. 7.3 Estimating the systolic BP by palpating the brachial artery.

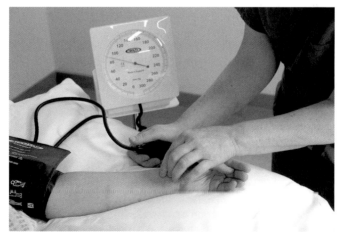

Fig. 7.4 Estimating the systolic BP by palpating the radial artery.

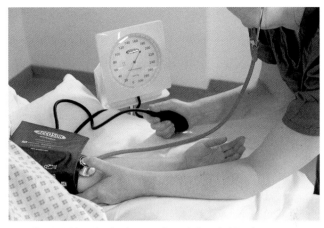

Fig. 7.5 Listening for the systolic and diastolic blood pressure.

7. If using a communal stethoscope, clean the stethoscope including the earpieces with an alcohol-impregnated swab. Curving the ends of the stethoscope slightly forward, place the earpieces in your ears.
8. If the stethoscope has two sides, check that it is turned to the diaphragm side.
9. Palpate the brachial artery.
10. Place the diaphragm of the stethoscope over the artery and hold it in place with your thumb while your fingers support the patient's elbow and ask the patient to relax their arm. You will not hear anything until the cuff is being deflated.
11. Check that the valve on the bulb is closed and inflate the cuff to 30 mmHg above the level noted in step 6. Slowly open the valve to allow the needle of the dial to drop **slowly and steadily** (2 to 3 mm per second). The arm should not be held rigid as muscle tension may cause a false reading (Fig. 7.5).
12. While observing the needle of the dial as it falls, listen for Korotkoff (thudding) sounds:
    ▪ **Systolic** pressure is the level where these are first heard.
    ▪ **Diastolic** pressure is the level where the sounds disappear.
13. Once the sounds have disappeared, open the valve fully to completely deflate the cuff. If you do not hear the systolic or diastolic pressure accurately, you will need to re-inflate the cuff and repeat the procedure. If still unclear, you should allow the patient to rest before repeating the procedure, as repeated attempts may affect the accuracy of the reading.
14. Remove the cuff from the patient's arm. Replace the clothing and ensure that the patient is comfortable. If recording lying and standing blood pressure, do not remove the cuff between recordings. The doctor may request that the patient be standing for at least 5 minutes before the standing blood pressure is recorded. Be aware that patients may feel dizzy on getting out of bed (postural hypotension).
15. Document the findings according to local policy and report any abnormalities. Report variations from previous recordings. The optimal BP in adults is a systolic pressure of <120 mmHg and a diastolic pressure of <80 mm Hg (BIHS, 2021).
16. Clean the stethoscope and sphygmomanometer and replace equipment. If using an electronic machine, plug it into the mains to charge.
17. Deconatminate hands.

Measuring Capillary Refill Time

Capilliary refill time (CRT) refers to the time it takes for blood refill compressed capilliaries and is used to assess dehydration and the haemodynamic status of the patient. It is a simple test that can be performed quickly; however, many factors can affect the result such as ambient (external) temperature and patient temperature.

CRT should be used in conjunction with other cardiovascular observations (e.g. blood pressure and pulse measurement, urine output etc.) (Resuscitation Council, 2021). The test is sometimes performed centrally, over the sternum (breastbone) or forehead.

PROCEDURE

1. Explain the procedure to gain consent and co-operation
2. Decontaminate hands.
3. Holding the patient's hand above the level of their heart, press on a finger nail for 5 seconds – this forces the blood out of the capilliaries and causes 'blanching' where the tissue beneath the finger nail looks pale.
4. After 5 seconds remove the pressure and count the number of seconds it takes for the normal nail bed colour to return.
5. The capilliary refill should take 2 seconds. It can take longer, i.e. is delayed, if the patient is hypovolaemic (blood or fluid loss), dehydrated or has peripheral vascular disease. A delayed capilliary refill time should be reported as it may indicate a problem with the patient's blood volume. Other cardiovascular observations should be performed as necessary.

Cardiac Monitoring

Continuous ECG monitoring is used to detect a change in clinical condition to help with the assessment of responses to therapy in real-time. Cardiac monitors have alarms that can be set to identify any significant changes in condition. They must be checked and set to safe physiological limits for each patient. Three or five lead ECG (Fig. 7.6) monitoring provides tracing of the cardiac conduction system. Lead II offers the best view and should be used as the default setting for monitoring.

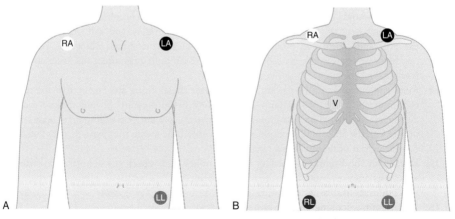

Fig. 7.6   (A) Three-lead electrocardiographic (ECG) monitoring system. (B) Five-lead monitoring system. (Sole, M. L., Klein, D. G., & Moseley, M. J. (2021). *Introduction to Critical Care Nursing*. Elsevier Inc.)

In the acute situation, most patients with cardiac monitors are required to rest in bed. However, patients undergoing investigations for cardiac rhythm abnormalities may be assessed via a 24-hour tape (Holter monitor) or ambulatory monitoring system (telemetry). The patient can be mobile with these systems, and the rhythm is analysed retrospectively. With telemetry, a transmitter sends signals to a central monitoring system, and the trace can be viewed in real time, though the patient may become 'disconnected' if the patient moves beyond the area where the signal can be picked up. It is vital to know where the patient is at all times in case of serious arrhythmias.

KEY POINTS

- Patients requiring continuous cardiac monitoring must be nursed in an area where they can be observed in case of sudden deterioration.
- Alarm limits should be checked at the start of every shift and should not be silenced.

PROCEDURE

1. Many acute clinical areas will have wall-mounted cardiac monitors. If using a portable monitor, place it on a firm surface, close to an electrical socket. Do not put anything on top of the monitor and keep sources of fluid away from it.
2. Raise the bed to a safe working height.
3. Expose the patient's chest and examine the sites that will be used for the electrodes.
4. If the chest is very hairy, shave or clip a small patch of hair at each site to allow good contact and adhesion of the electrodes.
5. Check the expiration date of the electrodes and check that the gel has not dried out.
6. If the electrode has a small raised patch on the back, use this to roughen the skin slightly where the electrode will be placed. This improves adhesion and contact.
7. Removing the backing paper and taking care not to touch the gel in the middle, stick the electrodes firmly to the chest. The electrodes should be placed over bone and not muscle, avoiding areas that may be used for the placement of defibrillator pads. Electrodes can usually remain in place for 24 to 72 hours but may need replacing more frequently if the patient sweats a lot, if the gel dries out or if the patient's skin shows signs of sensitivity.
8. Connect the leads to the electrodes. This is usually by means of a small clip or press stud. The leads are labelled or colour coded. If using a three-lead system, place the red electrode on the right shoulder, the yellow electrode on the left shoulder and the green electrode on the left lower abdomen. If using a four-lead system, the additional black lead is placed on the lower right side of the abdomen. If a five-lead system is used, place the first four leads as detailed above, and the white lead is placed in the middle of the chest.
9. Turn on the monitor and select lead II, which should produce the most positive (upright-looking) display. If lead II does not produce a good display, try lead I or lead III. If necessary, adjust the 'gain' or size on the monitor to make the display larger and easier to see.
10. Set the alarms to safe parameters, according to the patient's condition and local protocol.
11. Replace the patient's clothing and ensure that the leads are not pulling on the electrodes and that the cables are not under tension or trapped, e.g., in bed rails.
12. Explain/demonstrate what will happen if the patient moves or disturbs the electrodes (i.e. abnormal-looking pattern) to prevent unnecessary concern.
13. Lower the bed, adjusting the height for the patient's safety and convenience.
14. Remove apron and decontaminate hands.

15. Document the rhythm shown on the monitor and report any abnormalities as appropriate. Some monitors have the facility to digitally record abnormal rhythms, and record the rhythm whenever the alarm is triggered. If the monitor does not have this facility, it is good practice to print out a rhythm strip at the beginning of each shift and when any abnormal rhythms are noted. The printout should be labelled and signed before being stored in the patient's notes. Some specialist units also have monitors that enable ST-segment monitoring.

Recording a 12-Lead Electrocardiography

A 12-lead ECG is used to assess and diagnose patients with suspected arrhythmias, hypertension, coronary heart disease or heart failure (Menzies-Gow, 2018).

KEY POINTS

- Correct positioning of the electrodes using anatomical landmarks is essential for an accurate and high-quality ECG recording.
- Skin preparation is essential as it may affect the quality of the ECG recording.

PROCEDURE

1. Explain the procedure to gain consent and cooperation.
2. Close curtains or screens to ensure privacy.
3. Ask/assist the patient to lie in a recumbent or semi-recumbent position. Explain the need to lie still during the recording in order to gain a good trace.
4. Hands should be clean, and an apron should be worn. Additional protective clothing may be necessary if indicated by the patient's condition.
5. Raise the bed to a safe working height.
6. Expose the patient's ankles, wrists and chest area.
7. Apply the electrodes to the patient's ankles and wrists.
8. Apply the electrodes to the chest wall as shown in Fig. 7.7. If necessary, shave the area to ensure good contact/adhesion. In women with large breasts, it is sometimes difficult to place the chest leads under the breast. The electrodes may be placed over the breast in the appropriate position if this is the case.
9. Connect the ECG leads to the electrodes as labelled or colour coded.
10. Press 'start' on the ECG machine. All 12 leads (views of the heart) will print out on one page. Add the patient's name, ward and hospital number to the printout. It is usual to note whether the patient has chest pain or is pain-free at the time of the ECG recording. In some hospitals, it is policy for the person recording the ECG to date and sign the printout.
11. Remove the leads and electrodes, wiping away any traces of gel left on the skin.
12. Help the patient to replace their clothing and ensure they are comfortable.
13. Lower the bed to a safe level.
14. Remove apron and decontaminate hands.
15. File the ECG in the patient's notes and inform the requesting practitioner that it has been completed.
16. Leave the ECG machine clean, tidy and stocked, ready for the next user. Do not tie the leads together as this damages them. Plug the machine into the mains to charge if required.

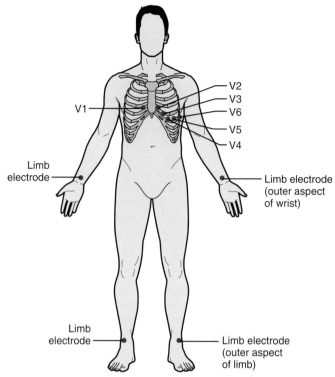

Fig. 7.7 Electrode positions for 12-lead electrocardiography. (Ignatavicius, D. D., Workman, M. L., Heimgartner, N.M. & Rebar, C. (2021). *Medical-Surgical Nursing: Concepts for Interprofessional Collaborative Care*, 10th ed. Elsevier.)

Temperature

Temperature constantly alters within a normal range. In normal circumstances, it will fall to its lowest in the morning and rise to its highest point in the evening. Measuring core body temperature is part of assessment for the presence and prognosis of disease. Cell metabolism operates at maximum efficiency when the body temperature is within normal limits, and adjustment mechanisms exist to maintain the temperature at its correct value.

When leucocytes, or white blood cells, become damaged in their work against invading organisms, they release pyrogens. Pyrogens affects the body temperature control in the hypothalamus resulting in a higher core temperature, which stimulates a process to either conserve or manufacture body heat. Temperature can be measured using the oral, axilla or tympanic route.

KEY POINTS

- A body temperature above 41°C (hyperthermia) will damage brain cells and blood vessels. A measured temperature below 35°C is described as hypothermia.
- A temperature lower than 32°C will become fatal if not treated.
- National Institute for Health and Care Excellence (NICE, 2016) recommends when using a temperature recording device, nurses are appropriately trained in their use in accordance with the manufacturer's instructions and local infection control policies.

PROCEDURE

1. Explain the procedure to gain consent and cooperation.
2. Assess the patient regarding a suitable site for temperature recording. If the patient is unconscious, extremely breathless (mouth breathing), confused, prone to seizures, has mouth sores or has undergone oral surgery, the oral site should not be used for temperature measurement. The temperature in the axilla is 0.5° lower than the oral temperature. The rectal site is only used for continuous temperature monitoring in some critical care areas, where a small electronic probe is inserted into the rectum. Tympanic thermometers measure the temperature by inserting a probe into the outer ear, adjacent to (but not touching) the tympanic membrane. An infrared light detects heat radiated from the tympanic membrane and provides a digital reading. This provides an accurate measure of body core temperature as it is close to the carotid artery.
3. Hands must be clean, and an apron should be worn.
4. Additional personal protective clothing may be necessary if indicated by the patient's condition.

ORAL

1. Patients should be rested and not have had a hot or cold drink or smoked a cigarette within the previous 20 minutes when using the oral site (McCallum and Higgins, 2012).
2. On the electronic thermometer, select the 'oral' site.
3. Cover the probe with a disposable cover to prevent contamination.
4. Place the covered probe under the tongue in the same way as a disposable thermometer (Fig. 7.8). When the audible signal is heard, remove the probe from the mouth.
5. The temperature is shown in the digital display box.

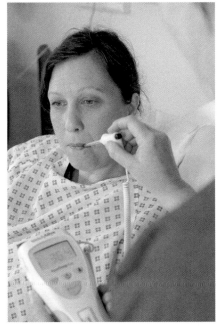

Fig. 7.8 Taking an oral temperature.

6. Using a non-touch technique, discard the cover into the locker bag or clinical waste. Most electronic thermometers have a mechanism to eject the probe cover without handling it.

Axillary

1. On the electronic thermometer, select the 'axilla' site.
2. Cover the probe with a disposable cover.
3. Insert the probe horizontally and hold the patient's arm close to the chest to ensure good contact with the skin.
4. When the audible signal is heard, remove the probe from the axilla. The temperature is shown in the digital display box.
5. Using a non-touch technique, discard the probe cover into the clinical waste.

Oral and Axillary

1. Check patient comfort and answer any questions regarding the recording.
2. Return the thermometer to the charging point/storage area as appropriate.
3. Document the temperature according to local policy. Report any abnormality. The normal range for adults is 36.0°C to 37.2°C.
4. Use an alcohol rub or wash and dry your hands.

Tympanic

1. Switch on the thermometer
2. Use a non-touch technique to fit a disposable cover.
3. Gently place the covered probe into the ear canal. Check for a snug fit.
4. When the audible signal is heard, remove the probe from the ear. The temperature is shown in the digital display box.
5. Use a non-touch technique to discard the cover into the clinical waste bag.
6. Document the findings according to local policy and report any abnormalities. The normal range for adults is 36.0°C to 37.2°C.
7. Return the thermometer to the charging point/storage area as appropriate.
8. Use an alcohol rub or wash and dry your hands.

Neurovascular Assessment

Neurovascular observations are undertaken on patients with an acute limb injury, post limb surgery, or treatment resulting in limb compression/constriction (such as casts, skin traction, circumferential bandaging) to reduce the risk of developing acute limb compartment syndrome (ALCS) (Royal College of Nursing, 2014). Patients at high risk include those with tibial, forearm or high-energy distal radius fractures, orthopaedic injury/intervention combined with known coagulopathies/patient taking anticoagulants, crush injuries and those who have sustained high impact trauma, including open fractures (Royal College of Nursing, 2016).

KEY POINTS

- Neurovascular observations should be performed hourly for the first 24 hours and then every 4 hours for the first 24 to 48 hours. However, monitoring should be increased to hourly if there are clinical concerns.
- When observing limb perfusion, movement and sensation, this should be compared to the other limb if that is unaffected.
- Changes in pulse, sensation and skin colour are late symptoms of neurovascular compromise and should not be relied upon to diagnose compartment syndrome.

PROCEDURE

Explain the procedure to the patient to gain consent and cooperation. The frequency of observations should also be explained.

To perform a neurovascular assessment:

1. **Movement** – ask the patient to move the toes/fingers and ankle/wrist of the affected limb if possible. If the patient is unable to do so, undertake the movement passively and note any pain that occurs with movement or rest. It is important to see all fingers/toes move as each digit has a separate nerve supply, which may be damaged or compressed.

2. **Sensation** – without letting the patient see which toes/fingers you are touching, touch the toes/fingers randomly and ask the patient to tell you which one you are touching. Ask the patient if they feel any altered sensation in the limb, such as numbness, tingling or 'pins and needles'.

3. **Perfusion** – in order to assess perfusion, observe and record the following:
   - Temperature – feel the warmth of the limb, both above and below the site of injury. It is best to do this using the back of the hand.
   - Colour – observe and record the colour of the skin and nail beds. Note any cyanosis, mottling or pallor.
   - Pulse – the pulse should be palpated distally to the injury. It may not always be possible to easily locate a pulse, particularly in the feet. Where possible, the pulse on the affected limb should be assessed on admission as a baseline for later comparison. Once located, it is helpful to mark the site to make it easier for subsequent checking. Note the strength of the pulse. If bandages or a splint prevent you from locating a pulse, this should be documented. If the dorsalis pedis pulse cannot be located, try to palpate the posterior tibial pulse. If recording 'pulse not felt', take care that it is not confused with 'pulse not able to be located' due to the bandage/splint, etc. If a pulse cannot be located due to a bandage or cast, capillary refill time may be measured to assess perfusion,

4. **Pain/swelling** – if the patient complains of pain or the toes/fingers are swollen, check the bandage, splint or plaster cast for tightness. Record the location, level and characteristics of any reported pain. If swelling is present, detail any increase since the last set of observations and consider the removal of tight-fitting jewelry and loosening of bandages. Elevation of the limb may help prevent swelling.
   - Pain should be assessed using a Numerical Rating Scale (see p. 111) or other alternative pain assessment tool. Severe pain and pain on passive movement of the muscles are key clinical findings. Pain at rest on passive extension of the limb or when passively extending the fingers or toes of the affected limb, or if not controlled by regular or appropriate analgesia, is an important clinical finding for potential ACLS.
   - Patients who have had an anaesthetic nerve block or epidural may not be able to report the pain associated with compartment syndrome. In addition, pain may be difficult to report, particularly if the patient has an impaired ability to report this symptom, for example, when the patient is unconscious.

5. If the patient has a bandage/dressing/splint/plaster cast – check for bleeding under or around these.

6. Following the procedure, check that the patient is appropriately covered and comfortable.

7. Remove apron and decontaminate hands prior to completing relevant documentation according to local policy.

References

BIHS, 2021. Blood Pressure Management. https://bihsoc.org/resources/bp-measurement/measure-blood-pressure/.

Care Quality Commission, 2021. Hypothermia. https://www.cqc.org.uk/guidance-providers/learning-safety-incidents/issue-8-hypothermia.

McCallum, L. and Higgins, D., 2012. Measuring body temperature. Nursing times, 108(45), pp. 20-22.

Menzies-Gow, E., 2018. How to record a 12-lead electrocardiogram. Nurs. Stand. doi:10.7748/ns.2018. e11066.

National Institute of Health and Care Excellence (NICE), 2016. Hypothermia: prevention and management in adults having surgery. Clin Guidel. (CG65). Available at: https://www.nice.org.uk/guidance/cg65/chapter/Recommendations#perioperative-care.

Royal College of Nursing, 2014. Peripheral neurovascular observations for acute limb compartment syndrome RCN consensus guidance. Publication code: 004 685.

Royal College of Nursing, 2016. Acute Limb Compartment Syndrome Observation Chart. Publication code: 005 457.

Tanner, J., Kay, J., Chambers, K., 2016. Avoiding inadvertent peri-operative hypothermia. Nurs. Times 112 (35), 10–12.

Williams, J. and Edwards, S., 2019. A Nurse's Survival Guide to Critical Care-Updated Edition. Elsevier.

CHAPTER 8

Neurological Assessment and Management

Neurological Assessment

AVPU ASSESSMENT

AVPU stands for Alert, Voice, Pain and Unresponsive. The scale has a simple structure, which is easy to apply and has been incorporated into the Early Warning Score assessment (see p. 18; Resuscitation Council (UK), 2021). This is in recognition of the fact that many patients who are acute and critically ill will have altered levels of consciousness. The AVPU provides a rapid assessment of the patient's level of consciousness. This can then be followed with a formal assessment using the Glasgow Coma Scale (GCS) (Resuscitation Council (UK), 2021).

However, neurological conditions always require formal assessment using the GCS, formal neurological assessment using the GCS these include head-injured patients, those with neurological disorders such as a brain tumour, stroke, meningitis and/or a reduced level of consciousness following sedation, e.g., anaesthetic, opiate analgesia or drug overdose. In consequence, nurses will need to determine the most appropriate assessment method to use based on the clinical situation and patient's condition.

KEY POINTS

The AVPU method of neurological assessment is used by nurses to complete a rapid initial assessment of a patient's conscious level.
Any patient with a reduced level of consciousness must have their blood glucose level recorded to rule out hypoglycaemia.
The pupillary reaction must also be recorded as part of this assessment.

EQUIPMENT REQUIRED

- Personal Protective Equipment
- Vital signs chart
- A pen torch for assessing pupil size and reactions
- Sphygmomanometer, stethoscope, thermometer and a watch to complete vital signs.

PROCEDURE

1. AVPU assessment can be used to assess the conscious level of all patients; it is usually conducted on encountering the patient, noting their response to a greeting such as 'hello', or 'how are you feeling?'
2. Assess the patient to determine if they are:
   - Alert.
   - Respond to Voice.

- Respond to painful stimulus. A painful stimulus can be given by squeezing the trapezius muscle, or by applying supra-orbital pressure (at the supra-orbital notch).
- Unresponsive.

3. Document and act on your findings.

Glasgow Coma Scale

RATIONALE

The Glasgow Coma Scale is an internationally recognised objective tool used to assess and monitor a patient's level of consciousness (Waterhouse, 2017). It is used in a wide variety of clinical settings and is a recommended assessment and observation tool for all patients with head injuries (NICE, 2019). The patient's level of consciousness is assessed by monitoring their ability to open their eyes (eye-opening), talk (verbal response) and move their limbs (motor response). Each of these areas is allocated a score based on the patient's response. The lowest total score is 3, and the highest is 15 (Fig. 8.1) with the total score for each section, Eyes 4, Verbal 5, Motor 6. Any reduction in the score is a sign that the patient's consciousness level is deteriorating and should be reported immediately. A patient with a score of 8 or less will usually be in a deep coma.

KEY POINTS

Any patient with a reduced level of consciousness is at risk of airway compromise. Therefore, the neurological assessment must form part of the ABCDE assessment.

Clinical methods of assessing neurological status include measurement and interpretation of vital signs (respiratory rate, pulse, blood pressure, and temperature), arterial blood gases, level of consciousness and pupillary response.

Any patient with a reduced level of consciousness must have their blood glucose level recorded to rule out hypoglycaemia.

The pupillary reaction must be checked and recorded as part of this assessment.

EQUIPMENT REQUIRED

- Personal protective equipment
- A pen torch for assessing pupil size and reactions
- Sphygmomanometer, stethoscope, thermometer and a watch
- Neurological assessment chart (Fig. 8.1)

PROCEDURE

Assessment of Eye-Opening

Eye-opening demonstrates that the arousal mechanisms in the brain are functioning. When assessing this, the scoring system is used as follows:

- A score of 4 is given to patients who are conscious, who sense your approach and open their eyes spontaneously or patients who are asleep, but open their eyes in response to a brief verbal stimulus, such as 'hello' or light touch.
- A score of 3 is given to patients who open their eyes in response to a verbal stimulus such as 'can you open your eyes, please?'
- A score of 2 is given to patients who open their eyes only in response to a painful stimulus. This is best applied by a trapezium squeeze (pinching the muscle where the head

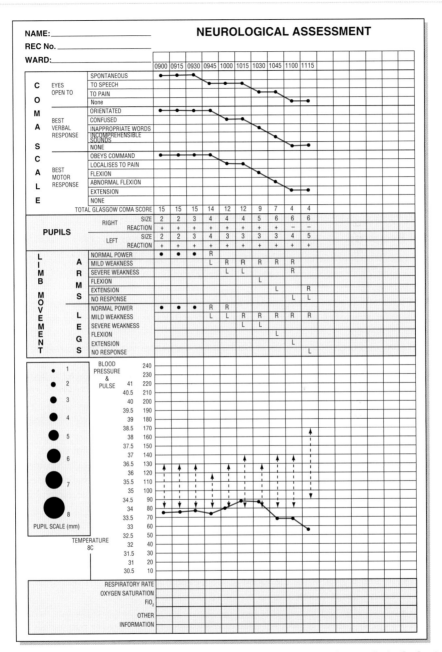

Fig. 8.1 Neurological assessment chart incorporating the Glasgow Coma Scale. (icol, M., Bavin, C., Cronin, P., Rawlings-Anderson, K., Cole, E., & Hunter, J. (2012). *Essential Nursing Skills*. Elsevier Inc.)

meets the shoulder) or supra-orbital pressure (firm pressure in the eye socket just above the eye) (DeSouza and Woodward, 2016). Response to centrally applied painful stimulus indicates that the motor pathways are still functioning to some extent (DeSouza and Woodward, 2016). Peripheral stimuli, although useful when assessing an individual limb that has not moved in response to a central stimulus, could also be a reflex activity. Other methods (e.g. rubbing the sternum with the knuckles or pressing on nail beds) are not recommended.

- A score of 1 is given where there is no eye-opening in response to verbal or painful stimuli.

Patients may not be able to open their eyes if there is damage to the oculomotor nerve, which is responsible for the movement of the eyelid, or if paralysing medication has been administered. In these situations, the nurse should gently open the eyelid (with assistance from another practitioner) when pupil response is to be assessed. If the patient is unable to open their eyes due to swelling, injury or an eye dressing, this is indicated using the letter 'C'.

Verbal Response

This assesses whether patients are aware of themselves and their environment. If the patient has a tracheostomy or an endotracheal tube, the letter 'T' can be used to indicate this. The score is used as follows:

- A score of 5 is given if the patient is orientated, i.e., able to tell the nurse who they are; where they are; what day, date, month and year it is; and why they are where they are.
- A score of 4 is given if the patient can hold a conversation, but not able to answer specific questions (i.e. they are confused and not orientated).
- A score of 3 is given when the patient can speak, but does so randomly and makes short verbal responses such as swearing or shouting.
- A score of 2 is given when the patients' speech is incomprehensible, they are grunting or groaning, and the nurse may have to use painful stimuli to get a response (as described previously).
- A score of 1 is given if the patient does not respond to verbal and painful stimuli.

Facial injuries, impairment to speech (e.g., following a stroke), cognitive difficulties (e.g., dementia) or language barriers all need to be considered when scoring the verbal response. Interpreters may be required, and the patient's normal cognitive state should be established as a baseline.

Motor Response

This assesses the patient's ability to move purposefully. When assessing motor response, scores are allocated as follows:

- A score of 6 is given when the patient can obey commands such as 'lift your arms' or 'squeeze my hands' (where there is no injury or weakness).
- A score of 5 is given when the patient can localise to pain. The pain stimulus (see 'Assessment of eye-opening' above) is used, and patients will usually respond by trying purposefully to remove the source of the pain (brush away the nurse's hand) or 'shrug off' the pain. Localising to pain means that the patient's brain is receiving sensory information regarding the process of feeling pain and therefore the reduced level of consciousness is not severe.
- A score of 4 is given when the patient withdraws from the painful stimulus or moves towards the source of the pain but does not attempt to remove it. Bending the arms and legs normally and fully in response to pain is known as flexion.
- A score of 3 is given when there is an abnormal bending movement such as wrist rotation or bending the ankle joints towards the knees. This is known as abnormal flexion

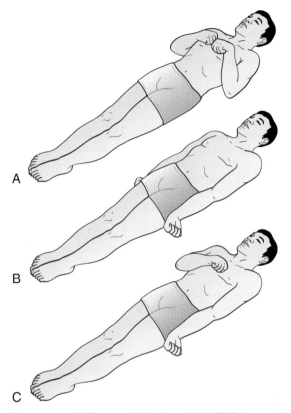

Fig. 8.2 Abnormal motor responses. (A) Flexor posturing (decorticate). (B) Extensor posturing (decerebrate). (C) Flexor posturing on right side and extensor posturing on left side. (Sole, M. L., Klein, D. G., & Moseley, M. J. (2021). *Introduction to Critical Care Nursing*. Elsevier Inc.)

and usually indicates that the nerve pathways are not functioning normally and in some cases is a sign of deterioration and a poor prognosis (Fig. 8.1)

- A score of 2 is given when the patient extends their limbs to pain. This may appear as if the patient is straightening or pointing their arms and legs in a rigid outwards or downwards position. This indicates damage to the brain stem, and the prognosis for the patient is very poor (see Fig. 8.2).
- A score of 1 is given where there is no response to painful stimuli.

Pupil Response

The pupillary response should be assessed and documented, as outlined on page 96.

Vital Signs

These are not part of the Glasgow Coma Scale itself, but because of their importance, they are usually included on the same chart (Fig. 8.1).

- **Temperature** – alterations in a patients' temperature may be due to damage to the thermoregulation centre of the brain. A rise in body temperature increases the demand for oxygen by the brain cells, which may already be compromised due to damage. It is usually desirable to keep the body temperature within normal limits, where possible.

This may require antipyretic agents such as paracetamol or active measures such as fan therapy. Patients with severe brain injuries may be kept mildly hypothermic to reduce metabolic demand in the brain tissue (Frank and Broessner, 2017).

- **Pulse rate and blood pressure** – in patients with severe raised intracranial pressure, the blood pressure rises, and pulse rate falls. As the brain becomes hypoxic and ischaemic, the body responds by attempting to increase the arterial blood pressure to increase oxygen flow to the brain. As a result, there is a need for more blood in each contraction of the heart. This results in a slowing of the heart rate (bradycardia). Respiration rate also decreases, and a change in the respiratory pattern occurs (see below). This is known as 'Cushing's reflex' and is a very late response to a deteriorating level of consciousness. Careful recording and charting are needed so that a trend in this direction is clearly detectable and reported urgently.
- **Respiration rate** – changes in respiration are a good indicator of the function of the brain stem. This is because there are four respiratory control centres in two parts of the brain stem. Monitoring of respiration rate and the pattern is essential as a sudden change, such as Cheyne–Stokes breathing (deep, sighing respirations followed by periods of apnoea for several seconds) or apnoea, is due to a significant rise in intracranial pressure.

Limb Movement

In addition to assessing motor response, as described previously, assessing limb movement can detect weakness in limbs or one side of the body. Assessing limb movement and motor power indicates the extent of the damage to the motor cortex that controls motor movement and is graded as follows:

- Normal power – the nurse applies resistance to any joint movement, and this can be matched by the patient, e.g., pulling or pushing while holding the hands
- Mild weakness – the patient is able to counter the resistance but is easily overcome
- Severe weakness – the patient is able to move the limb but not against resistance
- Flexion, extension or no response – there is flexion, extension or no movement in response to central or peripheral painful stimuli.

Assessing motor power requires knowledge of motor nerve anatomy (myotomes) and skill in performing the procedure. If the nurse is to assess more than the presence (or not) of limb weakness, then further training in this skill is required.

Measuring Pupil Reaction

RATIONALE

Assessing pupillary reaction is an integral component of both the AVPU and GCS assessment tools. Raised intracranial pressure causes changes in the size of the pupils and their response to light. Assessment of the pupils evaluates the function of the optic nerve, which causes a reaction to light being shone in the eye, and the oculomotor nerve, which constricts the pupil. A poor reaction in either of these assessments may indicate compression of the nerves and should be reported. When assessing the pupils, dim the light in the room and gently hold the eyelid open (you may need another practitioner to help with this).

KEY POINTS

- Pupil reaction should be used with either the AVPU or GCS method for neurological examination.

EQUIPMENT

- Personal protective equipment
- Pen torch
- Observation/GCS Chart

PROCEDURE

Explain procedure to patient.

Before you shine the light in the patient's eye, observe the following:

- The resting size of both pupils. The average size is 2 to 6 mm, but it varies according to the time of the day and the amount of light available.
- Whether both pupils are equal in size – inequality can be a severe sign of raised intracranial pressure (or the sign of previous eye injury).
- The shape of the pupils – they usually are round. Different shapes may indicate damage to the brain.

Bringing the light of the pen torch in from the side of the eye, observe:

- The reaction of each pupil to light (Fig. 8.3).
- The intensity of the reaction, i.e., whether it is brisk, sluggish or absent (Fig. 8.4).
- It is also important to note if the patient has a pre-existing abnormality, or irregularity of the eye/s, for example, cataracts, which will affect the response (Table 8.1). In addition, it is important to note any drugs or medications the patients may have had. Some cause dilation (e.g. atropine), while others (opiates, e.g. morphine) cause constriction. Prosthetic eyes will not elicit a pupillary response.

Document and act on your findings.

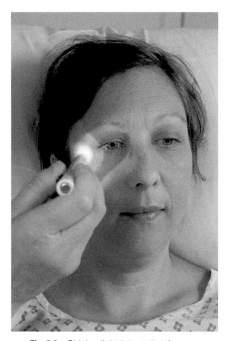

Fig. 8.3 Shining light into patient's eyes.

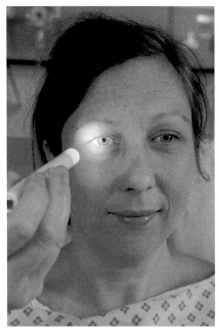

Fig. 8.4 Pupil reaction.

TABLE 8.1 ▪ **Potential Changes in Pupil Reaction**

Observation	Size	Reactivity	Possible Cause
Equal	Pinpoint	–	Opiates overdose
	Small	Reactive	Metabolic encephalopathy
	Mid-sized	Fixed	Midbrain lesion
		Reactive	Metabolic lesion
Unequal	Dilated	Unreactive	3rd nerve palsy
	Small	Reactive	Horner's syndrome

Measuring a Blood Glucose Level (BGL)

RATIONALE

Blood glucose testing is an example of a 'point of care test' (also termed 'near-patient testing'), which involves taking a blood sample but not sending it to the laboratory. This simple test is used to detect hyper or hypoglycaemia and to indicate whether a patient is able to maintain normo-glycaemia. Prior to undertaking the procedure, many clinical areas require nurses to have undergone formal training in the use of the glucometer. In addition, nurses must be able to interpret and act on the results within the context on the patient's situation (Dunning, 2015).

EQUIPMENT

- Gloves
- Access to soap and warm water

- Glucometer correctly calibrated
- Test strips appropriate for the glucometer
- Finger-pricking device or lancet
- Gauze
- Sharps box
- Clinical waste container

PROCEDURE

1. Explain the procedure to gain consent and cooperation.
2. Check that the patient's hands are clean. Avoid using alcohol wipes to clean the skin, as this may give a false reading and may harden the skin with frequent use. If necessary, assist the patient with washing and drying of the fingers/hands. The patient's hands should be clean and washing the hands in warm water will encourage blood flow. If the patient is unable to wash their hands, and there is any possibility that there may have been contact with substances such as fruit juice, the finger should be washed or wiped with a wet tissue and then a dry tissue before pricking.
3. Assemble the equipment (see Fig. 8.5). Preparation of the glucometer usually involves checking that it has been calibrated for the particular batch of testing strips that are being used. With some glucometers, the strip is inserted into the monitor after the blood is dropped onto it. Follow the manufacturer's instructions regarding timing and wiping prior to insertion into the machine.
4. Check the expiration date of the testing strips and prepare the blood glucose meter and insert the testing strip according to the manufacturer's instructions.
5. Using the appropriate device, prick the side of the patient's fingertip (see Fig. 8.6). Avoid frequent use of the thumbs, index and little fingers where possible. Before pricking the patient's finger, hold the hand downwards to encourage blood flow, and make a light tourniquet with your hand around the finger to ensure sufficient blood is present in the tip

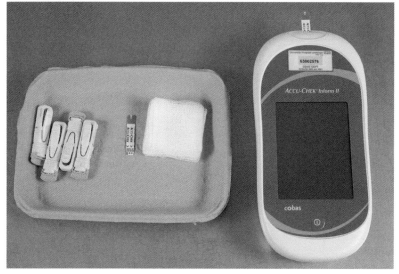

Fig. 8.5 Equipment assembled.

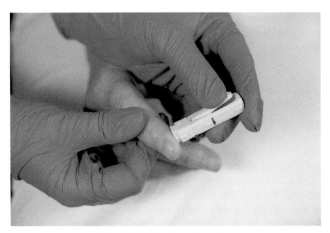

Fig. 8.6 Taking blood sample.

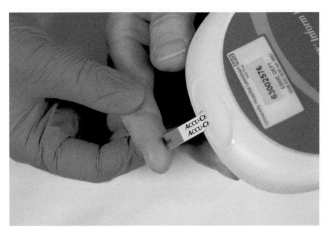

Fig. 8.7 Taking the blood glucose sample.

of the finger. Avoid 'milking' blood into the finger as the local blood composition may be disturbed by intermingling with tissue fluid. Taking time to encourage blood flow before pricking the finger will reduce the need for pricking again, which can be distressing for the patient.

6. Allow a drop of blood to fall onto the testing strip – do not smear it (Fig. 8.7), as this may lead to an inaccurate result. However, test strips do vary. Always check the manufacturer's instructions.

7. Ask the patient to press on the site, using the gauze swab, to stem bleeding and reduce the risk of bruising.

8. Wait for the meter to provide a digital display of the result.

9. Read and document the results according to local policy or use the monitor memory system (if available). Report any abnormalities.

10. Inform the patient of their blood glucose level.
11. Check the patient is comfortable and that bleeding has stopped
12. Dispose of all sharps and contaminated waste appropriately and return equipment as appropriate.
13. Remove gloves and apron and decontaminate hands.
14. Document and act on your findings.

Care of a Patient With Hypoglycaemia

RATIONALE

Hypoglycaemia is often a complication of diabetes but can also occur in people without diabetes, e.g., fasting hypoglycaemia comma, after excessive alcohol and the stomach is empty or after eating post gastric surgery (Smyth, 2018). It occurs when the blood glucose level is less than 4mmol/L. This is caused when any insulin in the body has moved too much glucose out of the bloodstream (Royal College of Nursing, 2019). In consequence, blood glucose levels must be taken in all patients with an altered level of consciousness to rule out hypoglycaemia.

Hypoglycaemia is categorised as:
- Mild: the person is conscious, orientated and able to swallow.
- Moderate: the person is conscious and able to swallow, but confused, disorientated or aggressive.
- Severe: the person is unconscious, seizure or aggressive.

(Joint British Diabetes Societies for Inpatient care, 2018).

Depending on the severity, signs of hypoglycaemia may include:
- Feeling shaky
- Irritability
- Sweating
- Feeling weak
- Hunger
- Nausea
- Slurred speech
- Confusion and disorientation
- Aggression
- Unconsciousness

(RCN, 2019).

TREATMENT OF HYPOGLYCAEMIA

Clinical areas may have 'hypo boxes' (Fig. 8.8) which contain emergency treatment for patients with hypoglycaemia. This equipment must be checked regularly in accordance with the local policies.

Mild to Moderate Hypoglycaemia

Treatment includes consuming one quick-acting carbohydrate immediately, such as 150 mL (a small can) of a non-diet fizzy drink, 200 mL (a small carton) of smooth orange juice, 4 to 5 GlucoTabs, 5 to 6 dextrose tablets, four large jelly babies (Trend UK). If the individuals do not feel better after 10 to 15 minutes or their BGL remains <4 mmol/L, a quick-acting carbohydrate should be repeated. The individual should be observed and monitored until their BGL improves.

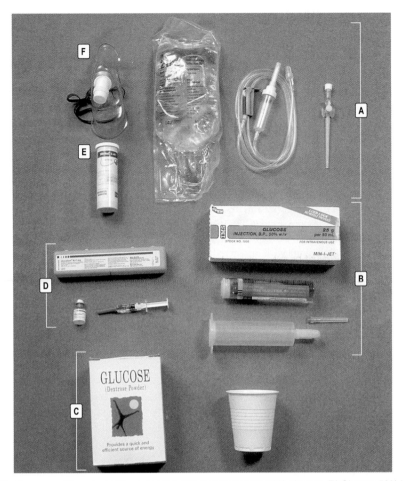

Fig. 8.8 Emergency Hypoglycaemia equipment: (A) Infusion set with 20% glucose. (B) Glucose 50% in Min-I-Jet format. The yellow plastic cover is removed from the back (left-hand end) of the syringe barrel and front of the glass cartridge and the cartridge is screwed into the syringe barrel. Available in two types, with needle fitted and with Luer lock fitting for a conventional needle (shown). After removing the front cover and fitting needle, if required, use it as a conventional syringe. (C) Glucose powder, dissolve 20 g in up to one cup of water. (D) Glucagon emergency set with a vial of lyophilised powder. Dissolve by injecting water for injection already in the syringe, and draw up for injection. (E) Blood glucose dipstick test strips. (F) Oxygen mask, give 5 L/min. (Thavaraj, S. & Banerjee, A. (2021). *Odell's Clinical Problem Solving in Dentistry*, 4th ed. Elsevier Ltd.)

Moderate to Severe Hypoglycaemia

A semi-conscious/unconscious patient will not have a sufficient swallow reflex. Therefore, no food or fluids should be given orally. Initially, they should be placed in the recovery position (p. 103), and an emergency team or ambulance called.

Glucagon IM should be given initially. Glucagon can be stored in the refrigerator between +2°C and +8°C or at room temperature provided it does not exceed +25°C.

Alternatively, once intravenous access has been secured, 50 mL of 10% glucose solution should be given. If necessary, further doses should be given every 1 minute until the patient is fully conscious or 250 mL of 10% glucose has been given (Resuscitation Council (UK), 2021).

Following administration of Glucagon and/or IV glucose BGL should be repeated.

Care of a Patient With a Reduced Level of Consciousness

RATIONALE

Reduced level of consciousness (LOC) may occur due to a variety of situations, e.g., following a head injury, stroke, hypoglycaemia, overdose of opiates or induced following administration of an anaesthetic. A patient with a GCS<8 is as risk of being unable to maintain and patent airway.

KEY POINTS

- Emergency help must be called for any patient with an acute deterioration resulting in a reduced level of consciousness.
- Patients should be assessed using the A–E Approach.
- The recovery position, the use of airway adjuncts and oxygen may be appropriate for patients with a GCS <8.

PROCEDURE

Airway:
- Use of airway opening procedures, e.g., head tilt, chin lift or jaw thrust.
- Use of airway adjuncts.
- Consider 3/4 prone position (recovery position).
- If a patient has a GCS ≤8, they will be unable to maintain their airway effectively, and intubation should be considered.

Breathing:
- Respiratory assessment.
- In an emergency, high-flow oxygen should be administered via a non-re-breath mask, and then titrated accordingly.
- Continuous pulse oximetry monitoring should be commenced.
- If there is any concern regarding the patient's swallow, they must be nil by mouth and a swallow assessment performed to avoid aspiration.

Circulation:
- Monitor pulse and blood pressure.
- Monitor temperature.
- IV fluids may be required to maintain hydration.
- Fluid balance monitoring, including urine output, should be maintained.

Disability (Neurological Assessment)
- Perform a GCS and check pupillary function.
- Check blood glucose level, if BGL <4 mmol/L treat, e.g., intramuscular (IM) glucagon or IV dextrose.
- Check the patient's drug chart for any drugs which may have affected their LOC.

Exposure:
- Observe for any bruising, injuries or rashes.

RECOVERY POSITION

1. Stand or kneel beside the person.
2. If the person is wearing spectacles, remove these and place on one side.
3. Position the person's nearest arm at 90° to their shoulder with the elbow bent.
4. Hold the back of the person's other hand against their cheek that is nearest to you and keep holding it in position.
5. Take hold of the leg furthest from you at the knee and raise it until the foot is flat on the floor (Figs. 8.9).
6. Place your hand on the knee and pull towards you so that the person turns onto their side.
7. Draw the person's knee towards their chest to prevent them from rolling onto their stomach (Figs. 8.10).
8. Tilt the chin again to maintain an open airway.
9. Call for help and continue to observe the person closely to check that breathing and circulation are being maintained. Depending on the resources available, consider the use of an airway adjunct and high-flow oxygen.
10. In the pre-hospital environment, if the ambulance has not arrived by 30 minutes, turn the person to their other side to prevent pressure ulcers.

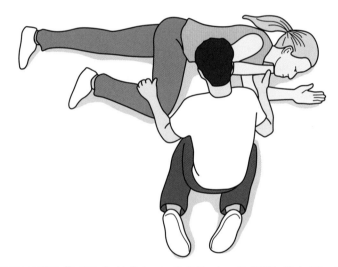

Fig. 8.9 Recovery position. (Renton, S., McGuinness, C. & Strachan, E. (2020). *Clinical Nursing Practices*, 6th ed. Elsevier Ltd.)

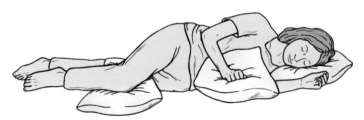

Fig. 8.10 Recovery position. (Perry, A. G., Potter, P. A., Ostendorf, W., & Laplante, N. (2022). *Clinical Nursing Skills and Techniques*. Elsevier Inc.)

OTHER CONSIDERATIONS FOR PATIENT'S WITH ONGOING NEUROLOGICAL IMPAIREMENT

- Always speak to the patient before touching them and explain what you are doing as hearing is thought to be the last sense to be lost.
- A nasogastric tube may be needed to provide nutrition and fluid.
- Mouth care to prevent complications.
- Eye care, particularly if the patient's GCS <8.
- Assess for signs of deep vein thrombosis (DVT). Anti-embolism stockings may be required.
- Assist with passive limb movements and liaison with a physiotherapist.
- When safe to do so, position the patient in bed at 30 degrees head up to reduce the risk of aspiration and intracranial pressure.
- Assess the patient's pressure areas and use an assessment tool, e.g., Waterlow Score to determine the risk and consider interventions, e.g., use of a pressure-relieving mattress.
- Reposition the patient regularly.
- Use appropriate moving and handling techniques, e.g., hoist, sliding sheets, to prevent complications for both the patient and practitioner.
- Assess the patient's ability to understand commands, their movement and strength in their limbs to determine the patient's ability to follow commands and other signs, e.g., poor balance, spatial awareness, etc.
- Use of bed rails (cot sides) should only be used following an appropriate risk assessment.
- Assess for bladder and bowel control and use of appropriate interventions, e.g., penile sheath to avoid urinary catheterisation, laxatives for constipation.
- Communication may be difficult and frustrating for the patient if they are not understood. Observe non-verbal signs and use verbal and aids, e.g., figure boards, writing boards to interact with the patient.

Care of a Patient Having a Seizure

RATIONALE

Seizures (previously termed 'fitting') may be due to a neurological condition, e.g., epilepsy, meningitis or traumatic brain injury. Seizures are a medical emergency and require prompt emergency care.

KEY POINTS

- During any seizure, the aim is to protect the patient's airway from injury and prevent complications, the individual should not be restrained and privacy and dignity maintained.
- Nurses must note the type, time and duration of each seizure.

EQUIPMENT REQUIRED

Personal protective equipment
Emergency oxygen
Non-re-breath mask
Emergency suction
Airway adjuncts

PROCEDURE

Maintain patient safety. Stay with the patient but do not place your fingers in the patient's mouth or try to restrain the patient. Personal protective clothing may be necessary if indicated by the patient's condition (chapter 2). This may entail clearing the environment or, on rare occasions, moving the patient from danger. Use pillows as necessary to pad hard surfaces, and remove non-essential furniture and equipment.

Administer high-flow oxygen via a non-re-breath mask. Be careful when applying the face mask; it may be necessary to lay the mask near to the patient's face.

Do not attempt to restrain the patient.

In status epilepticus, there may be three phases:

- During the tonic phase of the seizure, the patient will clench their jaw and may bite their tongue. Nothing should be inserted into the mouth to try and prevent this. This phase is also associated with rigidity of limbs and breath-holding. This phase may be brief.
- The second phase (clonic phase), there is rhythmical jerking of arms and legs. Characteristically, the jerks are unilateral; initially close together and then decreasing in frequency. Medications to terminate the seizure may be required.
- This phase is followed by a period of deep sleep when the patient is usually unarousable, and their body is limp. During this phase you may be required to:
  - Protect the patient from injury by turning them into the 3/4 prone position.
  - If the patient has bitten their tongue or if there is frothing of the mouth, suctioning of the oropharynx may be required.
  - Due to the fluctuating GCS during the postictal phase, a nasopharyngeal airway may be required. Oxygen should continue to be administered and titrated to the patient's condition.
  - During the period of deep sleep following the clonic phase, the patient should be left in the recovery position to maintain an airway and should not be disturbed, allowing the patient to recover in their own time. It can last up to 30 minutes.

Observe the patient continuously, noting the following:

- Duration of each phase of the seizure, including the recovery time (i.e. when able to resume normal activities).
- Limbs involved.
- Whether the movement is localised or general.
- Whether the jaw is clenched
- Whether the patient is frothing at the mouth (saliva)
- Whether the patient has been incontinent of urine or faeces.
- Breathing pattern – this will change. Patients are likely to hold their breath and may become cyanosed or looks pale. Loud breathing sounds may indicate the end of the seizure. (The breathing reverts spontaneously, and oxygen is not usually required).
- Time the seizure.

Following the seizure:

- Record the patient's vital signs and NEWS.
- Observe for any injuries.
- The patient may be disorientated and should be calmly reassured explaining what has happened. Check patient comfort and offer a wash, change of clothing, etc., as necessary.
- All seizures must be documented and reported.
- If seizures occur in rapid succession and last 30 minutes or longer, this is called status epilepticus, and requires urgent medical intervention.

References

DeSouza, J., Woodward, S., 2016. The Glasgow Coma Scale in adults: doing it right. Emerg. Nurs. 24 (8), 33–36.

Dunning, T., 2015. How to monitor blood glucose. Nurs. Stand. 30 (22), 36–39.

Frank, F., Broessner, G., 2017. Is there still a role for hypothermia in neurocritical care? Curr. Opin. Crit. Care. 23 (2), 115–121. doi:10.1097/MCC.0000000000000398. PMID: 28234783.

Joint British Diabetes Societies for Inpatient Care, 2018. The Hospital Management of Hypoglycaemia in Adults With Diabetes Mellitus, third ed. https://www.diabetes.org.uk/professionals/position-statements-reports/specialist-care-for-children-and-adults-and-complications/the-hospital-management-of-hypogly-caemia-in-adults-with-diabetes-mellitusresources-s3/2018-05/JBDS_HypoGuidelineRevised2.pdf%20 08.05.18.pdf.

National Institute for Health and Care Excellence, 2019. Head injury: assessment and early management. Clinical Guideline CG176. https://www.nice.org.uk/Guidance/CG176.

Resuscitation Council (UK), 2021. Recognising deteriorating and preventing cardiorespiratory arrest. In Immediate Life Support Course manual, eighth ed. London: Resuscitation Council.

Resuscitation Council (UK), 2021. Immediate Life Support Course, eighth ed. London: Resuscitation Council.

Royal College of Nursing, 2019. Emergency Treatment for Diabetes. https://rcni.com/hosted-content/rcn/diabetes/emergency-treatment-diabetes.

Smyth, T. 2018. Effective management of hypoglycaemia. Nurs. Stand. doi:10.7748/ns.2018.e11235.

Waterhouse, C., 2017. Practical aspects of performing Glasgow Coma Scale observations. Nurs. Stand. 31 (35), 40–46.

CHAPTER 9

Pain Assessment and Management

The Importance of Pain Assessment and Management

Almost three decades ago, pain was designated as the 'fifth vital sign' (American Pain Society, 1995), and today, elevated pain scores act as a 'red flag' to promote action (Levy et al., 2018). There are several definitions of pain; the most widely accepted definition within nursing practice is '*Pain is whatever the patient says it is and existing whenever the experiencing person says its does*' (McCaffery, 1968, p. 95). Another definition of pain frequently used is from the International Association for the Study of Pain (IASP) states that '*an unpleasant sensory or emotional experience associated with, or resembling that associated with actual or potential tissue damage*' (Raja et al., 2020). These two definitions recognise that pain as a complex and subjective phenomenon which can have harmful physiological, psychological and emotional effects (Wright, 2015).

The difficulties associated with defining and describing pain due to its complex and subjective nature mean it is a challenge to manage. When acute pain is not resolved after 3 months, it is referred to as chronic or persistent pain (British Pain Society, 2021). Chronic pain has been recognised as a long-term condition which can impact on the individual's mood and is associated with anxiety and depression and ability to sleep, communicate and work (RCN, 2015). Patients have a right to the best possible pain assessment and treatment, an integral aspect of nursing care and should involve patients and their family members (RCN, 2015). Therefore, it is essential that nurses have the knowledge and skills to assess and manage pain. There have been significant advances in the management of pain, with the development of acute and chronic pain services (acute and chronic). Improved techniques for administering analgesia, including patientcontrolled analgesia (PCA) and epidural analgesia. There is also a greater recognition of the role of nonpharmacological strategies such as transcutaneous electrical nerve stimulation (TENS), physiotherapy, heat pads, massage, relaxation, reflexology, acupuncture and, in some cases, cognitive behavioural therapy (CBT) in the management of pain (Dougherty et al., 2015. Tola et al., 2021)

Article three of the IASP Declaration of Montreal (IASP, 2010) identifies that pain management is a fundamental ethical right and that appropriately trained healthcare professionals have an obligation to ensure that patients in their care have their pain relieved. Thus pain management is a human right, and failure to treat it is considered unethical and a breach of these rights (Royal College of Nursing [RCN], 2015). In consequence, nurses must have the skills to assess and manage pain as essential to safeguarding patients (Nursing and Midwifery Council, 2018).

KEY POINTS

- Pain is an individual, multi-faceted, complex aspect of patient care.
- Acute pain left untreated can cause longer term problems and complications.
- Nurses must follow the Nursing and Midwifery Council (NMC) Code and be able to assess and manage both acute and chronic pain.
- Self-report pain assessment tools are gold standard.

Pain Management Services

Specialist pain management services aim at diagnosing and managing complex pain disorders through a multidisciplinary approach across both hospitals and the community (National Health Service (NHS) England, 2013; Faculty of Pain Medicine, 2015). The Core Standards for Pain Management Services in the UK (Faculty of Pain Medicine 2015) recommendations the management of acute and chronic pain include a range of techniques for administering analgesia, e.g. oral, intravenous, PCA and epidural analgesia. PCA and epidural analgesia. There is increasing recognition of the role of nonpharmacologic strategies which may include complementary and alternative medicine (CAM) therapies, transcutaneous electrical nerve stimulation (TENS). TENS, physiotherapy, heat pads, massage, relaxation, reflexology, acupuncture and, in some cases, Cognitive Behaviour Therapy (CBT) (Cox, 2010; Peate, 2019).

Effective pain management depends on good interprofessional team working, with nurses playing a significant role in managing a patient's pain. Nurses must be able to deliver evidenced, informed pain management appropriate to their level of practice and the setting in which they work, this includes understanding the complexities of pain (RCN, 2015). Successful pain management is a continuous process dependent on assessment and re-assessment of the patient's perception of their pain and includes the recognition of all aspects of the physical, psychological and social impact. (British Pain Society, 2021b).

Nurses with specialist pain management skills are employed across all clinical settings. Their roles range from clinical nurse specialist to a consultant nurse, with advanced practical and theoretical knowledge in pain management (RCN, 2015).

Role and responsibilities as follow:

1. To develop nurse-led services, which can inlcude acupuncture clinics, medication review clinics, and some senior nurses take on their own caseload.
2. To work across the interface between primary and secondary care, providing specific services for selected client groups with persistent pain.
3. Formulate treatment plans for patient centred-care, using a holistic approach that encompasses the patient's physical, psychological and social needs (RCN, 2015).
4. Offer advice to the multidisciplinary team as they have the extended knowledge and skills of medicine and non-pharmacological interventions.
5. Educate patients and their families, as well as members of the public, while at the same time teaching and supporting junior nurses and clinical colleagues, within their clinical setting (RCN, 2015).
6. Work within NMC Code (2018), which requires all nurses to recognise the limits of their clinical competence seeking appropriate support and advice when necessary.

Pain Assessment

Pain assessment should be a systematic process based on assessment, measurement and evaluation (Levy et al., 2018; Peate, 2019) and involves the following stages (Dougherty et al., 2015; Wright, 2015).

- Documentation of a pain history to identify any pre-existing conditions, medications (prescribed and nonprescribed medications used) and nonpharmacological methods used.
- Assessment of location and intensity of pain
- Assessment and documentation of physiological signs
- Use of appropriate pain assessment tools
- Evaluation and discussion of the findings to develop an individualised pain management plan in partnership with the patient with patients.

ASSESSMENT TOOLS

Self-reporting of pain is regarded as the gold standard assessment. Individuals' experiences and perceptions of pain are often undervalued, so listening and asking questions are the best ways know and understand the severity of pain the patient is experiencing. Nurses must observe changes in behaviour and physical signs of pain, such as grimacing, groaning or restlessness. (Ni Thuathail and Welford, 2011). Ethnic, religious and socioeconomic factors may affecting attitudes to and reporting of pain. Therefore it is the nurse's role to ensure that patients' pain is managed in a culturally sensitive way and to perceive pain management from the patient's perspective (Peate, 2019 Ni Thuathail and Welford, 2011).

Pain Measurement

Pain management requires the nurse to assess the amount of pain the patient is experiencing, and where possible, the patients' self-report of pain is regarded as the highest standard of pain assessment (Peate, 2019). Pain should be measured using appropriate tools, and variety exists for the nurse to competently manage a patient's pain and plan of care. The SOCRATES mnemonic is one of the strategies used by healthcare professionals to assess pain:

- S = Severity of pain: none, mild, moderate or severe
- O = Onset
- C = Characteristic (e.g., burning, aching, shooting)
- R = Radiation
- A = Additional factors (e.g., What makes it better?)
- T = Time (e.g., Is it associated with a particular time of day?)
- E = Exacerbating factors (e.g. What makes the pain worse?)
- S = Site: Where is the pain?

Encouraging patients to take an active role in understanding pain assessment tools helps them to feel part of the pain management process. However, the nurse must select the most appropriate measurement tool for a pain the patient is experiencing, and most pain assessment tools have numeric and visual dimensions (RCN, 2015). There are also, physiological measurements that relate to the objective measure of pain and the vital signs that are usually measured are temperature, pulse, respirations, blood pressure (BP) and oxygen saturation (RCN, 2015).

The frequency of pain assessment is dependent on individual circumstances. Factors to be considered when determining frequency include:

- The severity of the pain. Pain assessment is often carried out when the patient is resting, but a better indicator of the efficacy of analgesia may be achieved by asking the patient to cough, move or take a deep breath.
- Frequency of assessment should be increased if the patient reports their pain is poorly controlled or treatment regimens are changing.
- Regular pain assessments are important, particularly in a post-operative period. Patients with a PCA (see p. 116) should be assessed each time other vital signs are recorded. For patients with epidural analgesia (see p. 119), the sensory block should be checked approximately 20 minutes after administration of the analgesic or as per local policy.

There are multidimensional pain tools such as the McGill Pain Questionnaire (MPQ) which measure the various dimensions that make up the experience of pain and offer a framework for assessment of many of the key issues. These include the intensity, sensory, affective and evaluative elements of pain. No one tool is adequate for enabling the patient to describe the quality of their pain experience, and of equal importance enabling the patient to tell their 'story', through open questions, active listening and reflection (McLafferty and Farley, 2008). How questions are framed is crucial if the nurse is to understand the characteristics of the patients perception of their pain. Factors to consider are:

- **The location, duration, intensity and characteristics of the pain.** Defining the nature of a patient's pain is important because different types of pain are treated differently. The nurse should establish whether the pain is localised to a part of the body or whether it is more generalised. This includes asking whether the pain is 'sharp', 'dull', 'intermittent' or 'continuous', when it started, how long it lasts and if it is 'tolerable' or 'unbearable'.
- **The underlying condition.** The underlying diagnosis or cause of a patient's pain is central to determining whether the subsequent treatment is curative or palliative.
- **Acute, persistent (chronic) or referred pain.** It is important to establish the type of pain as this may influence the choice of treatment. Pharmacological interventions are usually the mainstay of acute pain management, whereas chronic pain may require a range of treatment options including pharmacological and nonpharmacological regimens. Referred pain is common in conditions that originate in the viscera, for example, the pain in a myocardial infarction is often referred to the left arm.
- **Medical/nursing treatment being given.** Any treatment currently being received by the patient should be reviewed to determine its effectiveness.
- **Precipitating or exacerbating factors (e.g. mobility/immobility, time of day, eating/ drinking).** Determining factors that precipitate or exacerbate the pain facilitates diagnosis and aids with identification of the goals of care. Time of day may also be significant; some patients report higher levels of pain at night.
- **Related symptoms (e.g. nausea, vomiting, breathlessness or sleeplessness).** Related symptoms, such as nausea and vomiting, are often significant in aiding diagnosis but are also important they may impact on the patient's ability to cope with pain. A score to indicate the level of nausea and vomiting is often used with patients receiving PCA. This should be assessed and recorded with other vital signs. Pain that causes sleeplessness significantly reduces the patient's ability to tolerate it.
- **Coping strategies used by the patient—pharmacological and non-pharmacological.** When determining the plan of care for a patient in pain, any coping strategies the patient may have developed must be considered. Medication used by the patient may indicate what 'works' and may subsequently minimise the risk of prescribing treatments that 'do not work'. Non-pharmacological coping strategies (e.g. use of heat pads or massage) should, whenever possible, be included in the plan of care. This will enhance the patient's perception of being involved in their plan of care.
- **Meaning or significance of the pain for the patient.** The patient's perception of the significance of their pain is a valid indicator. Pain creates fear, anxiety and a sense of loss of control, therefore, it is essential for the nurse to provide reassurance, support and escalate their concerns.

Self-Report Pain Assessment Tools

There are many self-report and observation methods for assessing pain intensity. Tools include Visual Analogue Scale (VAS), Numerical Rating Scale (NRS), Verbal Rating Scale (VRS), and Wong–Baker Face Pain Rating Scale (Bielewicz et al., 2022). These can be used in both initial and ongoing assessments.

Self-report scales:

- **VAS** is an instrument used for subjective rating of pain. It is most often used as a unidimensional measure of pain intensity, (The British Pain Society [BPS], 2021). The VAS

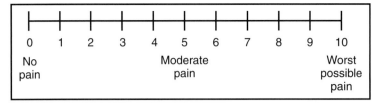

Fig. 9.1 Numeric Rating Scale. (Sarin, J., & Bhargavi, C. N. (2022). *Wong's Essentials of Pediatric Nursing:* 3rd South Asian ed. Elsevier.)

uses a 10-cm line with one end point indicating 'no pain' at one end and 'worst pain imaginable' at other end (Fig. 9.1). The patient points to the mark that best represents their pain. Some scales include words at set intervals (e.g. 'slight', 'moderate', 'severe'). The advantage of using this scale is that it is easy to use because the person in pain is not required to assign a numerical value or choose different words that describes the pain. However, this scale can be difficult to use for patients who have motor ability or visual acuity problems, because they must be able to indicate the point on the scale that represents their pain.

- **NRS:** This scale is the most used unidimensional pain scale and is similar to the VAS but has numbers added to aid description. This self report scale can be is used to measure pain in children who are 10 years or older. It uses a self-report scale, in which 0 is 'no pain' and 10 is 'worst imaginable pain', patients are asked to indicate the number that best represents their pain. This tool can be administered verbally, it is suitable for use with patients with motor ability or visual acuity problems.
- **VRS:** Ask the patient to consider a series of words that best describes the pain (e.g. 'none', 'mild', 'moderate', 'severe', 'very severe' and 'worst pain imaginable'). However, this scale uses words rather than numbers, and is dependent on the patient's understanding and/or interpretation of the words used to describe pain.
- **The Wong-Baker FACES® Pain Rating Scale** asks the patient to pick a face that best represents the level of pain from a series that ranges from happy and smiling to grimacing and crying. Each face is numbered, and they rise in increments of two, with 0 representing the happy face (no hurt) and 10 the saddest face (hurts worst) (Fig. 9.2) (McLafferty and

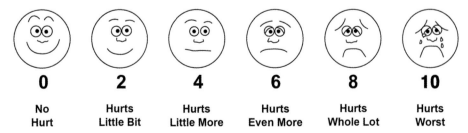

0	**2**	**4**	**6**	**8**	**10**
No Hurt	Hurts Little Bit	Hurts Little More	Hurts Even More	Hurts Whole Lot	Hurts Worst

Fig. 9.2 Wong–Baker FACES Pain Rating Scale. (Wong-Baker FACES Foundation (2022). Wong-Baker FACES® Pain Rating Scale. Retrieved 10-Jan-22 with permission from http://www.WongBakerFACES.org. Originally published in Whaley & Wong's Nursing Care of Infants and Children. © Elsevier Inc.)

Pain Assessment In Advanced Dementia (PAINAD) Scale

	0	1	2	Score
Breathing independent of vocalisation	Normal	Occasional laboured breathing, short period of hyperventilation	Noisy laboured breathing, long period of hyperventilation, Cheyne-Stokes respirations	
Negative vocalisation	None	Occasional moan or groan, low level of speech with a negative or disapproving quality	Repeated troubled calling out, loud moaning or groaning, crying	
Facial expression	Smiling or inexpressive	Sad, frightened, frown	Facial grimacing	
Body language	Relaxed	Tense, distressed pacing, fidgeting	Rigid, fists clenched, knees pulled up, pulling or pushing away, striking out	
Consolability	No need to console	Distracted or reassured by voice or touch	Unable to console, distract or reassure	
			TOTAL	

Fig. 9.3 Pain Assessment in Advanced Dementia Scale. (Jarvis, C., Eckhardt, A., Forbes, H., Watt, E. (2021). *Jarvis's Health Assessment & Physical Examination*, 3rd ed. Elsevier Inc.)

Farley, 2008). Although this type of rating scale was primarily used with children, it has now been adopted for use with those with communication and language difficulties.

- **The Pain Assessment in Advanced Dementia Scale (PAINAD):** A number of scales have been developed for specific use with cognitively impaired patients, (Fig. 9.3). Patients who are cognitively impaired may not be able to accurately convey their pain or its intensity, with the result that it may be untreated or undertreated. PAINAD uses five items: breathing independent of vocalisation; negative vocalisation; facial expression; body language and consolability (Warden et al., 2003). A score of 0, 1 or 2 is given to each item, with a possible score of 10 indicating severe pain.

Any of the above-described scales may be together with a body outline as that provides a good indication of pain sites. The advantage of having access to a range of measures is that it is possible to find a tool appropriate for each individual. They enable the patient to describe the intensity and location of their pain.

Care of Patient Using Patient-Controlled Analgesia (PCA)

PCA refers to method or route by which the patient self-administers analgesia (Allman et al., 2016). There is evidence to show that the use of PCA for postoperative pain improves patient's recovery time, thereby reducing length of hospital stay (LOS) (Peate, 2019). PCAs became popular as a method of managing postoperative pain in the early 1990s and are increasingly recognised as an ideal approach for postoperative pain management. They can be used for virtually any patient undergoing surgery who will experience postoperative pain of moderate or severe intensity. Usual routes include intravenous, subcutaneous or epidural.

When the patient feels pain, they press a button which releases a prescribed dose of analgesia, usually opioids, (National Institute for Health and Care Excellence [NICE], 2020). The underlying

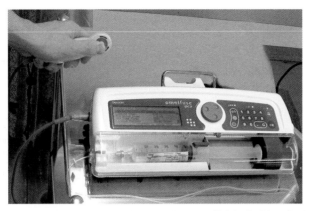

Fig. 9.4 Patient controlled analgesia with patient's control handset. (Quick, C., Biers, S., Arulampalam, T. & Deakin, P. (2020). *Essential Surgery: Problems, Diagnosis and Management*, 6th ed. Elsevier Ltd.)

principle of PCA is that while the patient controls the dose of analgesia there is a 'lock-out' etting which controls and regulates rate and dose of drugs being administered (Fig. 9.4). The use of the lock-out device allows time for the opioid to start working, and limits the amount of analgesia the patient can receive. During the interval lockout, if the patient triggers the button, they will not receive the medication. Which prevents the administration of an overdose of analgesic drugs.

Morphine is the most common opiate used, and a lock-out period of 5 minutes is normal when it is being administered intravenously. Subcutaneous administration requires a longer lock-out time of 10 minutes (NICE, 2020). Morphine administered in 1 mg boluses at 5-minute intervals will provide 12 mg per hour and will normally provide effective pain relief with minimal side effects. However, it is also important to note that patients' requirements for analgesia can vary considerably. Analgesia can also be provided via continuous infusion at a pre-defined rate.

The success of PCA is dependent on the patient being willing and able to use it. Therefore patient education is vital, and should occur pre-operatively, either in the pre-admission clinic or on the ward. The patient should be encouraged to handle the device and press the buttons etc., to familiarise themselves with the device. It is important that the nurse checks the patient's understanding and dexterity in handling the equipment because patients who are unable to manage the device may not receive any analgesia. If a patient is unable to use the system, nurse-administered analgesia will be required.

Patient-Controlled Analgesia Devices

There are a variety of battery or electrically operated PCA devices available. Most will include the following features:

- A lock-out device that prevents the syringe driver from delivering more than the maximum preset dose over a set period (e.g., 4 hours).
- Safety features that include alarms for occlusion (blockage), air in the line, low battery or empty syringe.
- A keypad lock and other locking devices that prevent unauthorised access and changes to the programme.
- An electronic microprocessor that allows the flow rate, bolus dose and lockout interval to be set. This will usually record the number of bolus doses requested and administered, which is important when determining the effectiveness of the PCA.
- Anti-syphon valves and anti-reflux valves should be used.

- An alternative is a mechanical system where a 'control module' is worn around the wrist with a connecting pocket-sized infusor. This is less flexible than the electronic pumps because it delivers only a preset, nonadjustable volume and has only one lock-out interval and no safety alarms. However, it is much cheaper than the electronic modes and affords the patient greater freedom of movement.

KEY FACTS

- Patient controlled analgesia gives the patient a sense of control, and they can receive pain relief when needed.
- It prevents the peaks and troughs associated with intermittent injection.
- Unlike the conventional system of intermittent injection, there is no delay between the request for analgesia and the provision of pain relief.

MONITORING THE PATIENT

Regular monitoring is essential for patients with a PCA. This includes the following:

Skill mix and nursing staff on the wards must be sufficient to provide safe care of the patient with a PCA. If there are any concerns about the safe staffing / skill mix this must be escalated.

Check and confirm the machine is placed at or below the level of the patient's heart to prevent any risk of siphoning.

Frequent monitoring of respiration rate is necessary.

  - Count respiratory rate for a full minute, particularly immediately after commencement, because respiratory depression is the main side effect of opiate analgesia. The local protocol should be consulted regarding the action to be taken if respirations decrease; a respiratory rate of less than 8 or 10 respirations per minute, requires intervention from the pain control nurse, the anaesthetist or doctor. Some protocols stipulate that patients should have oxygen administered while the PCA is in progress. Oxygen saturation levels should be recorded with respiratory rate.

Vital signs and National Early Warning Scoring (NEWS) should be recorded every 30 minutes for 2 hours initially, then every hour for the next 4 hours, then 2-hourly for the duration of the PCA; specific observations include (Anaesthesia UK, 2017):

The (volume to be infused) (VTBI) of the solution used must be recorded hourly as read from the pump display.

Pain should be assessed using a pain assessment tool to assess whether effective pain relief has been achieved.

The level of sedation must be monitored; opiates cause sedation, and it is important to ensure that the patient is still rousable. PCA documentation tends to incorporate a sedation score.

The incidence/severity of nausea and vomiting should be documented and managed.

Regular assessment of patients' use (i.e. how often they press the button) is essential to determine whether the pain control is effective.

The PCA must be attached to a dedicated intravenous cannula and must be clearly labelled as a PCA line. No other drugs or intravenous fluids should be administered via this line.

The prescribed settings for the PCA system must be checked regularly to check it is properly functioning.

Depending on local protocols, patients must have vital signs, sedation score and nausea assessment recorded hourly.

The nurse should monitor the infusion site for signs of inflammation, redness or tissue damage.

As with all controlled drugs, the nurse should prepare, administer and document the infusion in accordance with local policy. Where possible and to avoid errors, ready-made bags of opioids should be used.

No other opioid should be administered with a PCA.

Emergency Treatment

Depending on local policy, in the event of respiratory depression or other complication emergency treatment (e.g. naloxone, intravenous fluids) may be prescribed as required.

In the event of respiratory depression and/or reduced level of consciousness:

- If the respiratory rate is less than 8/min and reduced level of consciousness/unresponsive:
  - Immediately stop the PCA.
  - Emergency call an anaesthetist.
  - Assess airway, breathing and circulation (ABC)
  - Open the airway, and use airway adjuncts as appropriate.
  - Ventilate the patient using a bag, valve mask (p. 327) with high flow oxygen.
  - Administer naloxone. Note Naloxone has a short half-life, therefore, further doses may be required.
- Reversal of opioids with naloxone will also reverse all the analgesic effects. Therefore further appropriate analgesia will need to be prescribed. (Anaesthesia UK, 2017)

Care of Patient With an Epidural Analgesia

Epidural analgesia is commonly used for maternal analgesia during childbirth and patients who have undergone vascular surgery, thoracic or abdominal surgery or orthopaedic surgery to the lower limb. It is also used for patients with intractable cancer pain and those with persistent, neuropathic or visceral pain of a chronic nature (Allman et al., 2016). A fine-bore catheter is inserted into the epidural space, which is between the dura mater and the ligaments and bones of the spinal cord (Fig. 9.5). It can be inserted at any level of the spine but is most commonly at the lumbar or sacral level. However, the use of thoracic epidurals is increasing as evidence indicates it offers improved pain relief (NICE, 2020). (NICE, 2020). The catheter is usually secured to the patient's back using a sterile fixation device and a clear occlusive dressing and is then attached to the infusion device.

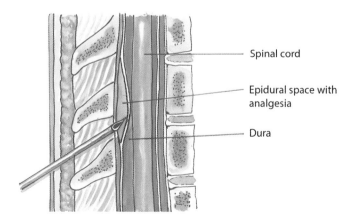

Fig. 9.5 Epidural analgesia. (Kumari, U. (2019). *Textbook of Obstetrics*. RELX India Pvt. Ltd)

The drugs most commonly used for epidural analgesia are opioids (e.g. fentanyl, diamorphine) and local anaesthetics (bupivacaine). Dosages vary according to the site of the catheter, the type of surgery, the age and medical condition of the patient. Administration as a continuous infusion is seen as the most effective in the management of postoperative pain. Bolus injections are used less commonly for postoperative pain but are used for the management of the pain of maternal labour. Patient-controlled epidural analgesia (PCEA) is used for postoperative or persistent (chronic) pain because it gives the patient control over the analgesia. It is most effective when used in combination with a low-dose background infusion (NICE, 2020. Allman et al., 2016).

KEY FACTORS

- Patients receiving epidural analgesia require close observation and monitoring for potential signs of complications (Boxes 9.1 and 9.2).
- Patients with epidural analgesia need to be nursed in specialist areas with immediate access to nurses and midwives who have undertaken additional training and education in epidural care.

MONITORING PATIENTS WITH EPIDURAL ANALGESIA

Careful monitoring of the patient is vital and includes the following:
- The prescribed settings on the epidural device or pump must be checked regularly to confirm it is functioning properly. The device should never be regarded as a fail-safe.
- Single Luer-lock connections must be used between the catheter and the administration set. Three-way connectors must not be used to prevent inadvertent administration of other medications.
- A bacterial filter must be in place at the end of the epidural cannula.

BOX 9.1 ■ Potential Drug Complications

■ Sedation	■ Urinary retention
■ Respiratory depression	■ Pruritus
■ Hypotension	■ Motor blockade
■ Nausea and vomiting	

Bird et al. (2013) and Allman et al. (2016).

BOX 9.2 ■ Potential Epidural Catheter-Related Complications

■ Dural puncture on insertion	■ Epidural abscess
■ Paraesthesia	■ Headache
■ Neurological damage	■ Nerve or spinal cord damage
■ Epidural haematoma	

Bird et al. (2013) and Allman et al. (2016).

- The epidural cannula must be clearly labelled so that it cannot be confused with an intravenous cannula.
- The dressing over the epidural cannula site should be transparent and secure to prevent inadvertently dislodging the catheter and to minimise the risk of contamination. The inspection site should be inspected daily.
- Close monitoring of sedation levels, because sedation and respiratory depression are known side effects of opioids. The use of a sedation score is recommended to assist in the early detection of respiratory depression. If the score signifies the patient is becoming unacceptably sedated, the infusion should be stopped and oxygen administered while medical or anaesthetic intervention is sought.
- Close monitoring of respirations should be undertaken alongside sedation scores. Oxygen saturation levels are recorded with respiratory rate, although they should not be used as the primary or only indicator of respiratory depression.
- The BP and pulse rate should be recorded hourly. Hypotension is associated with the use of local anaesthetics in epidural analgesia and can also occur if the epidural catheter migrates into the subarachnoid space. This would be accompanied by light-headedness, tachycardia (raised pulse) and difficulty with movement. The infusion should be stopped, and medical assistance sought immediately if any of these symptoms occur. However, it is essential to remember that in postoperative patients hypotension may be due to blood loss.
- Local anaesthetics can also be toxic to the central nervous systems. The nurse should assess the patient for excitation, numbness of the tongue and mouth, slurred speech, twitching, light-headedness and tinnitus (buzzing or ringing in the ears). If central nervous system toxicity occurs, the patient may experience respiratory depression or convulsions and is at risk of cardiac arrest. If toxicity is suspected the infusion must be stopped. The priority of medical intervention is the patient's ventilation and oxygen needs.
- Fluid intake should be monitored to ensure that any reduction in BP is not associated with dehydration. Where possible, oral fluids must be encouraged and intravenous infusion considered.
- Urinary output must be monitored, particularly in those patients with lumbar epidural analgesia, because it is commonly associated with urinary retention. If the patient has a urinary catheter, hourly measurements should be undertaken. Accurate recording on a fluid balance chart is essential.
- The height of the epidural block can be assessed by the application of cold to the skin surface. If the patient reports pins and needles in the fingers, this should be reported. The hourly rate of the infusion may need to be reduced.
- Pain should be assessed using a pain assessment tool to ensure effective pain relief is being achieved. Pain should be controlled sufficiently to enable the patient to cough, breathe deeply and mobilise. If the patient reports pain at the site of the infusion, medical staff should be informed because infection or haematoma may be present.
- Nausea and vomiting (often using a scoring system) should be recorded and managed.
- Patients receiving opioids can develop pruritus (itching) that is distressing and does not always respond to antihistamines. If the itching does not respond to intervention, the opioid may need to be discontinued.
- All of the above-described points should be monitored simultaneously and hourly for the duration of the epidural analgesia in accordance with local policy. Some clinical areas use a specially designed epidural assessment tool.
- As with all controlled drugs, the nurse must prepare, administer and document the medication according to the local policy. No other opiates should be prescribed or administered while epidural analgesia is in progress.

References

Allman, K., Wilson, I., O'Donnell, A., 2016. Oxford Handbook of Anaesthesia, fourth ed. Oxford University Press.

American Pain Society Quality of Care Committee, 1995. Quality improvement guidelines for the treatment of acute pain and cancer pain. JAMA. 274, 1874–1880.

Anaesthesia UK, 2017. Patient-Controlled Analgesia. https://www.frca.co.uk/article.aspx?articleid=101344.

Bielewicz J. Daniluk B. Kamieniak P. (2022). VAS and NRS, Same or Different? Are Visual Analog Scale Values and Numerical Rating Scale Equally Viable Tools for Assessing Patients after Microdiscectomy? Pain Research and Management. https://doi.org/10.1155/2022/5337483

Bird, A., Allcock, N., Cooper, J., 2013. Competency in managing care in epidural analgesia. Nurs. Times. 109 (5), 18–20.

British Pain Society, 2021. Useful Definitions and Glossary. https://www.britishpainsociety.org/people-with-pain/useful-definitions-and-glossary/#pain.

British Pain Society, 2021b. Pain Scales in Multiple Languages. https://www.britishpainsociety.org/british-pain-society-publications/pain-scales-in-multiple-languages/.

Cox, F., 2010. Basic principles of pain management: assessment and intervention. Nurs. Stand. 25 (1), 36–39.

Dougherty, L., Lister, S., 2015. The Royal Marsden Hospital Manual of Clinical Nursing Procedures. Blackwell, Oxford.

Faculty of Pain Management, 2015. Core Standards for Pain Management Services in the UK. https://fpm.ac.uk/sites/fpm/files/documents/2019-07/Core%20Standards%20for%20Pain%20Management%20Services.pdf.

International Association for the Study of Pain, 2010. Declaration of Montreal. Available from: www.iasp-pain.org/DeclarationofMontreal.

Levy, N., Sturgess, J., Mills, P., 2018. Pain as the fifth vital sign and dependence on the numerical rating scale is being abandoned in the US: why? Br J Anaesth. 120 (3), 435–438.

McCaffery, M. 1968. Nursing Practice Theories Related to Cognition, Bodily Pain, and Man-Environment Interactions. Los Angeles: UCLA Students' Store, CA.

National Institute for Health and Care Excellence, 2020. Perioperative Care in Adults. Evidence reviews for managing acute post-operative pain. https://www.nice.org.uk/guidance/ng180/evidence/n1-managing-acute-postoperative-pain-pdf-317993437913.

Ni Thuathail, A., Welford, C., 2011. Pain assessment tools for older people with cognitive impairment. Nurs. Stand. 26 (6), 39–46. doi:10.7748/ns2011.10.26.6.39.c8756.

NHS England, 2013. NHS England Commissioning for Specialised Pain Services. http://www.england.nhs.uk/wpcontent/uploads/2013/06/d08-spec.

Nursing and Midwifery Council, 2018. The Code. www.nmc.org.uk.

Peate, I., 2019. Fundamentals of Assessment and Care Planning for Nurses, first ed. Wiley Blackwell.

Raja, S.N., Carr, D.B., Cohen, M., et al., 2020. The revised International Association for the Study of Pain definition of pain: concepts, challenges, and compromises, PAIN. 161 (9), 1976–1982. doi:10.1097/j.pain.0000000000001939.

Royal College of Nursing, 2015. RCN Pain Knowledge and Skills Framework for the Nursing Team. Publication code: 004 984. www.rcn.org.uk.

Tola, Y.O., Chow, K.M., Liang, W., 2021. Effects of non-pharmacological interventions on preoperative anxiety and postoperative pain in patients undergoing breast cancer surgery: A systematic review. J Clin Nurs. doi:10.1111/jocn.15827. Epub ahead of print. PMID: 33942405.

Warden, V., Hurley, A.C., Volicer, L., 2003. Development and psychometric evaluation of the Pain Assessment in Advanced Dementia (PAINAD) scale. J Am Med Dir Assoc. 4 (1), 9–15.

Wright, S., 2015. Pain Management in Nursing Practice. SAGE publishing Inc.

CHAPTER 10

Sepsis Care

Sepsis Recognition and Causes

Sepsis is a life-threatening condition with a high in-hospital mortality rate, comparable with those of cancer and myocardial infarctions. The revised Surviving Sepsis Campaign (2021) makes evidenced-based recommendations for the management of those patients with sepsis and septic shock. As argued by Singer (2016), sepsis is not a specific illness, but a clinical syndrome characterised by severe inflammation, immunosuppression and altered activation of coagulation. Every system in the body may be affected by sepsis/septic shock; therefore a systematic assessment is vital to identify key clinical signs and symptoms. The pathophysiology of sepsis is still uncertain, and therefore management of sepsis/septic shock focuses on timely identification and appropriate supportive care while attempting to identify the source.

Sepsis is defined as 'a life threatening organ dysfunction due a dysregulated host response to infection' and septic shock as 'persisting hypotension requiring vasopressors to maintain a mean arterial pressure (MAP) of 65 mmHg or more and having a serum lactate level of greater than 2 mmol/l despite adequate volume resuscitation' (Singer et al., 2016. NICE, 2017). Whilst these definitions and changes in terminology have been in response to current evidence, they do not help with the early identification of sepsis at the bedside; subsequently clinical parameters are used to determine the severity of illness and potential organ dysfunction. Both NICE and the international consensus definitions have developed a range of simple tools which can be used in a variety of environments (NICE, 2017; Singer et al., 2016).

> **KEY POINTS**
> - Sepsis or septic shock is a life-threatening emergency and should be identified and treated as promptly as possible, with every hour treatment is delayed there is increased mortality.
> - Airway, Breathing, Circulation, Disability, Exposure (ABCDE) approach to assessing patients with potential sepsis or septic shock (see Chapter 3).
> - Nurses should be aware of, understand and be able to apply the Sepsis-3 definitions.
> - Knowledge and understanding of sepsis red flags are vital and should prompt urgent treatment.
> - Nurses should be aware of and aim where possible to use the 1-hour care bundle whenever sepsis is identified. Sepsis guidelines are continually evolving and nurses must keep abreast of the changing evidence.

CONDITIONS ASSOCIATED WITH SEPSIS

Sepsis is associated with a range of common infections, however, it important for nurses to recognise that an infection alone is not sepsis. Sepsis is a result of an individuals inability to maintain the physiological regulatory mechanisms due to an infection. Therefore, patients who are already immunosuppressed, critically ill or elderly (>65years) or have a particularly virulent pathogen increased risk of developing sepsis. It is important for the nurse to be alert to common conditions causing sepsis so that reversible causes can be identified and, where possible, treated.

Pneumonia

Pneumonia is an infection in the lungs which causes an inflammatory response and disrupts gaseous exchange. Patients commonly develop symptoms such as breathlessness, hypoxia, difficulty breathing and persistent productive cough. Pneumonia can be identified through chest x-ray, clinical signs and identification of patients of high risk, for example, individuals who are immobile or who have reduced mobility.

Urinary Tract Infections

Urinary tract infections (UTIs) are caused by a microorganism invading the usually sterile urinary tract. Symptoms include increased urgency in passing urine, offensive smelling or discoloured urine, pain on passing urine or urine samples where blood or protein is present. UTIs are more common in patients who have urinary catheters, which encourages the introduction of bacterial growth in the urinary tract, particularly those patients who have long-term catheters. UTIs can be identified through urine culture samples and clinical signs noted earlier.

Meningitis

Meningitis is inflammation of the layers surrounding the brain called the meninges. Children and young adults are at higher risk (UK Health Security Agency, 2022). The early signs and symptoms may be non-specific and include vomiting, nausea, stiff neck, confusion and photophobia. There may also be a rash if a specific type of bacteria is present called 'meningococcal bacteria', which does not blanch when a glass is rolled over it, however, a rash may not always be present. Definitive diagnosis is made through a lumbar puncture and clinical signs.

Line-Related Sepsis

Vascular access devices such as central lines, Peripherally Inserted Central Catheter (PICC) lines, Vascaths and peripheral vascular access devices are common sources of line-related sepsis. Those patients who have vascular access devices in for a long period are at high risk of developing bacteraemia; therefore lines should be removed when no longer necessary. If a line-related sepsis is suspected or no other source can be identified, the line should be removed and the tip sent for culture.

Sepsis Specific Scoring Systems

Sequential (or sepsis-related) Organ Failure Assessment (SOFA) score is a clinical criterion which predicts mortality in those infected patients most likely to have sepsis. The full SOFA score predominately used in critical care areas was not designed as a tool for patient management (Lambden et al., 2019).

There is a modified, short version of the full SOFA score to identify those patients at risk of a poor outcome which can be used outs where quick access to laboratory tests may not be available (Table 10.1). This score contains three elements: altered mental status (Glasgow Coma Scale < 15), fast respiratory rate (>22 breaths/min) and low blood pressure (systolic BP <100 mm Hg). Each element could potentially score one. More than two points is associated with the onset of infection and a higher mortality rate. Many early warning scoring tools (including the NEWS) incorporate q-SOFA.

TABLE 10.1 ■ q-SOFA Criteria

Respiratory rate ≥22/min
Altered mental state (Glasgow Coma Scale)
Systolic blood pressure ≤100 mm Hg

q-SOFA, Quick Sequential (or sepsis-related) Organ Failure Assessment.
Singer et al. (2016).

RECOGNITION OF SEPSIS

As part of a comprehensive ABCDE assessment, in addition, history and vital signs (NEWS-2 scoring), the nurse must look for any red or amber flags, which alert to potential life-threatening situations.

SEPSIS RED FLAGS

In any patient who presents with any red flags, acute deterioration is likely, and therefore nurses should act immediately using the sepsis management bundle (see p. 126) (UK Sepsis Trust 2022):

- Responds only to voice or pain/unresponsive
- Acute confusion
- Systolic BP ≤90 mm Hg (or drop of > 40 mm Hg from normal)
- Heart rate >130/min
- Respiratory rate ≥25/min
- Needs oxygen to keep SpO_2 ≥92% oxygen saturation (SpO_2)
- Nonblanching rash, mottled/ashen/cyanotic
- Not passed urine in past 18 h/urine output <0.5 mL/kg/h
- Lactate ≥2 mmol/L
- Recent chemotherapy

SEPSIS AMBER FLAGS

The absence of red flags does not necessarily indicate that a patient is well. Nurses should remain alert to the following amber flags which may indicate moderate to high risk of deterioration (UK Sepsis Trust).

- Relatives concerned about mental status
- Acute deterioration in functional ability
- Immunosuppressed
- Trauma/surgery/procedure in last 6 weeks
- Respiratory rate 21 to 24
- Systolic BP 91 to 100 mmHg
- Heart rate 91 to 130 OR new dysrhythmia
- Not passed urine in past 12 to 18 hours
- Temperature < 36°C
- Clinical signs of wound, device or skin infection

- Sepsis is a time critical condition, which can be life threatening.
- Patients should be assessed using the ABCDE approach.
- All patients with sepsis must have a management plan including an escalation plan.

SEPSIS MANAGEMENT

If the patient is acutely unwell and you suspect this could be due to infection, assess the patient for any red or amber flags. If the patient has any red flags you must initiate the Sepsis 6 within 1 hour (Sepsis Trust UK, 2022). If the patient has any amber flags it is still important to escalate your concerns and a senior clinical should review the patient within 1 hour. The sepsis six is intended for use across all healthcare settings, including community settings.

The Sepsis 6 includes:

- Ensure a senior clinician reviews the patient.
- Administer oxygen to maintain saturations > 94% (or 99-92% if risk of hypercarbia).
- Obtain IV access, take bloods including blood cultures, blood glucose levels, lactate levels, full blood count, renal profile, C-Reactive Protein (CRP), clotting and any other investigations as required.
- Give antibiotics as per local policy/protocols, considering any allergies.
- Give IV fluids in boluses of 20ml/kg for patients over the age of 16 years.
- Monitor the patient and escalate the patients care as required.

Treatment of Sepsis and Septic Shock

Delivering all elements of the sepsis care bundle within the specified timeframe is a challenge for nurses in busy clinical areas (McClelland and Moxon, 2014). The use of care bundles, helps practitioners to remain focused, to prioritise care and provide early treatment which is critical for successful outcome. The clinical setting and local guidelines will determine how you treat sepsis. Hospitals may use national and/or international guidelines to inform practice.

Recommended Ongoing Care

1. Regular reassessment/revaluation of interventions such as sepsis six.
2. Close monitoring (at least hourly) vital signs and NEWS.
3. Senior clinician review as soon as sepsis is identified.
4. Escalation to higher levels of care if interventions are not effective.
5. Microbiology teams should be involved as soon as sepsis is suspected, to identify correct antibiotic treatments.
6. Fluid balance monitoring.
7. Consider urinary catheter insertion.

References

Lambden, S., Laterre, P.F., Levy, M.M. et al., 2019. The SOFA score—development, utility and challenges of accurate assessment in clinical trials. Crit. Care. 23, 374. doi:10.1186/s13054-019-2663-7.

McClelland, H., Moxon, A., 2014. Early identification and treatment of sepsis. Nurs. Times. 110 (4), 14–17.

NICE, 2016. Sepsis: Recognition, Diagnosis and Early Management. Available from: www.nice.org.uk/guidance/ng51/resources/sepsis-recognition-diagnosis-and-early-management-1837508256709.

Sepsis Trust UK (2022). Screening and action tool for adults, children and young people aged 12 and over. https://sepsistrust.org/professional-resources/our-nice-clinical-tools/

Seymour, C.W., Liu, V.X., Iwashyna, T.J., et al., 2016. Assessment of clinical criteria for sepsis: for the Third International Consensus Definitions for Sepsis and Septic Shock (Sepsis-3). JAMA. 315, 762–774. doi:10.1001/jama.2016.0288.

Singer M, Deutschman CS, Seymour CW, Shankar-Hari M, Annane D, Bauer M, Bellomo R, Bernard GR, Chiche JD, Coopersmith CM, Hotchkiss RS, Levy MM, Marshall JC, Martin GS, Opal SM, Rubenfeld GD, van der Poll T, Vincent JL, Angus DC. (2016). The Third International Consensus Definitions for Sepsis and Septic Shock (Sepsis-3). JAMA. 315(8):801-10. doi: 10.1001/jama.2016.0287. PMID: 26903338; PMCID: PMC4968574.

Singer, M., et al., 2016. The third international consensus definitions for sepsis and septic shock (Sepsis-3). JAMA. 315 (8), 801–810. doi:10.1001/jama.2016.0287.

Society of Critical Care Medicine and European Society of Intensive Care Medicine, 2019. Hour-1 Bundle. Initial resuscitation for sepsis and septic shock. https://www.sccm.org/getattachment/SurvivingSepsis-Campaign/Guidelines/Adult-Patients/Surviving-Sepsis-Campaign-Hour-1-Bundle.pdf?lang=en-US.

Surviving Sepsis Campaign. (2021). Surviving Sepsis Campaign Guidelines 2021. https://www.sccm.org/Clinical-Resources/Guidelines/Guidelines/Surviving-Sepsis-Guidelines-2021#Recommendations

UK Health Security Agency. (2022). Meningococcal disease: guidance, data and analysis. https://www.gov.uk/government/collections/meningococcal-disease-guidance-data-and-analysis

UK Sepsis Trust. (2022). Clinical Tools. https://sepsistrust.org/professional-resources/our-aomrc-clinical-tools/

CHAPTER 11

Gastrointestinal Assessment and Management

Monitoring of Fluid Balance

In adults, the body comprises of 60% fluid for males and 55% for females. These fluids are a combination of water and electrolytes which maintain several key physiological functions, including temperature control, removal of waste products, maintenance of acid–base balance and the delivery of nutrients and diffused gases to the cells (Guest, 2020). Fluids are found in both intracellular (inside cells) and extracellular (outside cells) compartments. The extracellular compartment divides the interstitial compartment and intravascular compartment. The intravascular fluid is referred to as plasma. Plasma comprises 55% of the total volume of blood, with 45% being blood cells. In an adult, approximately 3 L of extracellular fluid is plasma, contributes to a total circulating volume of approximately 5 L. The walls of cells and capillary vessels are designed to separate the two compartments. A semi-permeable membrane can be found between the two compartments, which enables fluid to cross. The movement of fluids between the interstitial and intravascular space is maintained by physiologically controlled hydrostatic and osmotic pressures. The capillary vessel walls are permeable to water and small ions but impermeable to the large protein molecules found in plasma.

Homeostasis is maintained through the balance of fluid intake and excretion, with renal function a key activity (McLafferty et al., 2014). Therefore, a reduction in the circulating plasma volume, for example, due to hypovolaemia, affects oxygenation to tissues and cells and compensatory mechanisms are initiated to restore homeostasis. Physiological compensation mechanisms include the renin–angiotensin–aldosterone system (RAAS). Thus, a reduction in blood pressure triggers a series of renal, neural and adrenergic responses. The kidneys secrete renin into the blood, which activates the RAAS pathway. This then promotes the adrenal cortex to secrete the hormone aldosterone, which causes the renal tubules to increase the reabsorption of the sodium, which releases water back into the blood. This increases plasma volume and blood pressure. Aldosterone also regulates potassium levels; when potassium in the extracellular fluid increases, the aldosterone levels also increase, which results in additional potassium ions being excreted via the kidneys in the urine. This maintains electrolyte balance in the body.

Other compensatory mechanisms include vasoconstriction caused by the action of angiotensin II. This is a physiological response in which angiotensin I is converted by renin secreted by the kidneys, into angiotensin II by angiotensin-converting enzyme (ACE). ACE is secreted by the vascular endothelium, particularly in the lungs. Angiotensin II is a powerful vasoconstrictor and causes blood pressure to increase. Plasma volume is further regulated by the antidiuretic hormone (ADH), which is secreted by the posterior pituitary gland. When osmoreceptors and baroreceptors detect a decrease in osmolarity and blood pressure, ADH is released. In conscious patients, this results in increased thirst, which prompts an individual to improve their oral fluids, therefore increasing fluid body volume.

Fluid loss can be categorised as
- Sensible loss: urination, defecation, blood loss, burns, sepsis, wound and gastric drainage and vomiting.
- Insensible loss: perspiration and breathing.

Sensible loss is easier to measure than insensible loss (Guest, 2020). However, nurses need to remember that body's fluid balance can be altered by disease and injury. Although the body will attempt to maintain homeostasis; in ill health or if fluid lost is not replaced, compensatory mechanisms will ultimately fail. A decrease in the volume of circulating plasma will result in hypovolaemic shock, which is a state of impaired delivery of oxygen or use of oxygen by the cells. To restore tissue perfusion, rapid assessment and replacement of circulating plasma volume is needed. This can be achieved through controlling haemorrhage (e.g. direct pressure, replacement of circulating volume with intravenous fluids or blood and blood products).

Assessing Fluid Balance

Patients must be holistically assessed using the Airway, Breathing, Circulation, Disability and Exposure (ABCDE) approach (see p. 20), the use of an Early Warning Scoring tool (page 18), fluid input and output and examining biochemical markers.

Fluid charts provide crucial information, such as oral, intravenous and nasogastric (NG) intake. The output section must record all urine output, diarrhoea, stoma output, drains, NG aspirates and vomit. The fluid balance should be calculated every 1 to 2 hours to identify the ongoing balance. At the end of a 24-hour period, the total input and output over this period must be calculated, to ascertain whether the patient is in a positive or negative fluid balance.

Evidence suggests that in acute settings, fluid balance charting is often inaccurate (Jeyapala et al., 2015); in consequence, this has been identified as a patient safety concern (National Institute for Health and Care Excellence (NICE), 2017). Strategies to improve fluid balance documentation include regular audits to identify compliance, staff understanding the importance of correct and accurate fluid balance recording, appropriate identification of patient requiring monitoring and fluid charts which are easy to complete (Jeyapala et al., 2015).

KEY POINTS

- Fluid balance charts are an essential component of patient care and provide detailed information on the patients input, output and cumulative balance over set time period.
- If there is more intake than output, the patient is in a positive fluid balance. If there is more output than intake, the patient is in a negative fluid balance. In some patients, especially renal patients who do not pass urine, changes in weight will be used to calculate fluid loss or gain.

PROCEDURE

1. All oral, intravenous and NG intake should be recorded on the fluid intake side of the fluid balance chart (see Fig. 11.1).
2. In the output section, record: all urine output, diarrhoea or stoma output, NG aspirate and vomit. Any other output that can be measured or weighed (e.g. wound drainage) should also be documented.
3. The sections labelled 'Other' is included to enable annotation of individual fluid intake (Fig. 11.1).
4. Patients who are independent and able to drink, should be asked to record the nature and quantity of their oral fluid intake. For patients who require assistance with fluid intake, the nurse has the responsibility for completing the records. It is important to remember that, with the introduction of electronic patient notes, fluid balance charting is no longer charted on paper. This may prevent self-completion of the chart by the patient, increasing

Fluid balance chart

Hospital: _____	Reason for fluid balance chart __NBM__	Does patient require thickened fluids?	**NHS** Greater Glasgow and Clyde
Ward: __11B__	Is patient fluid restricted? Yes ☐ No ☐	Yes ☐ No ☐ Stage _____	
Date: __1/1/17__	If yes how many mL in 24 hours? _____	Is the patient on an oral supplement? Yes ☐ No ☑	
		If yes please indicate:	
		1. Type _____ circle how many daily 1 2 3	
	Fluid balance from previous 24 hours	2. Type _____ circle how many daily 1 2 3	
	+/− __+80__	Signature: _____ Designation: _____	

ONLY RECORD INTAKE CONSUMED NOT WHAT IS GIVEN TO PATIENT

Time	Input									Output								
	Oral Fluids		Enteral		IV/Other					Running total Input	Urine	Gastric/ vomit	Bowel	Type	Type	Type	Running total Output	Initials
	Type	Volume	Type	Volume	Type	Volume	Type	Volume										
00:00					IV	100	TPN	78										
01:00					Fluids	100		78										
02:00						100		78										
03:00						100		78		500	(e)							
04:00						100		78										
05:00						100		78										
06:00						100		78										
07:00						100		78										
08:00						100		78										
09:00						100		78		900	(e)							
10:00						100		78										
11:00						100		78										
12:00						100		78										
13:00			meds 420	200		100		78		500	(e)					1900		
14:00						100		78										
15:00								78										
16:00								78										
17:00								78										
18:00			meds 150 + 420					78	2592									
19:00								78										
20:00								78		1000						2900		
21:00								78										
22:00			meds + Flush	120				78										
23:00								78										
							*Total intake	3102				*Total output				2900	

*Transfer total intake/total output/24hours fluid balance to cumulative fluid balance on back of food, fluid and nutrition profile.

*24 hours fluid Balance+/− +202

Fig. 11.1 A completed fluid balance chart of a patient in the early postoperative period. (Murphy, M., Srivastava, R., & Deans, K. (2019). *Clinical Biochemistry: An Illustrated Colour Text*, 6th ed. Elsevier Ltd.)

the risk of inaccuracy and/or missed information. Therefore, the nurse must now gather and collate this information from the patient.

5. Patients who are independent must be asked to measure and chart their own urine output. If they are unable to do this themselves, they must be provided with a clearly labelled jug to leave in the sluice/toilet area for the nurse to measure and record.
6. It is important to individual needs, monitor and record input and output at regular intervals.
7. A new chart is needed for each 24-hour period. The fluid intake and output for the previous day is then totalled, and the balance is calculated.

Importance of Good Nutrition and Hydration: Nutritional Assessment

Good nutrition is essential to promote health and wellbeing and aid recovery from trauma, surgery or disease. However, there is evidence that malnutrition is common among those who are ill, whether they are in hospital or the community (British Association of Parenteral and Enteral Nutrition (BAPEN), 2018). Nurses need to recognise that people who are unwell may not eat or drink what they sufficiently or their ability to do so may be impaired due to the nature of their illness. In addition, it is accepted that at any one time, more than 90% of people at risk of malnutrition are living in the community.

Malnutrition is defined as a state in which a deficiency or excess or an imbalance of energy, protein and nutrients causes measurable adverse effects on body form and function and clinical outcomes (Johnstone, 2018). Although malnutrition or 'poor nutrition' associated with overeating are important issues for nurses undertaking nutritional assessment, the focus of much of the literature has been on undernutrition. However, it is important to note that patients who are overweight or obese may be malnourished. Also, that poor nutritional status is associated with a significant increase in hospital admissions and significantly longer length of hospital stay (Johnstone, 2018). Therefore, all patients must be screened at their first clinical appointment and on initial registration/admission (NICE, 2017). Screening should include assessment of body mass index (BMI), percentage unintentional weight loss, the time over which nutrient intake has been unintentionally reduced and/or the likelihood of future impaired nutrient intake.

In hospital and nursing home settings, screening should be repeated weekly or when there is clinical concern. In general practice (GP) settings, screening should be repeated during health checks, flu injections and other appointments etc. Nurses have an important role to play in the nutritional assessment of patients, and devising a plan of care that considers cultural and social preferences as well as specialist dietary needs (BAPEN, 2018). In addition, nurses must play a role in identifying and addressing malnutrition to improve the nutritional status and clinical and healthcare outcomes for each patient (BAPEN, 2018). Using a validated nutritional screening tools is a vital component of effective nutritional care (NICE, 2017). BAPEN's Malnutrition Universal Screening Tool (MUST) is a valid and reproducible tool that can be used in all adult-care settings in both primary and secondary care (BAPEN, 2016), through a five-step process which uses objective measurements to identify a risk category.

EQUIPMENT

Accurately calibrated weighting scales
Height measure
Tape measure

PROCEDURE

1. Explain the procedure, then gain consent and cooperation.
2. Obtain the patient's height and weight measurements using calibrated weighing scale and a height measure. Where this is not possible, obtain the patient's mid-upper arm circumference (MUAC) by measuring the ulna length and upper arm circumference with a tape measure (BAPEN, 2016).
3. Examine the patient for the following signs of malnutrition:
   a. Loose-fitting clothing which may indicate unintentional weight loss.
   b. Muscle wasting resulting in a skeletal appearance, due to the breakdown of muscle tissue. This may be more noticeable in the arms and faces, with prominent cheekbones and sunken eyes (Johnstone, 2018).
   c. Reduced skin elasticity due to the reduction of collagen in the skin.
   d. Hair loss.
   e. Brittle nails, indicating a diet lacking the main food groups, in particular protein.
4. Assess the patient's oral health.
5. Assess the patient's normal dietary intake, including portion size, frequency of intake and range of foods consumed.
6. Ask if the patient has noticed any changes in their weight recently.
7. Ask if the patient has experienced any changes to their appetite and/or sense of taste, smell or sight.
8. Ask the patient about his or her energy levels, mood and concentration.
9. Ask about access to food (e.g. whether they shop for groceries and if they have the ability to store food and cook).

10. Assess for any motor skills deficiencies which may be due to a CVA or caused by Parkinson's disease, multiple sclerosis or motor neurone disease, check if this has affected the ability to eat (e.g., holding cutlery).
11. Ask the patient about the ability to swallow food.
12. Observe the patient's ability to swallow saliva (e.g. drooling may indicate a swallow issue).
13. If appropriate, undertake a swallow assessment and implement an action plan to reduce the risk of aspiration.
14. Assess the patient using a validated nutritional screening tool such as MUST.
15. Document your findings.

NUTRITION ASSESSMENT TOOLS

The MUST nutritional screening tool (Fig. 11.2) is a rapid, simple and general tool that can be used by nursing, medical or other staff on first contact with the subject so that clear guidelines for action can be implemented and appropriate nutritional advice provided (BAPEN, 2016). It consists of a five-step process which uses objective measurements to obtain a risk category for individuals who are malnourished, at risk of malnutrition (undernutrition) or obese. It also includes management guidelines which can be used to develop a care plan. It is for use in hospitals, community and other care settings and can be used by all care workers (BAPEN, 2016). MUST is endorsed by the British Dietetic Association, The Royal College of Nursing (RCN), the Royal College of Physicians and the Registered Nursing Home Association and is approved for use by NICE and National Health Service (NHS) Quality Improvement Scotland.

Step 1: Calculating the BMI Score.

BMI is a tool for use with patients older than 18 years of age and enables determination of whether the patient has a normal weight, is underweight or is overweight (see Fig. 11.1). On its own it is not a good indicator of nutritional risk; but needs to be part of a comprehensive nutritional assessment. BMI is calculated by dividing the weight in kilograms (kg) by the height in metres squared (see later).

BMI is calculated by dividing the weight in kilograms (kg) by the height in metres squared (as follows).

$$BMI = \frac{\text{weight in kg}}{(\text{height in metres})^2} = \frac{60}{1.69 \times 1.69} = 20.01$$

A BMI of 20 to 24.9 indicates an average or desirable weight. A BMI of greater than 30 is classified as obese and greater than 40 as grossly obese. Patients with a BMI of less than 20 may show signs of undernutrition.

If it is not possible to obtain height and weight, there are alternative measurements which can be used alternative measurements. A frequently used method, uses the length of forearm (the ulna) to calculate height using Fig. 11.2. To estimate height from the ulna length, measure between the point of the elbow (olecranon process) and the midpoint of the prominent bone of the wrist (styloid process) (left side if possible), ideally use the left arm (BAPEN, 2016). Then using Table 11.1, convert the ulna length into the individual's estimated height. If this is not possible, alternative measurements include knee height and demi-span of the arm.

If MUAC is 32.0 cm, BMI is likely to be greater than 30 kg/m². The use of MUAC provides a general indication of BMI and is not designed to generate an actual score for use with MUST. For further information on use of MUAC, refer to the MUST Explanatory Booklet.

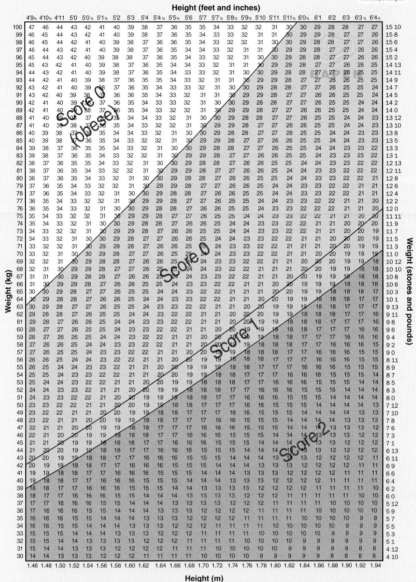

Fig. 11.2 (A) Malnutrition Universal Screening Tool (MUST). MUST is reproduced here with the kind permission of BAPEN (British Association for Parenteral and Enteral Nutrition). For further information on 'MUST' see www.bapen.org.uk Copyright © BAPEN 2012 (licence number LIC2206).

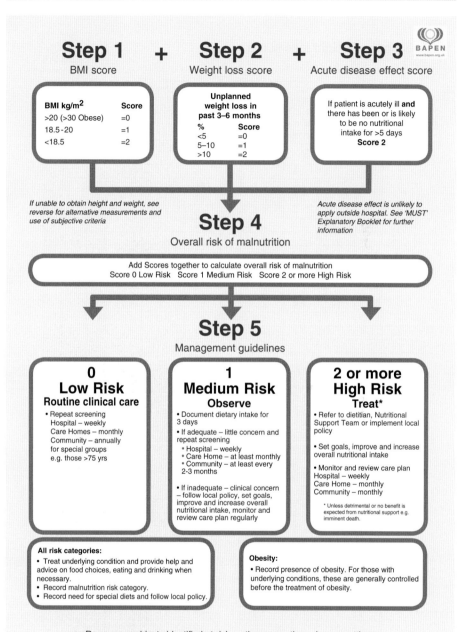

Step 1 + **Step 2** + **Step 3**
BMI score · Weight loss score · Acute disease effect score

BAPEN
www.bapen.org.uk

BMI kg/m^2	Score
>20 (>30 Obese)	=0
18.5-20	=1
<18.5	=2

Unplanned weight loss in past 3–6 months

%	Score
<5	=0
5–10	=1
>10	=2

If patient is acutely ill **and** there has been or is likely to be no nutritional intake for >5 days
Score 2

If unable to obtain height and weight, see reverse for alternative measurements and use of subjective criteria

Step 4
Overall risk of malnutrition

Acute disease effect is unlikely to apply outside hospital. See 'MUST' Explanatory Booklet for further information

Add Scores together to calculate overall risk of malnutrition
Score 0 Low Risk   Score 1 Medium Risk   Score 2 or more High Risk

Step 5
Management guidelines

0 Low Risk
Routine clinical care
- Repeat screening
  Hospital – weekly
  Care Homes – monthly
  Community – annually
  for special groups
  e.g. those >75 yrs

1 Medium Risk
Observe
- Document dietary intake for 3 days
- If adequate – little concern and repeat screening
  • Hospital – weekly
  • Care Home – at least monthly
  • Community – at least every 2-3 months
- If inadequate – clinical concern – follow local policy, set goals, improve and increase overall nutritional intake, monitor and review care plan regularly

2 or more High Risk
Treat*
- Refer to dietitian, Nutritional Support Team or implement local policy
- Set goals, improve and increase overall nutritional intake
- Monitor and review care plan
  Hospital – weekly
  Care Home – monthly
  Community – monthly

  * Unless detrimental or no benefit is expected from nutritional support e.g. imminent death.

All risk categories:
- Treat underlying condition and provide help and advice on food choices, eating and drinking when necessary.
- Record malnutrition risk category.
- Record need for special diets and follow local policy.

Obesity:
- Record presence of obesity. For those with underlying conditions, these are generally controlled before the treatment of obesity.

Re-assess subjects identified at risk as they move through care settings
See The 'MUST' Explanatory Booklet for further details and The 'MUST' Report for supporting evidence.

Fig. 11.2, cont'd (B) Body mass index (BMI) chart.

Step 2 – Weight loss score

BAPEN
www.bapen.org.uk

kg	Score 0 Wt loss < 5% Less than (kg)	Score 1 Wt loss 5 - 10% Between (kg)	Score 2 Wt loss > 5% More than (kg)	kg	Score 0 Wt loss < 5% Less than (kg)	Score 1 Wt loss 5 - 10% Between (kg)	Score 2 Wt loss > 10% More than (kg)
30	1.6	1.6 - 3.3	3.3	65	3.4	3.4 - 7.2	7.2
31	1.6	1.6 - 3.4	3.4	66	3.5	3.5 - 7.3	7.3
32	1.7	1.7 - 3.6	3.6	67	3.5	3.5 - 7.4	7.4
33	1.7	1.7 - 3.7	3.7	68	3.6	3.6 - 7.6	7.6
34	1.8	1.8 - 3.8	3.8	69	3.6	3.6 - 7.7	7.7
35	1.8	1.8 - 3.9	3.9	70	3.7	3.7 - 7.8	7.8
36	1.9	1.9 - 4.0	4.0	71	3.7	3.7 - 7.9	7.9
37	1.9	1.9 - 4.1	4.1	72	3.8	3.8 - 8.0	8.0
38	2.0	2.0 - 4.2	4.2	73	3.8	3.8 - 8.1	8.1
39	2.1	2.1 - 4.3	4.3	74	3.9	3.9 - 8.2	8.2
40	2.1	2.1 - 4.4	4.4	75	3.9	3.9 - 8.3	8.3
41	2.2	2.2 - 4.6	4.6	76	4.0	4.0 - 8.4	8.4
42	2.2	2.2 - 4.7	4.7	77	4.1	4.1 - 8.6	8.6
43	2.3	2.3 - 4.8	4.8	78	4.1	4.1 - 8.6	8.7
44	2.3	2.3 - 4.9	4.9	79	4.2	4.2 - 8.7	8.8
45	2.4	2.4 - 5.0	5.0	80	4.2	4.2 - 8.9	8.9
46	2.4	2.4 - 5.1	5.1	81	4.3	4.3 - 9.0	9.0
47	2.5	2.5 - 5.2	5.2	82	4.3	4.3 - 9.1	9.1
48	2.5	2.5 - 5.3	5.3	83	4.4	4.4 - 9.2	9.2
49	2.6	2.6 - 5.4	5.4	84	4.4	4.4 - 9.3	9.3
50	2.6	2.6 - 5.6	5.6	85	4.5	4.5 - 9.4	9.4
51	2.7	2.7 - 5.7	5.7	86	4.5	4.5 - 9.6	9.6
52	2.7	2.7 - 5.8	5.8	87	4.6	4.6 - 9.7	9.7
53	2.8	2.8 - 5.9	5.9	88	4.6	4.6 - 9.8	9.8
54	2.8	2.8 - 6.0	6.0	89	4.7	4.7 - 9.9	9.9
55	2.9	2.9 - 6.1	6.1	90	4.7	4.7 -10.0	10.0
56	2.9	2.9 - 6.2	6.2	91	4.8	4.8 -10.1	10.1
57	3.0	3.0 - 6.3	6.3	92	4.8	4.8 -10.2	10.2
58	3.1	3.1 - 6.4	6.4	93	4.9	4.9 -10.3	10.3
59	3.1	3.1 - 6.6	6.6	94	4.9	4.9 -10.4	10.4
60	3.2	3.2 - 6.7	6.7	95	5.0	5.0 -10.6	10.6
61	3.2	3.2 - 6.8	6.8	96	5.1	5.1 -10.7	10.7
62	3.3	3.3 - 6.9	6.9	97	5.1	5.1 -10.8	10.8
63	3.3	3.3 - 7.0	7.0	98	5.2	5.2 -10.9	10.9
64	3.4	3.4 - 7.1	7.1	99	5.2	5.2 -11.0	11.0

Current weight

Fig. 11.2, cont'd   (C) Estimating BMI category from mid upper arm circumference.

TABLE 11.1 ■ Using Ulna Length to Estimate Height

Ulna Length (cm)	32.0	31.5	31.0	30.5	30.0	29.5	29.0	28.5	28.0	27.5	27.0	26.5	26.0	25.5
Height (m) Men (<65 years)	1.94	1.93	1.91	1.89	1.87	1.85	1.841	1.82	1.80	1.78	1.76	1.751	1.73	1.71
Men (≥65 years)	1.87	1.86	1.84	1.82	1.81	1.79	1.78	1.76	1.75	1.73	1.71	1.70	1.68	1.67
Ulna Length (cm)	**32.0**	**31.5**	**31.0**	**30.5**	**30.0**	**29.5**	**29.0**	**28.5**	**28.0**	**27.5**	**27.0**	**26.5**	**26.0**	**25.5**
Height (m) Women (<65 years)	1.84	1.83	1.81	1.80	1.79	1.77	1.78	1.75	1.73	1.72	1.70	1.69	1.68	1.66
Women (≥65 years)	1.84	1.83	1.81	1.79	1.78	1.76	1.75	1.73	1.71	1.70	1.68	1.66	1.65	1.63

Ulna length (cm)	25.0	24.5	24.0	23.5	23.0	22.5	22.0	21.5	21.0	20.5	20.0	19.5	19.0	18.5
Height (m) Men (<65 years)	1.69	1.67	1.66	1.64	1.62	1.60	1.58	1.57	1.55	1.53	1.51	1.49	1.48	1.46
Men (≥65 years)	1.65	1.63	1.62	1.60	159	1.57	1.56	1.54	1.52	1.51	1.49	1.48	1.46	1.45
Height (m) Women (<65 years)	1.65	1.63	1.62	1.61	1.59	1.58	1.56	1.55	1.54	1.52	1.51	1.50	1.48	1.47
Women (≥65 years)	1.61	1.60	1.58	1.56	1.55	1.53	1.52	1.50	1.48	1.47	1.45	1.44	1.42	1.40

If the weight and height cannot be measured, and when screening patient groups in which extra care in interpretation is needed (e.g. those with fluid disturbances, plaster casts, amputations, critical illness and pregnant or lactating women).

Step 2: Assess the percentage of unplanned weight loss using Table 11.2.

Step 3: If the patient has been acutely ill and there has been or unlikely to have been no nutritional intake for more than 5 days, add a score of 2. These patients include:

- Those who are unable to take oral food or fluids following surgery involving the gastrointestinal tract or who have conditions that affect it, or those who are critically ill, have swallowing difficulties (e.g. after stroke) or have head injuries.
- Deterioration in mental state or conscious level is likely to affect the patient's desire and ability to eat and drink independently and so will increase the risk of malnutrition.

Step 4: Establish overall risk of malnutrition after considering all relevant factors. Add scores together from steps 1, 2 and 3 to calculate overall risk of malnutrition.

0 = low risk, 1 = medium risk, 2 or more = high risk

If neither BMI nor weight loss can be established, assess overall risk category using the following 'subjective criteria'

- Person looks thin, underweight, an acceptable weight or overweight.
- Obvious wasting (very thin) and obesity (very overweight) or unplanned weight loss
- Obvious signs that clothes and/or jewelry have become loose fitting (weight loss)
- Signs of physical disability such as manual dexterity and if the patient has the manual dexterity to eat and drink independently
- Unplanned weight loss as discussed in step 4.

Estimate a malnutrition risk category (low, medium or high) based on your overall evaluation.

Step 5: Ongoing assessment and evaluation.

TABLE 11.2 ■ Recent Weight Loss Score

BAPEN — Step 2 – Weight loss score

Weight loss in last 3 to 6 months. Score 0: Wt loss < 5%. Score 1: Wt loss 5 - 10%. Score 2: Wt loss > 10%.

kg	Less than (kg)	Between (kg)	More than (kg)	st lb	Less than (st lb)	Between (st lb)	More than (st lb)
30	1.6	1.6-3.3	3.3	4 10	0 3	0 3-0 7	0 7
31	1.6	1.6-3.4	3.4	4 12	0 4	0 4-0 8	0 8
32	1.7	1.7-3.6	3.6	5 1	0 4	0 4-0 8	0 8
33	1.7	1.7-3.7	3.7	5 3	0 4	0 4-0 8	0 8
34	1.8	1.8-3.8	3.8	5 5	0 4	0 4-0 8	0 8
35	1.8	1.8-3.9	3.9	5 7	0 4	0 4-0 9	0 9
36	1.9	1.9-4.0	4.0	5 9	0 4	0 4-0 9	0 9
37	1.9	1.9-4.1	4.1	5 12	0 4	0 4-0 9	0 9
38	2.0	2.0-4.2	4.2	6 0	0 4	0 4-0 9	0 9
39	2.1	2.1-4.3	4.3	6 2	0 5	0 5-0 10	0 10
40	2.1	2.1-4.4	4.4	6 4	0 5	0 5-0 10	0 10
41	2.2	2.2-4.6	4.6	6 6	0 5	0 5-0 10	0 10
42	2.2	2.2-4.7	4.7	6 9	0 5	0 5-0 10	0 10
43	2.3	2.3-4.8	4.8	6 11	0 5	0 5-0 11	0 11
44	2.3	2.3-4.9	4.9	6 13	0 5	0 5-0 11	0 11
45	2.4	2.4-5.0	5.0	7 1	0 5	0 5-0 11	0 11
46	2.4	2.4-5.1	5.1	7 3	0 5	0 5-0 11	0 11
47	2.5	2.5-5.2	5.2	7 6	0 5	0 5-0 12	0 12
48	2.5	2.5-5.3	5.3	7 8	0 6	0 6-0 12	0 12
49	2.6	2.6-5.4	5.4	7 10	0 6	0 6-0 12	0 12
50	2.6	2.6-5.6	5.6	7 12	0 6	0 6-0 12	0 12
51	2.7	2.7-5.7	5.7	8 0	0 6	0 6-0 12	0 12
52	2.7	2.7-5.8	5.8	8 3	0 6	0 6-0 13	0 13
53	2.8	2.8-5.9	5.9	8 5	0 6	0 6-0 13	0 13
54	2.8	2.8-6.0	6.0	8 7	0 6	0 6-0 13	0 13
55	2.9	2.9-6.1	6.1	8 9	0 6	0 6-0 13	0 13
56	2.9	2.9-6.2	6.2	8 11	0 6	0 6-1 0	1 0
57	3.0	3.0-6.3	6.3	9 0	0 7	0 7-1 0	1 0
58	3.1	3.1-6.4	6.4	9 2	0 7	0 7-1 0	1 0
59	3.1	3.1-6.6	6.6	9 4	0 7	0 7-1 0	1 0
60	3.2	3.2-6.7	6.7	9 6	0 7	0 7-1 1	1 1
61	3.2	3.2-6.8	6.8	9 8	0 7	0 7-1 1	1 1
62	3.3	3.3-6.9	6.9	9 11	0 7	0 7-1 1	1 1
63	3.3	3.3-7.0	7.0	9 13	0 7	0 7-1 1	1 1
64	3.4	3.4-7.1	7.1	10 1	0 7	0 7-1 2	1 2

kg	Less than (kg)	Between (kg)	More than (kg)	st lb	Less than (st lb)	Between (st lb)	More than (st lb)
65	3.4	3.4-7.2	7.2	10 3	0 8	0 8-1 2	1 2
66	3.5	3.5-7.3	7.3	10 6	0 8	0 8-1 2	1 2
67	3.5	3.5-7.4	7.4	10 8	0 8	0 8-1 2	1 2
68	3.6	3.6-7.6	7.6	10 10	0 8	0 8-1 3	1 3
69	3.6	3.6-7.7	7.7	10 12	0 8	0 8-1 3	1 3
70	3.7	3.7-7.8	7.8	11 0	0 8	0 8-1 3	1 3
71	3.7	3.7-7.9	7.9	11 3	0 8	0 8-1 3	1 3
72	3.8	3.8-8.0	8.0	11 5	0 8	0 8-1 4	1 4
73	3.8	3.8-8.1	8.1	11 7	0 8	0 8-1 4	1 4
74	3.9	3.9-8.2	8.2	11 9	0 9	0 9-1 4	1 4
75	3.9	3.9-8.3	8.3	11 11	0 9	0 9-1 4	1 4
76	4.0	4.0-8.4	8.4	12 0	0 9	0 9-1 5	1 5
77	4.1	4.1-8.6	8.6	12 2	0 9	0 9-1 5	1 5
78	4.1	4.1-8.6	8.7	12 4	0 9	0 9-1 5	1 5
79	4.2	4.2-8.7	8.8	12 6	0 9	0 9-1 5	1 5
80	4.2	4.2-8.9	8.9	12 8	0 9	0 9-1 6	1 6
81	4.3	4.3-9.0	9.0	12 11	0 9	0 9-1 6	1 6
82	4.3	4.3-9.1	9.1	12 13	0 10	0 10-1 6	1 6
83	4.4	4.4-9.2	9.2	13 1	0 10	0 10-1 6	1 6
84	4.4	4.4-9.3	9.3	13 3	0 10	0 10-1 7	1 7
85	4.5	4.5-9.4	9.4	13 5	0 10	0 10-1 7	1 7
86	4.5	4.5-9.6	9.6	13 8	0 10	0 10-1 7	1 7
87	4.6	4.6-9.7	9.7	13 10	0 10	0 10-1 7	1 7
88	4.6	4.6-9.8	9.8	13 12	0 10	0 10-1 8	1 8
89	4.7	4.7-9.9	9.9	14 0	0 10	0 10-1 8	1 8
90	4.7	4.7-10.0	10.0	14 2	0 10	0 10-1 8	1 8
91	4.8	4.8-10.1	10.1	14 5	0 11	0 11-1 8	1 8
92	4.8	4.8-10.2	10.2	14 7	0 11	0 11-1 9	1 9
93	4.9	4.9-10.3	10.3	14 9	0 11	0 11-1 9	1 9
94	4.9	4.9-10.4	10.4	14 11	0 11	0 11-1 9	1 9
95	5.0	5.0-10.6	10.6	14 13	0 11	0 11-1 9	1 9
96	5.1	5.1-10.7	10.7	15 2	0 11	0 11-1 10	1 10
97	5.1	5.1-10.8	10.8	15 4	0 11	0 11-1 10	1 10
98	5.2	5.2-10.9	10.9	15 6	0 11	0 11-1 10	1 10
99	5.2	5.2-11.0	11.0	15 8	0 11	0 11-1 10	1 10

© BAPEN

It is important to monitor for clinical factors that may contribute to an increase in patients' weight, such as fluid overload related to the patients' clinical diagnosis (e.g. heart failure, by observing for oedema or fluid collection in the patient's ankles and reporting same).

Patients who have been identified as being at risk of malnutrition should be monitored on a regular basis to check that their care plan continues to meet their needs. Patients with a high or medium risk score require treatment of underlying condition. If patients are unable to maintain nutritional requirements orally, they may require artificial nutritional support (e.g. enteral or parenteral nutrition) (BAPEN, 2016).

NUTRITIONAL SUPPORT

NICE (2017) recommendations for nutritional support in hospital and the community should be considered for patients who are malnourished, as defined as the following:

1. a BMI of less than 18.5 kg/m^2
2. unintentional weight loss greater than 10% within the last 3 to 6 months
3. a BMI of less than 20 kg/m^2 and unintentional weight loss greater than 5% within the last 3 to 6 months.

Patients at risk should be referred to a dietician, and nutritional support should be considered. The frequency of further assessments will be determined by the result of the initial assessment. Nutritional support may include oral, enteral (e.g. NG tube (NGT) or percutaneous endoscopic gastrostomy (PEG)) or parenteral (intravenous) nutritional support, either alone or combined and should be considered for those who are malnourished or at risk of malnourishment.

Assisting Adults With Eating and Drinking

The NHS Hospital Food Survey found approximately 65% of patients felt that hospital food had a direct impact on their overall hospital experience (Patients Association, 2020). All hospital wards should have a policy of protected or supported mealtimes to facilitate the optimum nutrition of all patients (DH, 2017). During protected or supported mealtimes, all non-urgent clinical activity ceases, patients can eat their meals without interruption and staff are available to assist patients who need help to eat and drink.

Risk of malnutrition is defined as:

- Having eaten little or nothing for more than 5 days and/or likely to be eating little or expected not to eat for the next five days.
- Where there is increased nutritional need, where the capacity for absorption is reduced or where there is a high nutrient loss.

KEY POINTS

- Assist patient to make appropriate menu choices. Do not choose for the patient; if they are unable to, enlist the help of a relative or carer.
- Note any special dietary requirements or cultural practices.
- Encourage the patient to sit in a chair if able, and assist upright in bed and use pillows to support if required.
- Use red trays to highlight patient who requires assistance with eating and drinking.
- Offer the patient the opportunity to wash hands.
- Check the patient is comfortable (i.e. has an empty bladder).
- If the patient has dentures, check these are in place before eating and mouth is clean.
- Check the patient is able to swallow, to prevent choking and aspiration into the lungs.

PROCEDURE

1. Aim to make mealtimes a pleasant experience for the patient.
2. In some hospitals, different-coloured aprons are used for activities, such as serving meals, washing patients and doing dressings. Obtain the correct food and drink, cutlery and napkin.
3. Arrange food attractively on the plate.
4. Take the tray to the bedside. If supervising the patient rather than assisting them with eating and drinking, place all food and drink within easy reach of the patient. Always inform the patient about the food on the plate, especially if they are partially sighted or the food is texture-modified.
5. Always discuss with the patient the level of help required. Assist with opening food packaging or cutting up food, as necessary. Encourage/support patients to feed themselves if possible, using special cutlery where appropriate.

If full assistance is required with eating and drinking, sit at eye level next to the patient to communicate effectively.

The use of red trays and jugs or specially marked equipment can help to highlight patients who are risk of dehydration or nutritionally vulnerable and who require assistance with eating and drinking. This allows staff to plan care at mealtimes. Patients who require help at mealtimes may also require help throughout the day to drink. Staff need to monitor nutritionally vulnerable patients and check they receive help at all drinks rounds as required and during interim periods to provide adequate hydration. All patients should have access to fresh water to maintain hydration and improve wellbeing (RCN, 2019).

If the patient is able to use only one hand, a plate guard and non-slip mat may help. If they are unable to grip ordinary cutlery, large-handled cutlery can usually be obtained from the occupational therapy department.

6. If the patient is unable to see the food, explain to the patient the food that is on the plate and ask for preference as to what they wish to eat first.
7. Ask patients for preferences for food flavouring they require with their meal (e.g. sauces)
8. Using appropriate cutlery, offer bite-size meal portions, and tell patient what it is.
9. Check that patient has enough time to chew and swallow, and offer drinks between each mouthful of food to facilitate eating. Care should be taken with hot drinks. When the patient has had enough of main course, offer dessert, which can provide a good energy source.
10. If the patient has swallowing difficulties, they may need thickened fluid to assist with swallowing. If the patient shows any signs of problems with swallowing, such as persistent coughing or difficulty clearing the mouth, refer them to a speech and language therapist urgently.
11. Respect the patient's dignity, and use the napkin to remove food or drink that has not been swallowed.
12. Respect the patient's wishes but do not press patients once they have indicated that they have had sufficient. Small amounts taken more frequently may be more successful.
13. Encourage the patient to eat a full meal for a balanced nutritional intake.
14. Avoid asking questions while the patient is eating.
15. Once meal is completed, provide the opportunity for the patient to clean their teeth or dentures and assist with mouth care as required.
16. Check the patient is comfortable and that their personal belonging and call bell are within easy reach.
17. Dispose of apron, and decontaminate hands by washing with soap and water or use alcohol-based sanitiser.
18. Nurses must complete relevant documentation such as fluid or food chart. An accurate and comprehensive record needs to be maintained because this forms part of the nutritional assessment. Any abnormal occurrences such as nausea, vomiting or food refusal require documentation and reporting.

Nausea and Vomiting

The causes of nausea and vomiting are often multifactorial; therefore it is important to identify the primary problem. A thorough patient history and assessment of precipitating, aggravating and relieving factors are key to identifying effective strategies for management of symptoms. Gan et al. (2014) advocate nurses and doctors using risk assessment tools to identify and manage a patient's nausea and vomiting symptoms.

A patient who vomits may be at risk of aspiration, in consequence, emergency equipment must be available. Where nausea and vomiting are causing considerable distress, the patient must be assessed, the cause identified and treated, escalate care as necessary. Causes of nausea and vomiting may be associated with medication (e.g. analgesic), surgery, and type of food or other cause. A prolonged period of starvation or an inadequate period of fasting can cause postoperative nausea and vomiting (PONV). PONV remains a common complication in the first 24 hours following surgery and is usually exacerbated by inadequate pain relief (Gan et al., 2014). This may be reduced by a combination of prophylactic antiemetics medication (Gan et al., 2014). Patients who experience PONV are at risk of developing complications such as aspiration, dehydration and electrolyte imbalance. In those who are receiving palliative care, antiemetics are an important intervention, but their cause should be carefully assessed (Webb, 2017).

KEY POINTS

- Respond promptly to calls for assistance (e.g. patient call bell within easy reach).
- Ensure patient safety: in clinical settings, emergency suction should be available at every bed space.

1. Check the patient is in a safe position to avoid injury or fall, and remain with patient.
2. Provide privacy and dignity to avoid any unnecessary embarrassment and distress.
3. If appropriate, remove the patient's dentures (where applicable) and store them safely.
4. Ask/assist the patient to sit forward, or if lying down or semiconscious, place in the lateral position to reduce the risk of aspiration into the lungs.
5. Support the patient's forehead.
6. Encourage the patient to breathe more deeply if possible.
7. Provide tissues, and promote comfort and dignity by cleaning the patient's mouth and face.
8. Assist the patient into a comfortable position once the episode has passed to ensure comfort.
9. Provide a second clean vomit bowl before removing the used one, even if the patient feels the episode has passed.
10. Offer a mouthwash or perform mouth care if the patient is too weak.
11. Offer the patient a bowl of warm water for face and hand washing to prevent cross-contamination.
12. Take the vomit bowel to the dirty utility area (sluice), measure volume and note colour, characteristics and smell. The vomit may contain undigested food or be watery (gastric juices only) or a green/brown fluid (indicates presence of bile). If the vomit is brown and foul (faecal) smelling, this may indicate that there is an obstruction in the large intestine.
13. O bserve for signs of blood, this is termed haematemesis. Bright red, indicates fresh blood from the stomach or upper gastrointestinal tract; dark brown and 'coffee ground' in appearance, indicates older blood that has been partially digested.
14. Document each vomiting episode, making a note of nausea, frequency, amount.
15. Report if vomiting is a new occurrence or if the vomiting has altered in any way.

16. Ascertain the cause of vomiting if possible, and take appropriate action.
17. Return to the patient, and assess nausea and vomiting at regular intervals to maintain patient safety.
18. If appropriate, administer antiemetic drugs as prescribed, and monitor the effect.

Subcutaneous Fluids or Medications (Hyperdermoclysis)

Fluids and some medications can be administered via the subcutaneous route (underneath the skin) if the patient is unable to take them orally. The following procedure describes how to insert a subcutaneous needle/infusion set and administer the prescribed fluid or medication via a gravity flow infusion. The healthcare professional carrying out subcutaneous infusion should be trained and competent in the use of medications, solutions and subcutaneous administration procedures (RCN, 2016).

The subcutaneous route is regarded as being just as effective at delivering fluid and electrolytes as the intravenous route for patients who are mild to moderately dehydrated (Dougherty & Lister, 2015). Currently it is mainly used for patients within the palliative care settings (NICE, 2015). Other indications for subcutaneous infusion include the continuous infusion of insulin (NICE, 2008) and the care of patients who have vomiting, diarrhoea or dysphagia and who cannot tolerate oral medication (Dougherty & Lister, 2015). Drugs administered by subcutaneous infusion include opioid analgesics, antiemetics, anxiolytic sedatives, corticosteroids, nonsteroidal anti-inflammatory drugs and anticholinergic drugs (Dougherty & Lister, 2015).

The subcutaneous route can also be used for patients who have poor venous access or where there is infected or broken skin at intravenous sites. The enzyme (hyaluronidase) which causes more rapid diffusion of the fluid by reducing normal interstitial barriers may be prescribed. It can be administered by injection into the site via the cannula prior to commencement of the infusion or added to the infusion bag. However, there is still conflicting evidence regarding its effectiveness, and reported side effects (discomfort and site irritation). Local guidelines should be followed regarding its use (Bowen, 2014).

A maximum volume of 2000 mL can be given over a 24-hour period continuously or intermittently, with a maximum bolus dose of 500 mL over 1 hour (Radcliffe, 2017). Subcutaneous administration of fluids must not be undertaken when rapid fluid replacement is needed. It is also contraindicated in patients who have clotting disorders, cardiac or renal disorders or peripheral vascular disease of the lower extremities (Radcliffe, 2017).

KEY POINTS

- Only registered healthcare professionals who are competent in the use subcutaneous administration procedures may insert the cannula and administer subcutaneous infusions nurse.
- Dextrose saline and 0.9% sodium chloride are the solutions most commonly administered subcutaneously. It is not suitable for the administration of colloids, blood or total parenteral nutrition.
- The device selected should be of the smallest gauge and shortest length necessary (Royal College of Nursing [RCN], 2016). The choice of cannula may vary according to local policy or practice guidelines; smaller needles may cause less pain for subcutaneous infusions (RCN, 2016).

PROCEDURE

1. Check the prescribed fluid, and prepare the administration set to expel all air. In most cases, all subcutaneous fluids must be checked by a registered healthcare professional, although

this may vary according to local policy. Check the fluid prescription, and ensure it is the correct fluid, strength and volume in accordance with the patient's prescription. Check that the medicine dose, volume, concentration and rate are suitable for the clinical need and appropriate for the condition of the patient's subcutaneous tissue (RCN, 2016). Calculate the drip rate.

2. Make sure the patient understands what is going to happen and obtain their consent. If the patient lacks mental capacity to consent to treatment, it is important to seek advice (Mental Capacity Act, 2005). At the bedside, ask/assist the patient to move into a suitable position to allow access to the site. Check the patient's name band against the prescription. Any site with sufficient subcutaneous tissue may be used, but oedematous areas, areas with infected, broken, or inflamed skin, bony prominences or sites near a joint and the patient's waistline must be avoided (RCN, 2016). The nurse should consider patient comfort, mobility, ease of access and skin condition when choosing the site. The abdomen and thighs are commonly used, although the areas over the scapula and anterior chest wall can also be used.

3. Remove the infusion device from its packaging and prepare to insert it in the subcutaneous tissue. Follow the manufacturer's instructions. Depending on the equipment, you may need to grasp the wings of the cannula and bring them together, pinching firmly. Some devices may need to be primed before insertion.

4. If possible, ask the patient to adjust or remove clothing to expose the insertion site.

5. Clean the site with a swab saturated with 2% chlorhexidine/70% alcohol and allow to dry, following local policy (Dougherty & Lister, 2015).

6. Maintaining asepsis, remove the protective cover from the cannula and hold it with the bevelled edge facing upwards. When inserting a subcutaneous needle, pinch the skin between the thumb and first finger of nondominant hand, to ensure that the subcutaneous tissue is separated from the skeletal muscle below. Failure to pinch the skin could result in inadvertent intramuscular injection (Fig. 11.3). The fold of pinched-up skin should be approximately double the length of the needle.

7. Insert the full length of the catheter and needle into the subcutaneous tissue at an angle of 45 degrees. If blood appears in the tubing, withdraw the cannula, and repeat the process at another site using a new cannula.

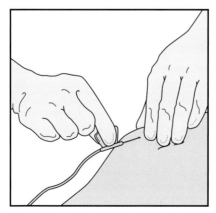

Fig. 11.3 Inserting the butterfly cannula for hyperdermoclysis. (Nicol, M., Bavin, C., Cronin, P., Rawlings-Anderson, K., Cole, E., & Hunter, J. (2012). *Essential Nursing Skills*. Elsevier Ltd.)

8. Close the clamp after removing the needle and dispose the needle in sharps bin.
9. Cover the area with the sterile transparent occlusive dressing to prevent catheter movement and for visual inspection for signs of for redness or infection. Date the dressing.
10. Set the infusion to the rate calculated, and label on the infusion set, stating the date and time the administration set was changed
11. Check the patient is comfortable.
12. Dispose of all clinical waste appropriately, and decontaminate hands.
13. Complete all necessary documentation for the infusion. Record needle insertion in the appropriate documents according to local policy. Line labels that indicate the time and date of insertion should be used. Documentation in the patient's notes should include an outline of the need for subcutaneous infusion, the insertion site and device used, any directions for monitoring of the infusion and the patient's response to therapy (RCN, 2016).
14. Record/monitor fluid balance according to local policy.
15. Observe the cannula daily site for redness, swelling or discomfort.
16. Change the infusion site regularly, according to local policy. Monitor insertion site every shift. Ideally the insertion site should be rotated at least every 3 days (Bowen, 2014; RCN, 2016). The administration set should be changed at least every 72 hours (RCN, 2016).

Naso-gastric Tube Insertion

A naso-gastric tube (NGT) is inserted through the nose, into the stomach via the oesophagus for the purposes of (a) enteral feeding, (b) administration of medication and (c) gastric aspiration and decompression (BAPEN, 2020; National Nurses Nutrition Group (NNNG), 2020). The responsibility for the decision to place an NGT lies with the senior healthcare professional in charge of the patient's care (BAPEN, 2020).

KEY POINTS

- The purpose of a nasogastric tube procedure and risks associated with it should be discussed with the patient before the procedure takes place.
- Nasogastric tube of appropriate size and type (usually 6–12, Ryle type, fine bore).

PROCEDURE

1. Before undertaking this procedure, the practitioner should have completed training and demonstrated competency in NGT insertion in accordance with local policy (Nursing and Midwifery Council (NMC), 2018).
2. Review the patient's medical notes to assess for previous surgery or contraindications to NGT insertion or use, and ensure all relevant investigations are undertaken (where appropriate) (e.g. blood clotting tests) (BAPEN, 2020).
3. Where the patient has capacity to consent, their agreement must be obtained before the procedure is undertaken. Before giving consent, the patient must be given time to consider the decision so that he or she demonstrates an understanding and agreement of the NGT placement procedure (BAPEN, 2020).
4. Ensure the rationale for the decision and discussion with the patient to insert an NGT has been documented in the patient's notes (NMC, 2018).

5. Gather all equipment prior to approaching the patient to undertake the procedure, (NHS Improvement, 2016).

6. Use an NGT appropriate for intended purpose and in accordance with local policy (NHS Improvement, 2016). If the NGT is being inserted for the purpose of enteral feeding, a fine- or small-bore tube must be used. They are radio-opaque throughout their length and have externally visible length markings (NHS Improvement, 2016). They reduce patient discomfort and provide a decreased risk of aspiration. They are also less likely to cause complications such as gastritis, oesophageal and nasal irritation. The wide bore (Ryles tube) should be used only for gastric drainage, medication administration, gastric lavage and diagnostic testing.

7. Inform the patient about the procedure including agreeing on a signal to indicate a problem or the wish to stop (e.g. hand signal).

8. Draw screens to provide privacy. Check the patient is comfortable—sitting upright if possible, with the head neither tilted backwards nor forwards. Insertion of the NGT may be for feeding or for gastric aspiration. The upright position is best for NGT insertion because it facilitates easier insertion of the tube and avoids the tube being inserted to the trachea. If sitting upright is not possible, the patient should be lying on one side (Dougherty and Lister, 2015).

9. Protect the patient's clothing with a towel. A glass of water and a straw will aid swallowing during insertion.

10. Wash hands before putting on gloves and apron, and follow the five moments for hand hygiene. Additional protective clothing (PPE) may be necessary if indicated by the patient's condition.

11. Estimate the length of tube to be inserted by measuring the distance from the patient's nose to the tip of the earlobe (Fig. 11.4) and then to the xiphisternum, and make a note of where this is on the tube (Fig. 11.5). The practitioner may mark the tube with a pen directly for a clear indication of the required measurement during the insertion procedure. The measurement from the tip of the nose, to the earlobe and the xiphisternum is known as the NEX measurement (NHS Improvement, 2016). Having undertaken the measurement, record the amount that will remain outside the nose. The tube may have markings

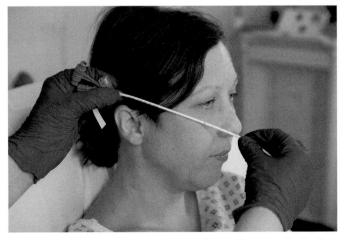

Fig. 11.4 Estimating the length of the nasogastric tube to be inserted by measuring the distance from the patient's nose to the tip of the earlobe.

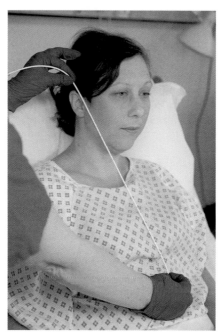

Fig. 11.5 Estimating the length of the nasogastric tube from the nostril to the xiphisternum.

on it to facilitate this. It is important to measure the tube to check that it does not pass through the stomach and into the duodenum. Once the tube is inserted, the amount of tube outside the nose must be recorded and confirmed before use, especially when feeding or giving medications. (NHS Improvement, 2016).

12. Clear the nose by asking them to blow their nose, if able to do so. If this is not possible, consider cleaning the nasal area.

13. Select the best nostril (not tender, no deviated septum, etc.).

14. Encourage the patient to relax as much as possible and to breathe steadily.

15. Remove the NGT from its packaging. If a guidewire is present, gently manipulate it to ensure it moves freely within the tube. Prior to inserting the NGT, ensure the guidewire is locked firmly into place. Lubricate the outside of the NGT as per manufacturers' guidance (BAPEN, 2020).

16. Pass the tube gently into the nostril, and pass backwards (not upwards) along the floor of the nose to the nasopharynx. (If a blockage is felt, change to the other nostril.)

17. Pause to allow the patient to draw breath and recover.

18. Ask the patient to breathe through the mouth and swallow. As the patient swallows, and while keeping the head level, gently advance the tube. When a patient is safe to swallow fluid and has capacity, offer a glass of water/squash with a straw, and ask patient to swallow some water. If it is not safe for the patient to swallow fluid but he or she has capacity, ask the patient to perform a dry swallow. In some instances, asking the patient to tuck the chin (chin tuck) down towards the chest may assist with tube insertion (BAPEN, 2020). Never force the NGT if resistance is felt, to minimise patient harm. A maximum of three attempts should be made at one time. If the procedure is unsuccessful after three attempts, stop and seek senior specialist advice (BAPEN, 2020).

19. Slowly, advance the tube to the predetermined measurement. If the patient starts to cough during the procedure, stop, pull the tube back slightly and wait for coughing to settle to minimise patient distress. Before continuing, ask the patient to open the mouth to check the NGT has not coiled up at the back of the oral cavity (BAPEN, 2020).

20. Once the NGT has been inserted to, or slightly beyond, the predetermined mark, leave the guidewire in position (if there is a guidewire).

21. Connect a 60-mL enteral syringe onto the end of the NGT. Using a larger syringe (60 mL) allows gentle pressure and suction. A smaller syringe may produce too much pressure and split the tube. Only appropriate oral/enteral syringes should be used (NHS Improvement, 2016).

22. When the tube has reached the measured distance, check it is in the stomach by one or more of the following methods:

    ■ Aspirate a small amount of stomach contents (0.5 to 1 mL) from the tube. Apply aspirate to a pH strip, leave for 1 minute and then compare with the colour bars to get a reading. A pH of 5.5 or less confirms gastric placement. A pH between 1 and 5.5 is considered safe when determining if the tube is in the stomach. The pH reading must be 5.5 or less before feed, fluid or medication can be administered via the NGT.

    ■ If unable to obtain any aspirate or the pH is greater than 5.5, injecting 10 to 20 mL of air using a 50-mL syringe will dispel any residual fluid. Advance the tube by 10 to 20 cm, turn the patient onto the side, leave for 15 to 30 min and try aspirating again. If the pH is still greater than 5.5, the position of the tube should be confirmed by x-ray. An x-ray should be used to confirm the position of the tube in all unconscious patients.

    ■ Once the NGT is inserted, gastric pH will need to be checked. If no aspirate can be obtained, try turning the patient on the side will enable the tube to enter the gastric fluid pool. Changes to the pH strip may not occur in some clinical conditions (e.g. pernicious anaemia or previous gastrectomy) or if the patient is receiving H_2-receptor antagonists (which decrease the secretion of gastric acid) or if the tube has passed through the pylorus. X-ray is only the second line method for testing the position of the NGT when no aspirate has been obtained or the pH indicator has failed to confirm the location (NHS Improvement, 2016). However, it is the method of choice in patients who are unconscious with no gag reflex. **The following methods are never used to test the position of the tube:** auscultation, litmus paper tests, the 'whoosh test' (injecting air and listening for a bubbling sound) and absence of respiratory distress in the patient (NHS Improvement, 2016).

23. Secure the tube with tape, ensuring that friction or pressure on the tip of the nose is avoided to avoid skin erosion and ensure the patient's vision is not obstructed. The pH of aspirate or an x-ray should always be used as a final means of confirming tube (NHS Improvement, 2016). The guide wire should not be removed until confirmation of its position in the stomach has been established. The guidewire is then removed by holding the tube at the nose with one hand and pulling the wire out with the other. If it is difficult to remove, then the tube should be removed as well. **Never** reinsert the guide wire after removal, because there is a risk of perforation of the oesophageal or stomach wall. To reduce displacement of the tube. Securing the NGT to the cheek rather than the nose using hypoallergenic tape reduces the risk of nasal erosion or ulceration. The tape/dressing should be checked daily and replaced if soiled or loose. The tape/dressing should be changed at least weekly but more frequently if it loosens or becomes.

24. Check the patient is comfortable and sitting in a position that is safe for the administration of feed, fluid or medication (i.e. greater than a 30 degree angle) (Oxford Medical Education, 2015).

25. Clear away the equipment, and dispose of waste appropriately.

26. Remove gloves and apron, and decontaminate hands.
27. Document NGT insertion. To reduce the risk of adverse events or outcomes, must be documented in the patient's medical records: Documentation is important to provide baseline information for subsequent tube insertions and, if trauma was experienced during tube insertion, to determine the need for specialist referral for NGT insertion in the future.
28. Documentation should include the following:
    ▪ The date and time tube inserted.
    ▪ The size and type of NGT used.
    ▪ External cm markings at the nostril.
    ▪ The result of pH testing including the pH if aspirate was obtained, the person who checked the pH and a confirmation as to the safety of commencing feed and/or medication.
    ▪ Details of the healthcare professional who inserted the tube including name and designation.
    ▪ Statement of how consent was obtained/patient agreement indicated. Fully document best interests' decisions.
    ▪ Any problems experienced during the procedure.
    ▪ Appropriate patient notes or bedside charts (as per local guidance).
29. The practitioner should also consider documenting the following:
    ▪ Patient tolerance to the procedure.
    ▪ The number of attempts undertaken to insert the NGT.
    ▪ In which nostril the tube is situated.
    ▪ The date a tube is due to be changed.

For ongoing safety, tube checks and minimising patient harm, pH testing and position of the tube must be checked and recorded at least once daily and before each feed, before administration of medicine or in the event of new or unexplained respiratory symptoms and following any incidences that may have affected the tube placement (coughing, vomiting, retching). Testing should not be undertaken within 1 hour of feeding or medication administration because it may affect the pH result. If the patient displays respiratory distress or becomes distressed, nothing should be administered via the tube. The NHS Improvement (2016) advises that NGT or securement devices are checked daily to ensure it is not causing pressure damage or excoriation externally or internally to the nostrils.

Enteral Nutrition

Do not undertake or attempt this procedure unless you are, or have supervision from, a properly trained, experienced and competent person in carrying out the procedure and using the medical device (BAPEN, 2020).

KEY POINTS

- Before giving feed via a nasogastric tube, it is vital to confirm the position of the tube prior to each feed (National Health Service (NHS) Improvement, 2016).
- The NGT can become occluded if not flushed between use. Most enteral feeding pumps have alarms that alert for occlusion, blockages or incorrect insertion of the giving set and when feeds have finished. (British Association of Parenteral and Enteral Nutrition (BAPEN) 2020).
- Sterile water should be used for patients who are immunosuppressed.
- If a second bottle of feed is due to commence, check that the first does not empty completely, allowing air to enter the administration set. If this does happen, the set will need to be disconnected and primed again before the second feed can commence.

PROCEDURE

1. Explain the procedure to the patient, and obtain consent in accordance with the Mental Capacity Act (2005) and local policy.
2. Decontaminate hands, and put on an apron and gloves. Place a pH stick in the receiver (Fig. 11.6).
3. Take the equipment to the bedside.
4. Before giving feed via an NGT, the practitioner must confirm gastric placement of the tube. Do not introduce any water or feed into the tube until the correct position has been confirmed (BAPEN, 2020).
5. Open the appropriate port on the end of the tube and attach a 50/60-mL enteral syringe to the port (Fig. 11.7). Do not use a smaller syringe, because it will create stronger suction, with the risk that the tube will collapse or cause gastric biopsy.
6. Slowly aspirate fluid. You need only a small amount, approximately 1 mL. Remove the syringe from the port, and close the end of the port (inset). Deposit one to two drops of aspirate onto pH paper or pH strip, ensuring you cover all the test pads. Read the result within the time specified on the product packaging: a pH of between 1 and 5.5 indicates gastric placement (NHS Improvement, 2016).
7. Flush NG feeding tube with freshly drawn tap water or sterile water (depending on local policy) (NICE, 2017) before beginning feeding, to check that the tube is patent before commencing any enteral feeding (NICE, 2017).
8. Remove gloves, and decontaminate hands.
9. Check the expiry date of the feed.
10. Attach feeding pump to a drip stand to hang up the feeding bottle or pack.
11. Decontaminate hands and put on nonsterile gloves.
12. Check that you have a clean area to work in, and prepare your equipment (NICE, 2017). Open the giving-set pack. If the giving set has a roller clamp or other type of clamp, close it.

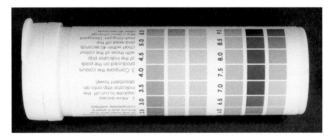

Fig. 11.6 pH test strips.

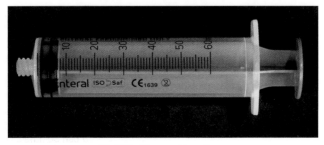

Fig. 11.7 Nasogastric syringe.

13. Remove the cap from the enteral feed pack or bottle. Most enteral feeds will have a foil seal beneath the cap, which is pierced as the giving set is screwed in. Screw the administration set firmly to the feed pack or bottle using an aseptic nontouch technique; check that it is not cross-threaded.

14. Allow the feed to run through the tubing to expel all air and then close the roller clamp.

15. Hang the feed on the drip stand. If there is a drip chamber on the administration set, position this in the appropriate place in the pump. At all times, keep hold of the connector on the other end of the administration set to avoid it touching anything.

16. Open any clamps that were previously closed, to allow the flow of feed and priming of the administration set. If there are no clamps, prime the set according to manufacturer's instructions.

17. Insert the administration set according to the manufacturer's instructions, and open the roller clamp. Attach the end of the administration set to the tube.

18. Switch the pump on. Ensure that the feed corresponds to the prescription, and check the feeding rate. The rate will normally be shown in millilitres per hour. Set the prescribed feeding rate on the pump according to the manufacturer's instructions.

19. Press the start button to allow delivery of the feed to commence.

20. Clear away the equipment and wipe up any spillages.

21. Remove apron and decontaminate hands.

22. Observe the patient for any signs of deterioration in respiratory function, such as shortness of breath or nausea and vomiting. These signs may indicate that the NGT has moved position. If these signs are present, stop the feed and reconfirm the position of the NGT before proceeding. Clearly document your concerns and your actions in the patient's records.

23. Check throughout that the feed is being administered at the correct rate. Check for signs of a blocked tube. Report any complications.

24. Attend to the patient's hygiene (mouth, lips and nostrils) as necessary.

25. Observe for diarrhoea or constipation.

26. When the feed has finished, detach the bottle from the administration set, and flush the NGT with at least 30 mL of sterile water to prevent stasis of feed and maintain patency of the tube. An NG spigot (Fig. 11.8) may be used to cover the NGT.

27. Change the administration set every 24 hours. Attach label indicating date and time commenced.

28. The practitioner must clearly document the following:
    - Gastric aspiration to confirm tube placement and pH of 3.0
    - Tube marking at the nostril is correct and as documented on insertion.

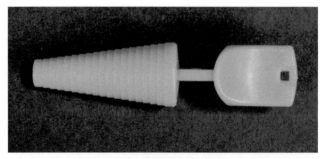

Fig. 11.8 Nasogastric spigot.

- The NGT was flushed with 50 mL water
- The feed was commenced as per prescription
- Record administration of feed and water flushed as part of the daily intake

Care of Gastrostomy Site

Gastrostomy feeding is used as an accepted method of placing a feeding tube in patients who are unable to swallow or where NG feeding is not possible likely to continue for a longer period (BAPEN, 2020). The selection of a patient for a gastrostomy tube is paramount for a good patient outcome. Multidisciplinary team assessment should be performed on all patients being referred for gastrostomy tube insertion. Best clinical practice guidelines emphasise the importance of patient consent, thorough assessment and counselling before the patient has a gastrostomy tube inserted (SIGN, 2020). Do not undertake or attempt any procedure related to gastrostomy care unless you are, or have supervision from, a trained experienced healthcare professional.

NURSING CONSIDERATIONS

- A gastrostomy is a tube placed directly into the stomach and is the most common type of enteral, long-term feeding device. It is introduced either endoscopically (PEG) or radiologically (radiologically inserted gastrostomy (RIG)) (Fig. 11.9).

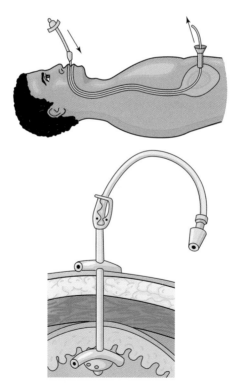

Fig. 11.9 (A) Diagram showing percutaneous endoscopic gastrostomy (PEG) tube inserted through mouth and exiting through stomach. (B) Cross-section of layers of body, with PEG tube anchored on skin, with other end of the tube holding a scope in the stomach. (Sorrentino, S. A., Remmert, L., & Wilk, M. J. (2022). *Canadian Textbook for the Support Worker*. Elsevier Inc.)

- A RIG is used for patients for whom an endoscopy is contraindicated, such as those whose airway would be compromised by an endoscope or patients who have an obstruction (e.g. tumour) that would make passing an endoscope difficult.
- There are different types of gastrostomy tubes, some of which lie flush with the skin and others that protrude. There are those that have a one-way valve to prevent reflux and a silicone dome that acts as an internal anchoring device. Most have both internal and external fixators, although low-profile balloon gastrostomy devices do not (SIGN, 2020). A RIG has stitches known as T-Fasteners, which help secure the stomach to the abdominal wall and facilitate the stoma tract to form. These stay in place for 10 to 14 days following insertion.
- The tube should be secure but not too tight. If the internal or external part of the tube is too tight against the abdominal wall, it can cause severe discomfort, cellulitis and bleeding.
- The main disadvantage of PEG is the risk of wound infection (Farrag et al., 2019). The site should be treated as a wound, and prophylactic antibiotic may be prescribed. The nurse should carefully observe the patient's vital signs in the postoperative period and for the first 7 days post insertion of the gastrostomy tube.
- RIG tubes have an increased risk of displacement due to the type of internal device (pigtail device with a string running through it) (Cherian et al., 2019).
- In the first 24 hours, the incision site should be monitored closely for redness, leakage of feed or swelling (Farrag et al. 2019). Should any of these occur, feeding should be stopped and medical advice sought.
- Until the site has granulated and healed, cleaning and dressing changes should be undertaken aseptically. Patients who have a RIG inserted should have their dressing changed aseptically (Dougherty & Lister, 2015).
- Although local practices vary, most policies recommend that the stoma site should be cleaned daily with sterile 0.9% sodium chloride or washed daily with warm water and a gauze swab, taking care not to undo the fixation site (NICE, 2017). Fold the gauze each time it meets the skin to ensure that a clean section is used each time. Clean and dry the external fixation with a gauze swab. Using a fresh gauze swab, dry the skin thoroughly. Inspect the stoma site for signs of leakage, redness or rashes.
- The sides of the external fixation device should be lifted gently to check the skin around the stoma, but the device itself should not be disturbed for the first 14 to 21 days to facilitate the formation of a stoma tract (Haywood, 2012). After this time, the stoma should be cleaned daily with lint-free gauze or a flannel cloth and mild soapy water depending on local policy. Secure the PEG tube to the flange using the external fixation device, in accordance with the manufacturer's instructions. Check that the device is comfortably positioned when the patient is in a sitting position.
- The external fixation device should be released regularly (10 to 14 days) to clean the skin around the stoma. Manufacturer guidelines should be referred to when releasing the tube from the external fixation device because the procedure differs for each tube.
- Once the PEG has been in place for more than 10 to 14 days, it is important to advance and rotate it regularly to prevent the internal fixation device from becoming embedded in the stomach wall. The frequency of this procedure will vary according to local policy and manufacturer's recommendations. However, for most types of PEG, it should be carried out at least weekly (BAPEN, 2020).
- Before replacing the external fixation device, the tube should be advanced (2 to 3 cm) and rotated completely (360 degrees). To reduce friction and make it more comfortable for the patient, carry this procedure out while the skin is wet (e.g. during cleaning) or apply a little lubricating gel to the site. If the centimetre marking on the tube is visible,

make a note of which marking shows at the level of the skin. If it is not possible to advance or rotate the tube, or you can feel resistance, you should discuss this problem with an appropriate medical professional. Note that tubes that have been sutured in place should not be advanced and rotated.

- For patients with a RIG, the external length of the tube should be recorded. If, on assessment, it appears to be moving too much or appears longer and the external fixator is in the correct position, medical assistance must be sought as the internal fixator may have broken. Check that the external fixation device is not too tight or too loose against the skin and that the patient is comfortable. Check this again when the patient is sitting up.

- If a patient is showering or bathing, the gastrostomy tube should be closed and the site dried thoroughly afterwards. Showering is preferred to bathing because the stoma site should not be immersed in water until site is healed. Creams and talcum powder should not be used around the site. Cream can impact on the grip of the fixation device and talcum powder and, when moist, can contribute to skin breakdown or infection.

- Check the stoma site for acid burn around the skin. If this occurs, ascertain that the patient is not constipated, as a full bowel may cause raised intragastric pressure and leakage around the stoma site. If this occurs, protect the skin with a relevant barrier cream as per local policy guidelines.

- Once the wound is healed, ongoing care of the site involves ensuring it remains clean and dry. If infection becomes evident, confirm same and treat in accordance to local policy guidelines.

- Feeding via a PEG can be commenced 4 hours after insertion when it is safe and well tolerated, although this may be longer if the patient has had a general anaesthetic as gastric function may be disrupted.

- Blockage may also occur when the external fixation device is incorrectly positioned, or if the patient is constipated and if there is a high concentration of gastric acid. The position of the external fixator can be checked by pulling gently on the feeding tube to ensure the internal device is against the stomach wall. The external device should be no more than 0.5 to 1 cm away from the skin to allow for slight movement. Observe the colour of the fluid, and look for signs of infection or overgranulation. Consider if the patient is constipated or has any other abdominal problems; if so, contact an appropriate healthcare professional for advice.

- Flushing should be carried out at least twice daily if the feeds are continuous, before and after feeds and the administration of drugs. Sterile water must be used for immunocompromised patients. While flushing, try to milk the feeding tube between thumb and forefinger to move any blockage. With this flushing technique, soda water may be used instead of water alone; however, do not use fruit juices or carbonated drinks (e.g. cola and lemonade), as these may curdle the occlusion further.

- In some instances, patients have a tube placed into the jejunum because they have had upper gastrointestinal surgery, or they have difficulties associated with gastric emptying. The care of a jejunostomy tube is like that of a PEG, with some notable exceptions. The lumen of the tube for a jejunostomy is much narrower than a gastrostomy, and particular care must be taken to maintain patency. Therefore 4-hourly flushing of the tube with sterile water is recommended. In addition, a jejunostomy tube must not be rotated, only advanced, as the jejunal extension may become dislodged. Following any aspect of PEG care, remove gloves and apron and decontaminate hands (Loveday et al., 2014).

Document care in the patient's records:

Feeding Via Percutaneous Endoscopic Gastrostomy/Radiologically Inserted Gastrostomy

Feeding via a PEG tube may be intermittent or continuous. Pump feeding can be administered continuously 24 hours or over a shorter 16- to 18-hour period. For patients in intensive care, continuous feeding may be of benefit in preventing a high level of gastric residue and stabilising blood glucose levels.

As eating and drinking are social activities as well as physical necessities, it is important to try and make gastrostomy feeds as pleasant and 'normal' as possible (e.g., if the feed is not continuous, by administering the feed when others are eating their meals).

KEY POINTS

- It is advisable for the patient to be sitting up (unless the feed is given very slowly).
- Individuals with a PEG/RIG should be encouraged to join in social activity associated with eating, such as eating as a family.

PROCEDURE

1. Put on an apron, decontaminate hands and put on nonsterile gloves according to local policy

2. Take the equipment and the feed to the bedside, and check the patient's name band.

3. Ideally, patients receiving enteral feeding should be semiupright or upright during the administration of the feed and should remain in this position for at least 30 minutes after the feed has finished. This is particularly important for patients who are receiving bolus feeds, to prevent reflux and possible aspiration of gastric contents. However, if this is not possible or if feed is being given overnight, then the patient's head and shoulders should be supported on at least two pillows, at a 45-degree angle to the bed. Always follow local policy, where it exists.

4. Check the gastrostomy tube is in the stomach, aspirating a small amount of stomach contents with a 20-mL oral/enteral syringe. Apply aspirate to a pH strip and then compare with the colour bars to get a reading. A pH of 5.5 indicates gastric placement.

5. Draw up 30 to 50 mL (depending on local policy) of fresh tap water, and flush the tube using the purple 50/60-mL enteral syringe. Avoid adding anything to the feed. If drugs are to be administered via the PEG tube, they must be soluble in water. Always flush the gastrostomy tube with 30 to 50 mL of freshly drawn tap water or sterile water according to local policy, before and after their administration, to prevent blockage.

6. Remove the seal or port of the feed bottle, but avoid touching to prevent contamination

7. Maintaining asepsis, open the enteral feed administration set, attach it to the bottle according to the manufacturer's instructions and close the flow control roller clamp. When flushing the PEG tube, care should be taken when attaching the syringe, to avoid damaging the connection. A 50-mL enteral syringe should be used to flush the tube, as the pressure exerted by smaller syringes is too great. If the PEG tube is not being used for feeding for a period, it should be flushed twice a day to maintain patency (Best, 2019).

8. Attach the hanger to the feed container and hang the feed container on the infusion stand.

9. Open the roller clamp on the administration set, allow the feed to run through to expel all air and then close the clamp. The plastic cap on the end of the administration set should remain in place so that the tube remains sterile.

10. Insert the administration set into the pump according to the manufacturer's instructions, remove the plastic cap at the distal end of it and attach it to the PEG tube.
11. Open the roller clamp and turn on the pump.
12. Set the flow rate as prescribed (e.g. 125 mL per hour), and start the pump.
13. Ensure that the feed corresponds to the patient's prescription before and after each bag of feed, and check the feeding rate.
14. Check that the feed is running, that it is not leaking at the connection with the PEG tube and that the tube is not kinked or blocked.
15. Check the patient is comfortable. Observe the PEG site for signs of leakage, swelling, skin irritation or breakdown, soreness or excessive movement of the tube.
16. Clear away equipment, and wipe up any spillages, especially on the pump.
17. Remove apron, and decontaminate hands.
18. Document the type of feed, time started, rate of flow and volume of water used to flush the tube.
19. Return regularly to check the feed is running as prescribed. The pump usually has alarms to indicate when the feed has finished or if the tube has become blocked or kinked. If there are no alarms, extra checking is required.
20. Observe the patient for nausea, vomiting or diarrhoea.
21. On completion of the feed, disconnect the administration set and flush the tube with sterile water according to local policy. The administration set must be changed every 24 hours and should be labelled to indicate the date that the change is due.

References

Best, C., 2019. Selection and management of commonly used enteral feeding tubes. Nurs. Times. 115 (3), 43–47.

Bowen, P., 2014. Using subcutaneous fluids in end-of-life care. Nurs. Times. 110 (40), 12–14.

British Association of Parental and Enteral Nutrition [BAPEN], 2020. A Position Paper on Nasogastric Tube Safety "Time to put patient safety first". https://www.bapen.org.uk/pdfs/ngsig/a-position-paper-on-nasogastric-tube-safety.pdf.

British Association of Parenteral and Enteral Nutrition [BAPEN], 2018. Managing Malnutrition to Improve Lives and Save Money. https://www.bapen.org.uk/resources-and-education/publications-and-reports/malnutrition.

British Association of Parenteral and Enteral Nutrition, 2016. The 'MUST' Toolkit. https://www.bapen.org.uk/screening-and-must/must/must-toolkit/the-must-itself.

British Association of Parenteral and Enteral Nutrition, 2016. A Position Paper on Nasogastric Tube Safety "Time to put patient safety first". https://www.bapen.org.uk/pdfs/ngsig/a-position-paper-on-nasogastric-tube-safety.pdf.

Care Quality Commission, 2014. Regulation 14: Meeting Nutritional and Hydration Needs. https://www.cqc.org.uk/guidance-providers/regulations-enforcement/regulation-14-meeting-nutritional-hydration-needs.

Cherian, P., Blake, C., Appleyard, M., et al., 2019. Outcomes of radiologically inserted gastrostomy versus percutaneous endoscopic gastrostomy. J. Med. Imaging Radiat. Oncol. 63, 610–616. https://doi-org.ezproxy.bcu.ac.uk/10.1111/1754-9485.12932.

Department of Health, 2017. Establishing Food Standards for NHS Hospitals. https://www.gov.uk/government/publications/establishing-food-standards-for-nhs-hospitals#history.

Dougherty, L., Lister, S., 2015. The Royal Marsden Manual of Clinical Nursing Procedures. Wiley-Blackwell, Oxford.

Farrag, K., Shastri, Y.M., Beilenhoff, U., et al., 2019. Percutaneous endoscopic gastrostomy: a practical approach for long term management. BMJ 364, k5311.

Gan, T.J., Diemunsch, P., Habib, A.S., et al. 2014. Consensus guidelines for the management of postoperative nausea and vomiting. Anesth. Analg. 118, 85–113.

Guest, M., 2020. Understanding the principles and aims of intravenous fluid therapy. Nurs. Stand. 35 (2), 75–81.

Haywood, S., 2012. PEG feeding tube placement and aftercare. Nurs. Times. 108 (42), 20.

Jeyapala, S., Gerth, A., Patel, A., et al., 2015. Improving fluid balance monitoring on the wards. BMJ Open Quality. 4, u209890.w4102. doi:10.1136/bmjquality.u209890.w4102.

Johnstone, C.C., 2018. How to undertake a nutritional assessment in adults. Nurs. Stand. 32 (2), 41–45.

Loveday, H.P., et al., 2014. National evidence-based guidelines for preventing healthcare associated infections in NHS hospitals. J. Hosp. Infect. 8651, S1–S70.

McLafferty, E., Johnstone, C., Hendry, C., et al., 2014. Fluid and electrolyte balance. Nurs. Stand. 28 (29), 42–49.

Mental Capacity Act, 2005. Mental Capacity Act 2005. https://www.legislation.gov.uk/ukpga/2005/9/pdfs/ukpga_20050009_en.pdf.

National Institute for Health and Care Excellence, 2017. Nutrition Support for Adults: Oral Nutrition Support, Enteral Tube Feeding and Parenteral Nutrition. Clinical Guideline 32. www.nice.org.uk.

National Institute for Health and Care Excellence, 2015. Care of Dying Adults in the Last Days of Life NG31. https://www.nice.org.uk/guidance/ng31.

National Institute for Health and Care Excellence, 2008. Continuous subcutaneous insulin infusion for the treatment of diabetes mellitus. Technology appraisal guidance (TA151). Overview | Continuous subcutaneous insulin infusion for the treatment of diabetes mellitus | Guidance | NICE.

National Nurses Nutrition Group, 2020. Nasogastric Tube Safety Position Paper. https://nnng.org.uk/2020/09/ng-tube-safety-time-to-put-patient-safety-first/.

NHS Improvement, 2016. Nasogastric Tube Misplacement: Continuing Risk of Death and Severe Harm. Alert reference number: NHS/PSA/RE/2016/006. https://www.england.nhs.uk/wp-content/uploads/2019/12/Patient_Safety_Alert_Stage_2_-_NG_tube_resource_set.pdf.

Nursing and Midwifery Council, 2018. Code. https://www.nmc.org.uk/globalassets/sitedocuments/nmc-publications/nmc-code.pdf

Oxford Medical Education, 2015. Nasogastric Tube Placement. https://oxfordmedicaleducation.com/clinical-skills/procedures/nasogastric-ng-tube/

Patients Association, 2020. NHS Hospital Food Survey. www.patients-association.org.uk

Radcliffe, C., 2017. Guideline for the Use of Subcutaneous Hydration in Palliative Care. https://www.palliativedrugs.com/download/180214_Subcutaneous_hydration_in_palliative_care_v2.4_Final.pdf.

Royal College of Nursing, 2016. Standards for Infusion Therapy, fourth ed. Publication code: 005 704. www.rcn.org.uk

Royal College of Nursing, 2019. Hydration Essentials. https://www.rcn.org.uk/clinical-topics/nutrition-and-hydration/hydration-essentials.

Scottish Intercollegiate College Guidelines. (2020). Management of Patients With Stroke: Identification and Management of Dysphagia. A National Clinical Guideline. www.sign.ac.uk

Webb A. (2017). Management of nausea and vomiting in patients with advanced cancer at the end of life. Nursing Standard, 32 (10), 53–63. doi:10.7748/ns.2017.e10993.

CHAPTER 12

Managing Safe Intravenous Therapy and Blood Transfusions

Venepuncture

Venepuncture involves inserting a needle into the vein and refers to the process of taking blood samples from a patient. In practice, these samples are taken to investigate and guide treatment. Blood samples can also be taken to monitor the effectiveness of treatments, i.e., when checking for therapeutic levels of medication.

EQUIPMENT

Wipeable tray, cleaned with the appropriate hard surface agent

Vacuum tube sampling system (includes tube holder and needle adaptor, usually 21-gauge or a winged infusion set)

Blood sample tube(s) as appropriate

Skin-cleansing agent (e.g., a swab impregnated with 2% chlorhexidine in 70% alcohol), in accordance with local policy

Tourniquet (single use, disposable)

Low-linting gauze swabs

Hypoallergenic tape or small self-adhesive dressing

Sharps container

PROCEDURE

1. Establish why you are taking the blood sample and if it is still required.
2. Fully discuss the procedure with the patient to gain informed consent (Nursing and Midwifery Council [NMC], 2018). This will also allow you to establish if the patient has a needle phobia, if there have been problems obtaining samples in the past and if they already have a device in place that a sample could be taken from.

   Discussing previous experiences can help you to ascertain which might be the best site for insertion. If there is a device through which samples can be taken this will reduce patient discomfort that occurs with venepuncture. A competent practitioner must take this sample and local policy must be adhered to.
3. The patient should be sitting or lying comfortably, with the appropriate arm supported. The patient's arm should be free of any tight or restrictive clothing.
4. Check the patient's identity with the blood test request form and ask the patient to confirm. Assist patient to adjust clothing, as necessary.
5. Assemble all equipment checking that it is intact and in date. Do not label the sample tubes until filled with the blood specimen in case of unsuccessful collection.

6. Adequate hand hygiene must have been performed prior to approaching the patient. Wear appropriate personal protective equipment. Non-sterile gloves (close-fitting to allow dexterity) and a single-use disposable apron are the minimal requirements. Additional protective clothing may be necessary if indicated by the patient's condition (see Chapter 2).

7. Adopt a comfortable position. Ideally sit on a chair to avoid stooping.

8. Apply the tourniquet using the quick-release method (Figs. 12.1 to 12.4) and inspect the arm to select a suitable vein, usually the median cubital, cephalic and basilic veins at the antecubital fossa (ACF). Palpate the vein to locate its position and ensure that it is not an artery (which will pulsate) or a tendon. Then release the tourniquet.

   The quick-release method when applying the tourniquet involves placing the band at the back of the arm and ensuring that the ends are equally placed around the arm. Then make a loop with the left end and cross over the right bringing the loop through. This will ensure that the ends are placed away from the site of collection. The tourniquet should only be used for 1 minute to avoid damage to the vessels and surrounding tissue (Brooks, 2017).

9. Clean the skin with the skin-cleansing agent using the cross-hatch technique (Brooks, 2017) ensuring that you clean for 30 seconds and leave it to dry for a minimum period of 30 seconds to ensure that it is completely dry and reduce the risk of any alcohol entering the skin and vein causing subsequent pain for the patient and potentially contaminating the sample. Do not touch the area once the skin is cleaned as if touched the area will be contaminated and will need to be cleaned again (Loveday et al., 2014).

10. Reapply the tourniquet.

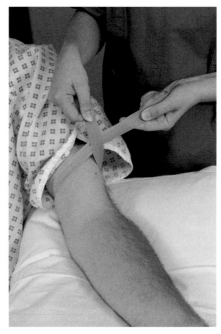

Fig. 12.1 Applying 'quick-release' tourniquet. Place the band at the back of the arm and ensure that the ends are equally placed around the arm.

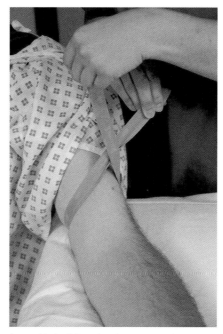

Fig. 12.2   Then make a loop with the left end and cross over the right bringing the loop through.

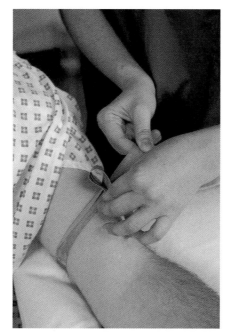

Fig. 12.3   Maintaining pressure, secure the tourniquet, so that the ends are facing towards the patient's head and not in the sterile field. The tourniquet should not be tied.

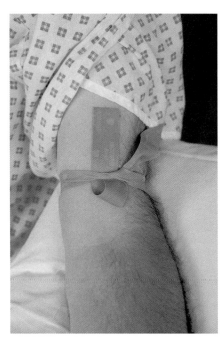

Fig. 12.4 Quick-release tourniquet in position. To release pull one of the ends.

11. Decontaminate hands and once dry, apply non-sterile gloves. With the patient's arm straight and well supported, ideally on a pillow, use your non-dominant hand to apply traction to ensure that the vein is straight and established. This traction, 'anchoring', should be applied just below the insertion site (Fig. 12.5) (Skarparis and Ford, 2018).

12. Take the vacutainer and needle in your dominant hand. Remove the needle sheath and inspect the device to ensure that it is working correctly. With the bevel of the needle upward and directly over the vein, insert the needle at an angle between 15 and 30 degrees through the skin and into the vein. When the vein is punctured, reduce the angle of the needle to avoid damaging the vein wall and insert 2 mm further (Fig. 12.6).
An appropriate angle is required to ensure that you enter the vein but do not pierce the outer edge of the vessel. Once the vein is punctured flash back will be seen in the winged infusion set. Inserting the needle 2 mms further post puncture will ensure that the needle is fully in the vein and that a sample can be easily achieved.

13. **Vacuum system**—hold the needle and plastic holder securely in place (no blood is visible until the sample tube is attached) and attach the sample tube by pushing it firmly onto the needle inside the vacutainer (Fig. 12.7). The tube will then automatically fill with blood to the required amount. If additional samples are required, remove the tube when full (no blood will leak out) and attach another ensuring that you follow the order of the draw (Skarparis and Ford, 2018).

14. Gently invert each blood bottle a few times, in accordance with manufacturer's guidance, to mix the blood sample with any additives. This should be done after each blood sample is taken.

15. Once the blood samples have been taken, remove the tourniquet, then hold the low-linting sterile gauze swab over the puncture site and remove the needle. Do not press

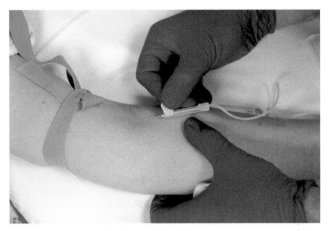

Fig. 12.5   Anchoring the skin.

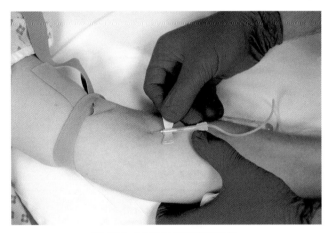

Fig. 12.6   Inserting butterfly needle.

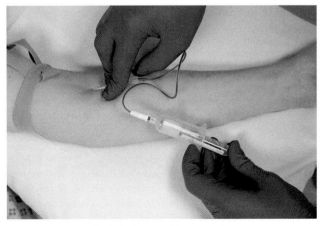

Fig. 12.7   Taking a blood sample.

until the needle is out of the vein as this is very painful (Shaw, 2018). Continue to apply pressure (or ask the patient to do this) for 2 to 3 minutes until the bleeding stops, to prevent bruising. Ask the patient not to bend their arm as this may cause a haematoma (Brooks, 2017).

16. **Vacuum system**—Activate the sharp safety mechanism and immediately dispose of the entire system into the sharps container.
17. Inspect the puncture site; once the bleeding has stopped, apply sterile low-linting gauze with hypoallergenic tape or a small self-adhesive dressing, if required.
18. Assist the patient to replace clothing as necessary; readjust the height of the bed.
19. Remove gloves and discard all other clinical waste. Decontaminate hands.
20. Label specimens with either an electronic printed adhesive label or hand write the details onto specimen bottle, as required in accordance with local policy. Ensure that the patient's surname, first names, hospital number, date of birth, ward/clinic and the date of the sample is provided.
21. Place samples in the appropriate collection point for transportation to the laboratory. If taking samples in someone's home return to the appropriate clinical setting for transfer.
22. Document the blood samples taken, the site of selection as well as the site of any failed attempts.

Special Considerations

When performing venepuncture on people living with diabetes, renal disease or the older adult the veins can become fragile and sclerosed. A full patient assessment must be undertaken prior to performing venepuncture on this client group (Gabriel, 2013) to avoid complications, such as haematoma. Avoid performing venepuncture when:

- There is an infusion above the site of insertion
- There is rash, bruising or oedema in the area
- The vein is tortuous, and feels hard under palpation

Cannulation

Cannulation is the process of inserting a flexible tube into a vein, and is performed in a clinical setting to give intravenous medication, fluids or for diagnostic processes (Ford, 2019). There is also some evidence to suggest that blood samples can be taken from a venous access device to reduce unnecessary pain to the patient, but this will be dependent on the recommendations within local policy (RCN, 2016).

When performing cannulation, it is necessary to know why the peripheral venous access device is being inserted. This will ensure that an appropriately sized cannula is inserted and will also reduce the likelihood of a device being inserted unnecessarily. The size of cannula required will be determined by the type of fluid to be infused and the size and condition of the patient's veins (Brooks, 2017). The smallest gauge capable of achieving the required flow rate should be used (RCN, 2016).

It is imperative that a patient-focused approach is taken and that the patient is aware of any additions that may improve the process. Whilst most adult patients will not require it, local anaesthetic may be desirable with patients who are extremely anxious or needle phobic. This local anaesthetic cream must be applied at least 1 hour in advance to be effective and the possibility of allergy must be considered (Bond et al., 2015).

EQUIPMENT

- Wipeable tray, cleaned with the appropriate hard surface agent
- Skin-cleansing agent (e.g. a swab impregnated with 2% chlorhexidine in 70% alcohol), (Loveday et al., 2014) in accordance with local policy
- Tourniquet (latex-free, single use, disposable)
- Cannula of appropriate size—check the expiration date and that the packaging is intact
- Sterile cannula dressing pack if available
- 10 mL of 0.9% sodium chloride to flush the device after insertion (this may come prefilled)
- A connection extension set as required
- Disposable pad or towel to place under the arm to protect the patient's clothes or bed linen
- Low-linting gauze swabs (for unsuccessful attempts)
- Hypoallergenic tape
- Sharps container

PROCEDURE

1. Establish why you are cannulating and if a peripheral venous access device (PVAD) is still required.
2. Fully discuss the procedure and rationale with the patient to gain informed consent (NMC, 2018). This will also allow you to establish if the patient has a needle phobia, if there have been problems with cannulation in the past and if they already have a PVAD in place that could be used.
3. Ask the patient to provide their name, date of birth and allergy status and check the patient's identity on the name band before proceeding. Assist the patient to adjust clothing, as necessary.
4. Assemble all equipment ensuring that it is both intact and in date. Out-of-date or tampered-with equipment will no longer be sterile (Fig. 12.8).
5. Appropriate Personal Protective Equipment (PPE) should be applied. This is usually non-sterile gloves (close-fitting to allow dexterity) and a single-use disposable apron. Additional protective clothing may be necessary if indicated by the patient's condition (see Chapter 2). Adopt a suitable position to avoid stooping; ideally use a chair.

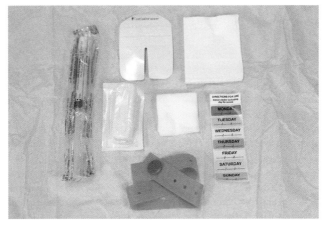

Fig. 12.8 Equipment assembled.

6. If possible, choose the patient's non-dominant arm for cannulation for comfort. Place the sterile towel under the arm to protect the patient's clothes and surroundings. If the cannula is for an intravenous infusion or the clothing is tight or restrictive, remove the arm from the sleeve.

7. Local anaesthetic cream, if used, must be applied at least 60 minutes prior to the procedure (Bond et al., 2015).

8. Apply the tourniquet 8 to 10 cm/3 to 4 inches, above the proposed site of cannulation, using the quick-release knot, and check for arterial blood flow (as outlined on p. 161–162). If the tourniquet is so tight that it prevents arterial blood flow, the veins will not fill.

9. Ask the patient to clench and unclench their fist several times to encourage venous filling. It may also help to lower the arm below the heart level.

10. Select a vein by palpation, not just visually, to ensure that it is suitable (i.e. bouncy not hard) and is not an artery (which will pulsate) or a tendon. Release the tourniquet.
    The tourniquet should only be used for 1 minute to avoid damage to the vessels and surrounding tissue (Brooks, 2017).

11. Clean the skin with the skin-cleansing agent using the cross-hatch technique (Brooks, 2017) ensuring that you clean for 30 seconds and leave it to dry for a minimum period of 30 seconds. Do not touch the area once the skin is cleaned.
    Leaving the skin to dry ensures that it is completely dry and reduces the risk of any alcohol entering the skin and vein causing subsequent pain for the patient and potentially contaminating the sample. If the skin is touched once the skin has been cleaned it has been contaminated and will need to be cleaned again.

12. Reapply the tourniquet.

13. Decontaminate hands and once dry apply non-sterile gloves. With the patient's arm straight and well supported, ideally on a pillow, use your non-dominant hand to apply traction to ensure that the vein is straight and established. This traction, 'anchoring', should be applied just below the insertion site.
    Avoid palpating the vein prior to inserting the device as this will contaminate the area.

14. Take the PVAD in your dominant hand and check that the needle can be removed easily but do not remove it fully. Hold the device with the bevel facing upwards, so that is can pierce the skin easily. This will cause less pain for the patient.

15. Holding the PVAD at an angle of 20 to 30 degrees either directly over the vein or just to one side of it (Ford, 2019), insert the device through the skin and into the vein (Fig. 12.9).
    The correct angle must be used to ensure that the device is inserted into the vein. If a higher angle is used the needle could enter the vein and then pass through the vein (Fig. 12.10).

16. Stop advancing the device as soon as blood appears at the end of the PVAD, which indicates that it has entered the vein. Lower the angle and using the one-hand technique insert the cannula and remove the needle simultaneously.
    While maintaining traction with one hand, advance the cannula and remove the needle with your other hand (Fig. 12.11).

17. Once in place hold the PVAD to prevent dislodgement and release the tourniquet. Place a piece of sterile low-linting gauze under the end of the device if using an open system to contain any drops of blood during removal of the needle.

18. With your other hand, apply pressure to the vein immediately above the end of the cannula to minimise blood flow.

19. Remove the needle and if applicable apply the connection extension set (Fig. 12.12). This must be flushed with 0.9% sodium chloride before attachment.

20. Discard the needle into the sharps container.

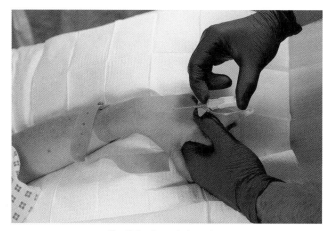

Fig. 12.9 Cannula insertion.

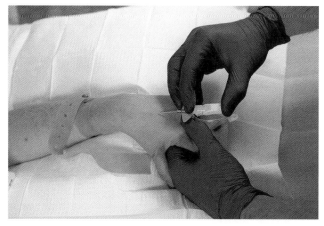

Fig. 12.10 Flash back in the cannula.

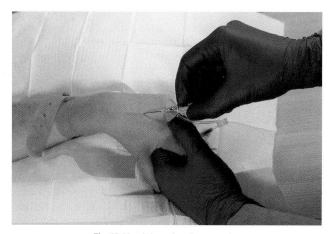

Fig. 12.11 Advancing the cannula.

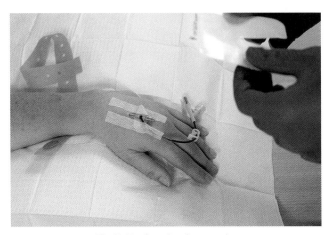

Fig. 12.12 Securing the cannula.

21. Clean any blood and apply the semi-permeable transparent dressing. Ensure that the device is secure and that the site of insertion is clear underneath the transparent dressing (Fig. 12.13).
22. Flush the cannula with 0.9% sodium chloride to ensure patency (Fig. 12.14).
23. Discard all clinical waste separately and appropriately, including gloves and apron.
24. Decontaminate hands.
25. Return any unused equipment and sharps container to the appropriate place.
26. Document the date and time of cannulation, the location, type and gauge used, site of insertion and any failed attempts in the nursing records. Apply a sticker to indicate date of cannulation on the dressing.
27. Check the patient is comfortable and explain any restrictions to mobility and the need to protect the PVAD site. Ask the patient to report any swelling, redness or pain.

Special Considerations

There are certain contraindications for insertion of a peripheral venous device. A device should not be inserted if:
- There is a rash, bruising or oedema in the area
- The patient has weakness or paralysis in the arm, often because of a cerebrovascular accident
- The patient has had lymph nodes previously removed from that arm
- The patient has an arteriovenous fistula in that arm

  In certain conditions such as diabetes, renal disease and aging the veins can become fragile and sclerosed. A full patient assessment must be undertaken prior to performing cannulation on this client group (Gabriel, 2013) to ensure that an appropriately sized cannula is used and complications are minimised.

Visual Infusion Phlebitis Score

When a peripheral intravenous cannula (also known as a peripheral vascular access device) is inserted there are many local complications that can occur. These complications include:

1. **Infiltration**: occurs when non-irritant fluids or medication accidentally leak out of the vascular system into the surrounding tissues

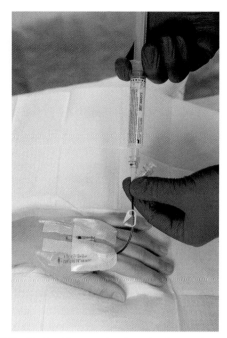

Fig. 12.13 Flushing the cannula using a 'push pause' technique.

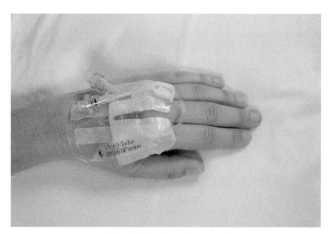

Fig. 12.14 Cannula secured.

  2. Extravasation: occurs when irritant fluids or medications infiltrate the surrounding tissues, causing tissue damage and necrosis
  3. Phlebitis: occurs when the wall of the vein becomes inflamed
  4. Infection: of the vein or surrounding tissue; redness or pain at the site may indicate infection
As a result of these potential complications peripheral venous access devices must be assessed at least once per shift (RCN, 2016) and must be removed if no longer required. It is also important for the site to be assessed before administration of any intravenous medications, fluids or blood products and before changing the intravenous administration set, or regulating the

intravenous flow rate (RCN, 2016). The nurse's role in assessing the venous access device (VAD) site is to observe for any signs of infiltration, extravasation, inflammation and infection whilst confirming the VAD and dressing is dry and secure. For safe and accurate practice, it is widely recognised that the VIP score introduced by Jackson (1998) helps nurses to assess and monitor the VAD site.

PROCEDURE: USING THE VISUAL INFUSION PHLEBITIS SCORE

1. Inspect the cannulation site for signs of swelling, redness, erythema (redness and flushing of the skin), induration (abnormal hardening of the tissues) and a palpable venous cord (a hard inflamed vein is felt along the vein path with your fingertips). Ask the patient how the site feels, e.g., does the insertion site feel sore? Does it hurt to move their arm?
2. Look at the VIP score (see above) and compare your findings with the descriptors to identify the condition of the site, and the score. For example: slight redness around the intravenous site indicates a score of 1 and indicates that the first signs of phlebitis may be present. Pain at the intravenous site and swelling alongside redness (a score of 2) indicates signs of early phlebitis.
3. To complete an accurate assessment, look at the next highest score to the one you have identified and compare your findings to the descriptors. If your findings do not fit those descriptors you have the correct result. Refer to the VIP score to determine the required action for the score; for example, if the score is 1, the device will need observing. If the VIP score is 2, the VAD will need to be removed and a new site established for insertion.
4. Document the VIP score, and any actions taken, according to local policy. Escalate as appropriate. For care of and removal of the peripheral venous access device see below.

Special Considerations

- The VIP scoring is important due to the risk of infection, even if the device is not being used.
- When infiltration is present the arm is often oedematous and cold to touch. This indicates the device has moved out of the vein and into the surrounding tissue. The device should be removed immediately, and local policy guidance followed to care for the limb.
- If the patient complains of pain at the site but there are no signs of phlebitis, consider what the device is being used for. Extravasation is not initially seen at the site of insertion due to damage occurring in the tissue local to the vein. If in doubt remove the VAD.
- Some patients may not be able to verbalise pain. In these instances, look for non-verbal signs of pain.

Removal of a Peripheral Venous Access Device

A PVAD should be removed once intravenous treatment is complete, if there are signs of infection, extravasation, infiltration, or inflammation and if it was inserted but not used. Removal of the PVAD involves removing the dressing, removing the device and applying an appropriate covering. The patient must be fully informed of the process and the reason why the device is being used.

EQUIPMENT

- Sterile low-linting gauze squares
- Small self-adhesive dressing, or hypoallergenic tape and sterile low-linting gauze

- Clinical waste bag
- Sharps container

PROCEDURE

1. Decontaminate hands.
2. A single-use disposable apron and non-sterile gloves should be worn. These should be close-fitting to enable manipulation of adhesive dressings and tape. Additional protective clothing may be necessary if indicated by the patient's condition (see Chapter 2).
3. Explain the procedure, to gain informed consent and co-operation.
4. Carefully remove the old dressing, leaving the PVAD in place.
5. If using large sterile gauze fold a piece of gauze three or four times to create an absorbent pad. If using smaller sizes 3 to 4 pieces should be used to create the absorbency.
6. Place the gauze over the PVAD insertion site. Gently withdraw the device and immediately apply firm pressure over the insertion site.
7. Continue to apply pressure until the bleeding has stopped (about 3 minutes) to prevent haematoma formation. Holding the arm vertically may assist with this.
8. Apply a small dressing or use hypoallergenic tape and a piece of low-linting sterile gauze over the site.
9. Discard all waste, including the plastic PVAD, into the clinical waste bag.
10. Remove gloves and apron, discard in clinical waste and decontaminate hands.
11. Check the patient is comfort and advise them to report any bleeding or discomfort at the site.
12. Document removal of cannula and report any abnormalities.

Special Considerations

Clinical judgement has to be used when considering removal of a VAD. The device should be removed if there is any sign of infection, infiltration, extravasation and inflammation at the site (RCN, 2016) and if the device is no longer in use. It is usually recommended that the PVAD is removed and re-sited every 7 days (Loveday et al., 2014) but this varies with some local policies advising of 72 hrs and some 96 hrs. The key is to follow local Trust policy and if unsure to seek further guidance.

If the device is removed due to possible phlebitis, infiltration or extravasation local policy must be followed. An adverse incident form should also be completed to prevent repetition of such instances.

Preparing An Infusion

People admitted to the secondary care setting may require an intravenous infusion (National Institute for Health and Care Excellence [NICE], 2017). This can be routine maintenance, because of fluid redistribution or for fluid resuscitation (NICE, 2017). For each person receiving an intravenous infusion there must be a clear indication (RCN, 2016) and the infusion should be reviewed every 24 hrs (NICE, 2017).

EQUIPMENT

- Appropriate intravenous infusion fluid according to the prescription
- Appropriate intravenous administration set
- Intravenous infusion stand
- Sterile low-linting gauze squares

PROCEDURE

1. Check that you are aware of why the intravenous infusion is being administered and that you explain this fully to the patient prior to commencing the safety checks and commencing the infusion. To gain informed consent and maintain patient safety.
2. Explain the reasons for intravenous infusion to gain informed consent and highlight limitations to mobility that may result.
3. Decontaminate hands and put on a single-use, disposable apron.
4. Non-sterile gloves should be worn when connecting the infusion to the cannula to ensure that the key parts (see Chapter 2) are not touched. Additional protective clothing may be necessary if indicated by the patient's condition (see Chapter 2).
5. Check the '9 rights' as described on page 195–196. Follow local Trust policy regarding prescription checks. In most cases the prescription requires checking of a registered nurse but in some instances two registered nurses may be required to check. Blood transfusions require special checking procedure (see p. 178).
6. Check the outer wrapper is intact, not damaged in any way, and in date.
   An out-of-date infusion is no longer sterile and thus should not be used. If the outer wrapper is no longer intact it is also not sterile and could have been tampered with. This will need to be reported.
7. Open the outer wrapper and remove the bag.
8. Check the fluid bag for leakage, particles, cloudiness, expiration date and batch number. Document the relevant details either electronic or paper hard copy.

Administration Set

1. Check that the contents are sterile, i.e., the outer wrapper is not damaged or wet.
2. Check the expiry date/date of sterilisation. There will always be two dates. If the set is out of date it will no longer be sterile.
3. Open the packaging and remove the administration set. Both ends should be covered with protective caps to maintain sterility.
4. Close the flow control clamp on the administration set. This can be done by moving it gently. It is imperative to ensure that it is functioning effectively before attaching to the infusion.

Assembly

1. Remove the protective cap from the insertion port on the bag of fluid and hold carefully to maintain sterility.
2. Remove the protective cover from the spike of the administration set (just above the drip chamber).
3. Taking care to maintain sterility, insert the spike into the bag, pushing and twisting until fully inserted (Fig. 12.15).
4. Hang the bag on the infusion stand. Squeeze and release the drip chamber until it is half-full of fluid.
5. To expel the air from the administration set, partially open the roller clamp to allow fluid to run through the set. Do not do this too quickly or it will draw in air from the drip chamber. When all the air has been expelled, close the roller clamp. The infusion is now ready for use.

Connecting the Infusion

1. Inspect the PVAD site using a VIP (see p. 168–170). Do not continue with administration if complications are noted.

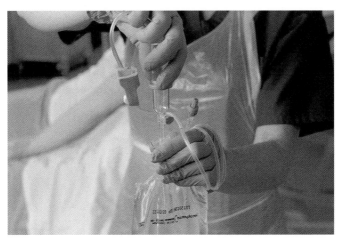

Fig. 12.15 Spiking an infusion bag.

2. If the PVAD is in good condition, scoring 0 on VIP, put on non-sterile gloves and place a folded gauze square under the end of the cannula to catch any spillage.
3. Clean the end of the PVAD, or connection, set using the appropriate cleansing agent (Loveday et al., 2014). The site should be cleansed for 30 seconds and allowed to dry for 30 seconds using the aseptic non-touch technique (Loveday et al., 2014).
4. Taking care to maintain sterility, remove the protective cap from the administration set and connect the set by 'locking' into place. All administration sets should be fitted with a Luer-Lok device that can be twisted to lock the tubing in place. This is to prevent an accidental disconnection and prevent the entry of micro-organisms. The administration set can then be changed every 72 hrs (Loveday et al., 2014).
5. Adjust the roller clamp to set the infusion to the prescribed rate. Infusions requiring great accuracy will be controlled through an intravenous pump or syringe driver. A burette may be used to administer small amounts of fluid or drugs.
6. Check the patient is comfortable and understands why they are having the infusion and how it may limit mobility. Instruct the patient to report any swelling, redness or pain.
7. Discard all packaging and remove gloves and apron, discard in clinical waste and decontaminate hands.
8. Record the date and time that the infusion started, the batch number of the intravenous fluid and any other details required according to local policy.
9. Document the infusion and monitor fluid balance according to local policy.

Special Considerations

Always consider whether the intravenous infusion is required. Ask if the medication could be given orally or whether there are other methods of providing fluids which are less invasive.

It is imperative to consider wellbeing of the patient who may not be able to give informed consent. In this instance the multi-disciplinary team will need to take a best interest approach (NMC, 2018). The situation needs to be reviewed once if the patients condition changes (MCA, 2005).

Changing An Infusion Bag

Patients requiring intravenous therapy may need a regimen of different types of fluid. This means that the fluid bag must be changed in line with the prescription, as the infusion set only needs to be changed every 72 hrs (RCN, 2016). The procedure below advises on how to change the infusion bag only. Information on how to set up an infusion set is provided on p. 171–174, and for blood transfusions see p. 180

EQUIPMENT

- Intravenous infusion fluid as prescribed

PROCEDURE

1. Explain the procedure to the patient to ensure that informed consent is obtained.
2. Check that the fluid has been checked following safe medication administration principles (Elliot and Liu, 2010) and that you have considered if the fluid is still required. Make the patient aware of the need to change the bag and explain the procedure fully to gain informed consent (NMC, 2018).
3. Decontaminate hands.
4. Ensure that the infusion fluid check has followed the 9 Rights of medication administration (Elliot and Liu, 2010) and is in line with local policy.
5. Inspect the cannula site using a visual infusion phlebitis score (see p. 168–170). If phlebitis is noted, do not continue with the administration.
6. Remove the infusion fluid from its outer wrapper and check the fluid bag for leakage, particles, cloudiness, expiration date, volume and batch number.
7. Close the roller clamp on the administration set.
8. Remove the empty infusion bag from the stand and pull out the spike of the administration set, taking care not to contaminate it. Whilst this is a non-touch technique some clinical areas will require the use of non-sterile gloves for this procedure. Always follow local Trust policy.
9. Remove the protective cover from the inlet port of the new infusion bag and insert the spike of the giving set, twisting until fully inserted. Replace the bag on the infusion stand.
10. Adjust the roller clamp to the prescribed flow rate.
    Where possible use a pump for greater accuracy and safety.
11. Discard the used infusion bag and packaging into the clinical waste.
12. Document the infusion (amount, type of fluid, time commenced, batch number and signature of the nurses) according to local policy.
13. Record the infusion completion and commencement on the fluid balance chart according to local policy.
14. Check at least hourly that the infusion is running as prescribed and the patient is not complaining of pain or discomfort at the site.
15. Observe the patient for signs of fluid overload (rising pulse and respiratory rate).

Special Considerations

The patient must be monitored and medically reviewed every 24 hrs when receiving intravenous therapy and it is usual for urea and electrolytes to be monitored through blood sampling.

It is important to check the rate and volume of fluid being administered are appropriate for the patient's current health status. It is likely that doses and volumes will need to be adjusted for those people living with heart failure.

Giving an Intravenous Fluid Challenge

An intravenous fluid challenge is used during fluid resuscitation when fluid replacement is urgently needed to correct severe hypovolaemia (Cathala and Moorley, 2018). Common causes of hypovolaemia include sepsis, haemorrhage and dehydration due to diarrhoea and/or vomiting. Three types of fluids are used: crystalloids, colloids and blood products (Table 12.1). However, there is a lack of consensus on which fluid to use for treating fluid loss (Cathala and Moorley, 2018).

All IV fluids must be correctly prescribed and checked according to organisational policies. However, if the patient's condition is life-threatening, NICE (2016) recommends that nurses should be able to start IV fluids following organisational policy until these are prescribed by a practitioner.

KEY POINTS

- Patients should be assessed using an ABCDE approach (see chapter 3).
- Fluid loss can occur from sensible and insensible losses.
- Fluid resuscitation requires regular re-assessment and treatment of the underlying cause.
- This is likely to be an emergency situation, therefore, expert help should be sought early, e.g., Critical Care Outreach Team, Medical Emergency Team.

EQUIPMENT

IV drip stand
IV fluids (checked)
Fluid flush to check patency of IV access
Appropriate giving set
Infusion pump
IV access
PPE

TABLE 12.1 ■ **Types of Intravenous Fluids**

Type of Fluid	Examples
Crystalloids	Isotonic crystalloids, e.g., sodium chloride 0.9% (normal saline) Balanced isotonic crystalloids, e.g., Ringer's lactate and Hartmann's solution Hypotonic crystalloids, e.g., dextrose saline, 5% dextrose Hypertonic crystalloids, e.g., 3% NaCl, 20% dextrose and 50% dextrose
Colloids	Gelatins Dextrans Hydroxyethyl starches (HES)
Blood Products	Red blood cells Fresh frozen plasma (FFP) Cryoprecipitate Platelets Albumin

Cathala and Moorley (2018).

TABLE 12.2 ■ **Indications for Fluid Resuscitation**

- Systolic blood pressure <100 mm Hg
- Heart rate >90 bpm
- Capillary refill time >2 s or peripheries cold to touch
- Respiratory rate >20 breaths/min
- National Early Warning Score ≥5 or more
- Passive leg raising suggesting fluid responsiveness

NICE (2016).

PROCEDURE

Assess patient using A to E approach to identify the need for fluid resuscitation (Table 12.2). This includes identifying and responding to the causes of fluid deficit.

Check IV Access Patency

Run through IV fluids using an appropriate giving set and attach to an infusion pump if available.

Give prescribed fluid bolus (250 to 500 mL fluid bolus) of crystalloid in less than 15 minutes.

Reassess patient using A-E approach to determine if the patient continues to have signs of shock or signs of fluid overload.

Assess fluid balance; if < 2000 mL of fluid given, give another 250 to 500 mL fluid bolus.

Systemic observations should be undertaken frequently according to organisational policy.

Expert help must be sought as this is an emergency situation.

Document your actions including signing for fluids.

Regulation of Flow Rate

Intravenous devices (pumps and syringe drivers) to regulate infusions are increasingly being used in clinical practice, as they improve patient safety. Devices must be serviced regularly and the healthcare practitioner using them must have had the appropriate training. Whilst infusion pumps are common there are situations when a standard pump may have limitations or may be unavailable and as such it is imperative that the nurse knows how to administer infusions without a pump (Fig. 12.16). It is key that the infusion is calculated correctly to run at a constant rate over the prescribed time. This will also involve giving the patient key information on management of the infusion and checking the infusion regularly.

PROCEDURE: CALCULATING THE FLOW RATE IN 'DROPS PER MINUTE'

If it is a simple gravity infusion, or an infusion device that regulates the flow rate in 'drops per minute' is being used, calculation of the rate in drops per minute is required. The calculation used is as follows:

$$\frac{\text{volume of infusion in ml} \times \text{number of drops per ml}}{\text{time in minutes}} = \text{flow rate in drops per minute}$$

The number of drops per mL will be determined by the administration set being used and is indicated on the packaging:

1. Standard administration set = 20 drops per mL.
2. Blood administration set = 15 drops per mL.
3. Paediatric set (burette) = 60 drops per mL.

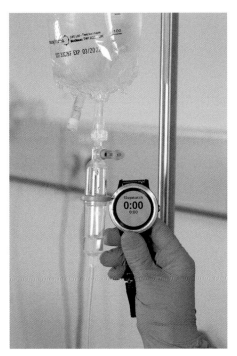

Fig. 12.16   Regulating flow rate.

Example: A patient has been prescribed 500 mL of 0.9% sodium chloride (normal saline) to be given over 6 hours using a standard administration set. The calculation is as follows:

$$\frac{500\,(\text{vol. of infusion}) \times 20\,(\text{No. of drops per ml})}{360\,(6\,\text{hours} \times 60\,\text{minutes})} = \frac{500 \times 20}{360} = \frac{10\,000}{360}$$

$$= 27.77\,\textbf{drops per minute}\,(\text{round up to 28 drops})$$

Example: A patient has been prescribed 420 mL of whole blood to be given over 4 hours using a blood administration set. The calculation is as follows:

$$\frac{420 \times 15}{220} = \frac{6300}{240} = \textbf{26.25 drops per minute}\,(\text{round up to 27 drops})$$

Calculating the flow rate in 'millilitres per hour'

$$\frac{\text{volume of infusion in ml}}{\text{No. of hours}} = \text{flow rate in millilitres per hour}$$

Example: A patient has been prescribed 1 L of 5% dextrose to be given over 8 hours. The calculation is as follows: ml per hour

$$\frac{1000}{8} = \textbf{125 ml per hour}$$

> **Special Considerations**
>
> A calculator for accuracy, but it is important that you check your answer for accuracy with another practitioner. All checks are dependent on the medication being administered and local policy.
>
> Remember that using the gravity and roller clamp method means that there are no alerts to occlusions in the line and proactive monitoring is essential.

Care and Management of the Blood Transfusion

Blood transfusions are frequently administered in clinical practice, there are multiple stages in the transfusion process, and the patient could be exposed to the risk of errors being made at each stage (Robinson et al., 2018). If incorrect blood is transfused the results can be fatal and the greatest risk is that patients either receive an infusion that is not meant for them or that is not suitable for them (SHOT, 2018). Traceability of each blood component transfused is therefore essential. There must be a clear audit trail of the collection, delivery, receipt (and return) of all blood components (Robinson, et al., 2018). Positive evidence of transfusion of each blood component must be kept for a minimum of 30 years.

The most important elements of the blood transfusion process are positive patient identification, meticulous documentation and communication (Robinson et al., 2018) The patient must wear an identification band that includes their first name, last name, date of birth and a unique identification number, e.g., their NHS number. All documentation relating to the patient must be clear and identical in every detail to the information on the patient's identification band.

Whenever possible prior to transfusion, the patient should be asked to state their full name and date of birth during the checking procedures. This information must match *exactly* the information on their identification band. It is imperative that repetitive patient checks are carried out at each stage of the blood transfusion process, namely: decision to transfuse, prescription; requests for transfusion; blood samples for cross matching; collection of blood and administration as even with these checks blood transfusion errors still occur (SHOT, 2018).

Documentation required for all stages of the blood transfusion process should be clearly outlined in local policies. Adverse reactions most commonly occur within the first 30 minutes of the transfusion and so it is vital that nurses continually observe the patient during this time. For this reason, it is advised that blood transfusions are not undertaken at night, unless clinically essential (NICE, 2015).

STORAGE AND COLLECTION OF BLOOD

Blood must be stored in a dedicated refrigerator at 2°C to 6°C to prevent contaminants reproducing. It must not be kept in a ward refrigerator. Blood for transfusion should be collected from the blood transfusion department or dedicated refrigerator no longer than 30 minutes before it is required by a trained member of staff (Robinson et al., 2018). This is because pathogens grow extremely quickly in blood at room temperature. As such it is the nurse's responsibility to check that the patient is ready to start the transfusion and has patent venous access prior to requesting blood collection.

If the transfusion has not commenced within 30 minutes, the blood bank must be informed and the blood may need to be discarded (Robinson et al., 2018). If the blood is stored in a special 'blood carrier' this time may be extended (see local policy). It is also recommended that transfusions are completed within 4 hours of removal from a controlled temperature environment (Robinson et al., 2018).

The staff member collecting the blood must take the authorised documentation containing the patient's core identifiers and check these with the label on the blood component. Many collection errors occur when the patient details on the laboratory-produced label attached to the blood component pack (compatibility label) are not checked against the patient's identification details (SHOT, 2018).

Unless large quantities of blood are required for rapid transfusion, only one unit of blood should be collected at a time. The identity of the person collecting the blood and the date and time of collection must be documented.

Administration Equipment

- A special blood administration set that incorporates a 170 mm filter chamber must be used. Patients who are receiving multiple blood transfusions or who have had febrile reactions in response to previous transfusions may require an additional filter. These are fine-mesh filters that are placed between the blood bag and the administration set to remove micro aggregates (e.g. fibrin and clots) formed during storage. The same filter can be used for up to four units of blood. If a filter is required, it is usually supplied with the blood and the team should be made aware of this before collecting it from the blood transfusion department.
- When rapid transfusion or transfusion via a central venous catheter is necessary, blood needs to warmed by using a blood warmer during administration. Direct heat must never be used as this can cause blood to haemolyse. The design of blood warmers will vary, but most incorporate a 'zig-zag' tube or coil through which the blood passes over a heater element and is warmed before reaching the patient.
- Be aware that some infusion pumps may damage blood cells and should only be used if the manufacturer's instructions specifically state that they are safe to use with blood transfusion.

PROCEDURE: BLOOD TRANSFUSION ADMINISTRATION

1. Check the patient's identity at the bedside. Where possible, positively identify patients by asking them to state their full name and date of birth. Check that these match the identification band.
2. Check the patient's surname, first names, date of birth, unique identification number, blood group and rhesus factor on:
   1. Patient's identification band
   2. Blood transfusion compatibility report form
   3. Compatibility label attached to the bag
   4. The blood bag
   5. Intravenous (IV) fluid/ blood prescription chart.
3. Check the expiration date of the unit of blood (and time if applicable, e.g. platelets) on:
   - Compatibility label on the bag
   - Blood bag
4. Check the blood group and unique component donation number on:
   - Blood bag
   - Compatibility label on the bag
5. Record this on the prescription chart. There is usually a peel-off section on the blood compatibility label for this.
6. Check any special requirements:
   - The unit of blood must comply with the prescription (e.g. gamma irradiated).

7. Record the date and time and signature of the nurse(s) on:
  - Blood transfusion compatibility report form.
  - Compatibility label.
  - IV fluid prescription chart.
8. Check the blood bag:
  - Inspect for any signs of leakage or damaged packaging
  - Inspect the blood for unusual colour, turbidity or clumping of the contents.
  - If any discrepancies are noted, the blood must not be transfused, the blood bank must be informed and the blood and blood transfusion compatibility form returned to the blood bank.

Special Considerations

Transfusions at night should only proceed when there is a clear clinical indication (SHOT, 2018). All transfusion decisions must consider all options available (SHOT, 2018).

Informed consent must be obtained from the patient. Where this is not possible it needs to be established if an advanced decision was made regarding blood products. If this information is not available the multi-disciplinary team must act in the patient's best interests (MCA, 2005).

Care and Management of a Transfusion

Once the blood products have been collected and the transfusion is ready to be commenced there are numerous actions detailed below that need to be taken. All the actions must be followed to avoid unnecessary error and to monitor the patient effectively. When administering blood products, the patient may be critically unwell and thus standard care of the critically unwell patient must also be provided. It is also imperative that all actions are communicated clearly to the patient to ensure that they understand the procedure and to provide reassurance.

It is important that the correct administration set is used. The administration set for blood transfusions has an additional chamber above the drip chamber, which contains a filter. This filters out debris (platelets and white cells). When administering platelets, a special administration set with no filter is required. Additionally, platelets must be administered rapidly (over 20 to 30 minutes) as soon as they are available.

EQUIPMENT

Blood administration set
Clinical thermometer and watch with second hand
Sphygmomanometer and stethoscope.
Observation chart, usually an Early Warning Score, i.e., NEWS 2 (RCP, 2017)
Fluid balance chart
Intravenous prescription chart
Infusion stand
Intravenous adrenaline (epinephrine) and chlorpheniramine should be available on the ward (in case of allergic reactions

PROCEDURE

1. Explain the procedure, to gain informed consent and cooperation.
2. Decontaminate hands.

3. Non-sterile gloves and a single-use, disposable apron should be worn. Additional personal protective clothing may be required, in accordance with the patient's condition (see Chapter 2).
4. The patient must be wearing an identification band.
5. Advise the patient not to leave the ward during the transfusion.
6. Unconscious and critically unwell patients require very close monitoring.
7. If an intravenous infusion is running to keep the vein open, this must be 0.9% sodium chloride.
8. Record baseline observations of temperature, pulse, respiration and blood pressure immediately prior to commencement of the transfusion (Robinson et al., 2018).
9. Whilst the evidence does not show a marked benefit to this it is recognised that regular monitoring will allow for early detection of acute transfusion reactions.
10. At the bedside, check the blood as described on p. 180 against the prescription and the patient's identification band.
11. Check the cannula site (see VIP score p. 171–173). Using an aseptic non-touch technique prepare the infusion as described on page 168–170 .
12. Calculate the rate of infusion and set the infusion to the required rate (see p. 177–178).
13. Observe the patient continuously for the first 30 minutes as this is when a reaction is most likely to occur (Robinson et al., 2018). Record the temperature, respiratory rate, pulse and blood pressure evert 15 minutes once the transfusion commences. If the observations alter significantly from baseline, these should be reported immediately. These should be repeated during the transfusion according to local policy and again at the end of the transfusion.
14. Be mindful that if the patient is critically unwell you will be undertaking the vital signs more frequently than outlined above.
15. Observe the urine output for volume and colour throughout the transfusion.
16. Reduced volume and changes of colour need to be noted and escalated as this could be a sign of deteriorating health. Absence of urine, oliguria and haemoglobinuria, blood in the urine, could be indicative of adverse haemolytic transfusion reaction and must be escalated immediately.
17. Throughout your observations look for and encourage the patient to report any of the following:
    - **Allergic reaction/anaphylaxis** (allergic reaction to 'foreign' plasma proteins):
      - Wheezing and shortness of breath
      - Hypotension
      - Urticaria on the chest or abdomen
      - Oedema of the eyes or face
      - Laryngeal swelling (a stridor could indicate airway obstruction)
    - **Febrile reaction** (reaction of the patient's antibodies to donor leucocytes):
      - Pyrexia (an increased temperature above 38°C or significantly raised from the baseline recording
      - Feeling hot and flushed or shivering
      - Rigors
    - **Adverse haemolytic transfusion reaction** (this is the most serious reaction, due to transfusion of incompatible blood):
      - Chest or abdominal pain, or pain in the extremities
      - Lumbar or loin pain
      - Oliguria
      - Hypotension and shock
      - Circulatory overload

⬚ Rising pulse and respiration rates
⬚ Dyspnoea or 'bubbly' respiration and frothy sputum
⬚ Hypotension

18. The transfusion should be stopped immediately, and care must be escalated to the nurse in charge and appropriate medical team if:
   ⬚ There is a rise in temperature of greater than 1°C
   ⬚ There is a significant rise or fall in blood pressure (≥20 mmHgs)
   ⬚ There is a significant rise in pulse rate (≥20 bpm)
   ⬚ Any of the above reactions occur.

19. If several units of blood are being transfused, the administration set should be changed every 12 hours to prevent bacterial growth.

20. The blood transfusion compatibility form must be readily available throughout the transfusion.

21. When the transfusion is complete, disconnect the infusion using an aseptic non touch technique. If an intravenous infusion is to follow, change to the correct administration set.

22. Check the patient is comfortable and knows to report any adverse reactions as noted above.

23. Replace equipment and discard waste appropriately.

24. Remove non-sterile gloves and single use disposable apron before decontaminating hands.

25. Document the time that the transfusion stopped in accordance with local policy.

Special Considerations

Nurses must be familiar with local policies relating to administration of blood products. Nurses must be competent in the delivery of blood transfusions, depending on local policies.

All blood products, including the administration set, should be kept after an adverse reaction occurs. It is imperative that local trust policy is followed in these instances.

References

Bond, M., Crathorne, L., Peters, J., et al., 2015. First do no harm: pain relief for the peripheral venous cannulation of adults, a systematic review and network meta-analysis. BMC Anaesthesiol. 16 (81), 1–11

Brooks, N., 2017. Venepuncture and Cannulation: A Practical Guide. MK Publishers, Kerswick.

Cathala, X., Moorley, C., 2018. Selecting IV fluids to manage fluid loss in critically ill patients. Nurs. Times [online]. 114 (12), 41–44.

Elliott, M., Liu, Y., 2010. The nine rights of medication administration: an overview. Br J Nurs. 19 (5), 300–5. doi:10.12968/bjon.2010.19.5.47064.

Ford, C., 2019. Cannulation in adults. Br. J. Nurs. 28 (13), 838–841.

Gabriel, G., 2013. Venepuncture and cannulation: considering the aging vein. Br. J. Nurs. 21 (S1), S22–S28.

Jackson, A., 1998. Infection control: a battle in vein infusion phlebitis. Nurs. Times. 94 (4), 68–71.

Legislation.gov.uk, 2005. Mental Capacity Act.

Loveday, H.P., Wilson, J.A., Pratt, R.J., et al., 2014. National Evidence-Based Guidelines for Preventing Healthcare-Associated Infections in NHS Hospitals in England. J. Hosp. Infect. 8651 (2014), S1–S70.

National Institute for Health and Care Excellence (NICE), 2015. NG24: Transfusion: Blood Transfusion. National Institute for Health and Care Excellence, London.

National Institute for Health and Care Excellence, 2016. Algorithms for IV fluid therapy in adults. https://www.nice.org.uk/guidance/cg174/resources/intravenous-fluid-therapy-in-adults-in-hospital-algorithm-poster-set-191627821

National Institute for Health and Care Excellence (NICE), 2017. CG174 Intravenous Therapy in adults in hospital. National Institute for Health and Care Excellence, London.

Norfolk, D., 2013. Handbook of Transfusion Medicine. TBA, Norwich.

Nursing and Midwifery Council (NMC), 2018. Professional Standards of Practice and Behaviour for Nurses, Midwives and Nursing Associates. Nursing and Midwifery Council, London.

Robinson, S., Harris, A., Atkinson, S., et al., 2018. The administration of blood components: a British Society for Haematology Guideline. Transfus. Med. 28 (1), 3–21.

Royal College of Nursing (RCN), 2016. Standards for Infusion Therapy. Royal College of Nursing, London.

Royal College of Physicians, 2017. National Early Warning Score (NEWS) 2. https://www.rcplondon.ac.uk/projects/outputs/national-early-warning-score-news-2

Serious Hazards of Transfusion, 2018. 2018 SHOT Annual Report. https://www.shotuk.org/shot-reports/report-summary-and-supplement-2018/2018-shot-annual-report-individual-chapters/

Skarparis, K., Ford, C., 2018. Venepuncture in adults. Br. J. Nurs. 27 (22), 1312–1315.

Shaw, S.J., 2018. How to undertake venepuncture to obtain venous blood samples. Nurs. Stand. 32 (29), 41–47

CHAPTER 13

Peri-Operative Care

Pre-Operative Care

There are three phases to the patient's surgical journey: pre-operative, intra-operative and post-operative. Together, these phases are known as the peri-operative period. Surgery can be classified as elective (planned) or emergency (unplanned). When patients are admitted for planned surgery (e.g. cholecystectomy, hysterectomy), a full assessment is undertaken in the pre-admission clinic, and any potential complications are addressed to optimise the patient's health before surgery. However, this is not the case for emergency procedures, where the time available to prepare the patient is usually short. Emergency surgery may be due to trauma and accidents (e.g., head injury or ruptured spleen), obstruction of the gastrointestinal tract (strangulated hernia, bowel cancer) or perforated viscera (e.g., ulcer, appendix).

There have been significant advances in surgical techniques with many procedures now undertaken using keyhole, robotic or laparoscopic approaches. The nurse has an important role in the physical and psychological preparation of the patient throughout the patient's peri-operative pathway. It is now accepted that patients who are well prepared for surgery will experience fewer postoperative complications and enhanced recovery (Dougherty et al., 2015). The following principles focus on the care of a patient undergoing elective surgery, although many of the principles are equally relevant to emergency procedures.

PRE-OPERATIVE CARE

When preparing the patient for surgery, the nurse must develop an individualised care plan, that takes account of general care needs and specific preparation required for the surgical procedure to be undertaken. As stated above, because elective surgery in planned in advance, preparation can be completed before admission. Patients may be required to attend a Pre-Operative Assessment Clinic (POAC) or Surgical Pre-Assessment Clinic (SPAC) before admission for surgery. This appointment involves an assessment of their physical, psychological and social needs, with the aim of reducing potential intra- and postoperative complications. In some instances, POAC may be conducted through telephone consultations (Johnstone, 2020; Dougherty et al., 2015). Before patients attend a POAC, they may complete a pre-surgical questionnaire, and this can act as a prompt during the consultation to ascertain more information. In addition, other assessment tools including baseline observations, body mass index (BMI), electrocardiogram (ECG), medication, family/social history will help the nurse to complete a holistic assessment (Johnstone, 2020).

In contrast, emergency surgery requires immediate admission to hospital, generally via the Emergency Department (Royal College of Surgeons [RCS], 2019). Therefore, preparation and planning are constrained, with a focus on stabilising the patient for theatre.

KEY POINTS

Peri-operative care involves three stages, the pre-operative, intra-operative and postopera-
tive phase (Dougherty et al., 2015).
Surgery can be planned or unplanned. The reason for surgery will determine how practitio-
ners prepare patients during the pre-operative phase.
Patients must be risk assessed prior to surgery using an approved tool, for example the
American Society of Anesthesiologist (ASA) Physical Status Classification System.

CONSENT

The surgeon is ultimately responsible for obtaining the patient's consent before any surgical
procedure (RCS, 2018). For consent to be valid, patients must have the capacity to understand
and retain information about the procedure to decide whether they wish to proceed with the
surgery. Patients must also be able to consider the consequences of the surgical procedure and
communicate their decision to the medical staff (Department of Health, 2009). Patients must
give their consent willingly, without influence or pressure from family, friends or medical staff.
Under no circumstances should any pre-operative medication be given before the consent is
confirmed (Department of Health, 2009). It is the nurse's responsibility to check that the patient's consent is completed correctly before they go to the theatre.

ANXIETY

It is generally accepted that undergoing surgery is an anxiety-provoking time that can make
patients feel vulnerable, nervous or distressed. Determining the factors that trigger such feelings helps the nurse to allay the patient's fears and concerns. These may include fear of the
unknown (what to expect, diagnosis), fear of the anaesthetic, fear of pain, feeling ill, dying,
changes in body image, separation from children and family, loss of security (Peate, 2016; Royal
College of Anaesthetists [RCA], 2019). Providing pre-operative education, information and
support is vital in helping the patients understand their surgery, what is expected of them and
what will happen post-operatively. It is crucial to describe the recovery phase including any
equipment to expect (e.g. catheter, IV fluids, nasogastric tube), the method of pain control (e.g.
PCA,), and information about mobility, when they can eat and drink, postoperative nausea and
vomiting and breathing exercises (RCA, 2019). This helps to reduce anxiety, stress and pain,
which may promote the patient's well-being (Peate, 2016). The information given at this stage
is dependent on the proposed surgical procedure.

Preparing for Surgery

Prior to surgery, a patient will need to be nil-by mouth for a period of time. Sweets and chewing
gum must not be eaten on the day of surgery as these stimulate gastric juices. This safeguards
the patient from the risk of regurgitation and aspiration of gastric contents while undergoing a
general anaesthetic. Certain medications may need to be stopped or withheld prior to surgery (e.g.
Warfarin); angiotensin-converting enzyme (ACE) inhibitors, with only medications deemed necessary administered during this period (Peate, 2016). If the patient is prescribed regular oral
medication, this can be given with a small amount of fluid 2 to 3 hours before surgery. However,
if the nurse is unsure of which medications to withhold or give, it is their responsibility to check
with the medical team or anaesthetist.

Effective hygiene before surgery reduces the number of microorganisms on the skin and
minimises the risk of a postoperative surgical site infection (Peate, 2016). Depending on the type
of surgery, patients will be asked to shower prior to surgery using an anti-bacterial solution the

night before and the morning of surgery. The patient will then need to change into a theatre gown as this allows access to the operation site. Some patients may be able to wear cotton or disposable underwear to maintain dignity according to the local hospital policy.

ANAESTHETIC AND AIRWAY ASSESSMENT

Patients who have had previous complications with an anaesthetic or who are identified as having a potential airway problem will need to be seen by an anaesthetist prior to surgery.

Questions may be used, to identify whether:

- Any problems with previous anaesthetics (The patient may have a letter, a Difficult Airway Society card, or a Medic-Alert bracelet).
- Family history of any problems with anaesthetics
- Any issues with their teeth, (e.g. dentures, loose teeth)
- Able to extend your neck and open their mouth, (e.g. scoliosis or arthritis of the neck)
- Able to lie flat, (e.g. those with shortness of breath may sleep semi-upright)
- Have a History of respiratory disease (e.g. asthma, Chronic Obstructive Pulmonary Disease COPD, sleep apnoea)
- Identification of any allergies.

RESPIRATORY ASSESSMENT

Identification of any respiratory condition (e.g. asthma, COPD).

- Respiratory rate (see p. 26)
- Pulse oximetry (see p. 36)
- Peak expiratory flow (see p. 35)
- Spirometry
- Medication history
- Complications with anaesthetics in the past.

CARDIAC ASSESSMENT

History of cardiovascular disease (e.g. clotting disease, hypertension or Myocardial Infarction MI).

- Blood pressure
- Pulse
- ECG
- Any risk of thrombosis, excessive bleeding.

NEUROLOGICAL ASSESSMENT

- History of neurological disease (e.g. epilepsy).
- Pain profile
- Mini-mental state assessment in patients over 65 years old.

GASTROINTESTINAL ASSESSMENT

- Digestive history
- Recent weight loss
- Nutritional and BMI status
- Hepatic function
- Renal function, including urination patterns
- Alcohol intake assessment.

MUSCULOSKELETAL

- Musculoskeletal history (e.g. arthritis).

FAMILY HISTORY

- Familial illnesses (e.g. hypertension, coronary artery disease, stroke, diabetes)
- Genetic problems (e.g. malignant hyperpyrexia or Suxamethonium apnoea).

SOCIAL HISTORY

- Home life
- Occupation
- Religious beliefs
- Smoking, drug and alcohol use
- Social situation (e.g. access to house, availability of carers to help with postoperative care).

INFECTION SCREENING

- Swabs for methicillin-resistant Staphylococcus aureus (MRSA)
- Midstream urine (MSU) as indicated.

MEDICATION ASSESSMENT

- Medication review to identify any that need to be stopped or adjusted preoperatively.

PSYCHOLOGICAL SUPPORT

- Undergoing surgery can be stressful and a frightening experience; therefore, the nurse must listen to patients' concerns and provide time for patients (and relatives) to discuss their concerns.
- Identification of any mental health support or specialist input that will be required.

On completion of this assessment, the nurse grades the patient using the ASA Physical Status Classification System (Table 13.1) to identify the risk.

TABLE 13.1 ■ American Society of Anaesthesiologists Physical Status Classification System

ASA Classification	Definition	Examples
ASA I	A normal healthy patient	Healthy, non-smoking, no or minimal alcohol use
ASA II	A patient with mild systemic disease	Hypertension, mild diabetes without end-organ damage
ASA III	A patient with severe systemic disease	Angina, moderate to severe COPD
ASA IV	A patient with an incapacitating disease that is a contact threat to life	Advanced COPD, cardiac failure
ASA V	A moribund patient who is not expected to live 24 hours without an operation	Ruptured abdominal aortic aneurysm
ASA VI	A declared brain dead patient whose organs are being removed for donor purposes	

ASA (2014) and Dougherty et al. (2015).

CHECKLIST

Surgical checklists are used to reduce the risk of errors by not missing vital information. The World Health Organization (WHO) Surgical Safety Checklist (2009) is a 19-item checklist aiming to decrease errors and adverse events, and increase teamwork and communication in surgery. The checklist is completed in three parts:

- Prior to induction of anaesthesia
- Prior to skin incision
- Prior to transfer to the recovery room.

A pre-operative checklist is completed by the nurse according to local policies before the patient is taken to the operating theatre department. This usually includes the following:

- Identification name bands: must contain the patient's full name, date of birth and NHS number (NHS Improvement, 2018). This information must agree with the patient's medical notes to ensure that the correct patient is identified. Many hospitals require two name bands (one on the wrist and the other on the ankle) so that the patient can still be identified if one is removed (e.g. when a cannula is inserted).
- Allergies: It is essential to ask whether the patient has any allergies (e.g. skin preparation solution (iodine), dressings and plasters, medications, antibiotics, and latex) to reduce any potential harm to the patient during surgery. If an allergy is known, the patient must wear an allergy alert name band, and any known allergies must be documented in the patient's notes (NHS Improvement, 2018). It is also important to indicate any adverse reactions to previous blood transfusions or blood products.
- Baseline observations: The patient's respiratory rate, pulse rate, blood pressure and temperature must be recorded to establish a baseline for intra and postoperative comparison. The patient's weight will be required by the anaesthetist to calculate the correct dose of anaesthetic medication.
- Pregnancy test: With the woman's consent, a pregnancy test should be performed on all women of childbearing age. An unknown pregnancy during the first trimester may pose an adverse risk to the woman and the foetus (NICE, 2016).
- Marking the operation site: It is the surgeon's responsibility to mark the operation site. The operation site must be marked with an indelible pen and matched with the patient's medical notes (WHO, 2009).
- Pre-operative fasting: The nurse must document when the patient last ate and drank. It is important that the patient has no food for at least 6 hours and no fluids for 2 hours before going to the theatre.
- Dental: The presence of dental crowns, caps, bridgework or loose teeth must be documented as these may obstruct the airway if they accidentally become dislodged and inhaled during the induction of anaesthesia. Dentures are normally removed and stored in a labelled denture pot.
- Jewellery and piercings: Body piercings and Jewellery must be removed or securely taped according to local policy. These may become dislodged and lost when the patient is moved, and the use of diathermy may harm the patient (diathermy burns) if wearing metal Jewellery. Wedding/partnership rings and other items of Jewellery that cannot be removed must be secured to avoid loss. Some local hosptial policies may allow certain items of Jewellery for cultural reasons if they do not compromise the patient's safety. These must be documented in the patient's notes.
- Nail varnish, false nails and make-up: Nail varnish and false nails must be removed as they will affect the accuracy of the oxygen saturation result (see p. 36–37). Make-up must also be removed, as this will make it difficult to assess the patient's skin colour.

- Spectacles, hearing aids, contact lenses and prostheses: The presence of any prosthesis must be documented and, if appropriate, removed. Contact lenses can become dry and cause corneal abrasions if left in place for prolonged periods. A hearing aid should remain in place to allow the patient to communicate and understand what is happening before they are anaesthetised. Spectacles should be removed when the patient is in the anaesthetic room. Prostheses such as false limbs should be removed before leaving the ward. Internal mechanisms such as pacemakers must be documented on the pre-operative checklist.
- Urinalysis and an empty bladder: NICE (2016) recommends not to routinely perform a urinalysis and to consider microscopy and culture of a midstream urine sample before surgery if the presence of a urinary tract infection would influence the decision to operate. Before surgery, check that the patient has passed urine to avoid urinary incontinence and contamination of the sterile field while anesthetised. This also prevents the bladder being accidentally damaged during surgery.
- A venous-thromboembolism risk assessment must be done to identify the patient's risk factors and determine the most appropriate treatment to reduce the risk of deep vein thrombosis (NICE, 2018). When anti-embolic stockings are used, these must be correctly measured and applied.
- Hair removal may be necessary when the surgeon's view of the operation site is restricted or where it is difficult to apply the ECG adhesive pads or dressings/plaster. The nurse should consult their local policy for the method of hair removal (e.g. shaving, electric clippers or depilatory creams. If shaving of the operation site is required, this is done as close as possible to the time of the operation).
- Medical notes, x-rays, blood tests etc. The nurse must ensure that the medical notes, x-rays, scans, blood results, consent form, prescription chart, observation chart, and any other relevant documents accompany the patient to the operating theatre department. This will facilitate a safe and accurate handover to the theatre staff and provide the surgeon with all the information necessary before the surgery begins.

INTRA-OPERATIVE CARE

This refers to the physical and psychological care given to the patient while in the anaesthetic room, operating theatre and recovery area, these are specialist areas and beyond the scope of this text. The nurse has a key role in accompanying the patient to the anaesthetic room and on collecting them from the recovery room. Before the patient returns to the ward, it is important that the nurse assesses the patient and receives a comprehensive handover from the theatre staff. This should include: the type of surgery, any concerns or complications, any blood transfusions, any medications administered in recovery, any special instructions (when they can eat and drink), vital signs, level of consciousness, pain management, wound and wound drainage, intravenous fluids, and the urine output. The patient must not be transferred to the ward until they are conscious, able to maintain their airway and their clinical observations are stable.

Postoperative Care

Once back in the ward it is vital that the nurse performs a full nursing assessment. Using the Airway, Breathing, Circulation, Disability (neurological), Exposure ABCDE approach enables the nurse to systematically assess the patient's condition, determine the priorities of care and recognise the early deterioration of the patient (see p. 18). These observations provide a baseline for the patient's postoperative care and should be compared with the pre and intra-operative recordings. The frequency of the observations will be determined by the patient's condition.

Many organisations have local policies that stipulate the frequency of postoperative observations, but it is important that nurses use professional judgement to interpret the observations to closely monitor the patient's condition. The use of an early warning score (see p. 18) will alert the nurse should the patient's condition start to deteriorate and can be used to escalate care if necessary.

ABCDE Assessment of a Postoperative Patient

Some specific aspects of this assessment will depend on the type of surgery. For example, following orthopaedic or vascular surgery assessment might include neurovascular assessment (see p. 87). The systematic ABCDE assessment on page 20 should be used for the postoperative evaluation. In addition, the following are important for most postoperative patients.

- **Level of consciousness should be assessed using AVPU.** When a more comprehensive neurological assessment is needed (e.g. following neurological surgery), the Glasgow coma scale should be used. Unconscious patients need careful monitoring. Snoring or noisy breathing indicates a partially obstructed airway and must be reported and appropriate interventions initiated.
- **Psychological support.** Although most patients will be prepared for surgery they are likely to feel anxious and will continue to need reassurance. Information relating to the outcome of the operation, any equipment, the use of PCA, or any other concerns or worries will need to be discussed (e.g. altered body image). The involvement of the family is important during the postoperative phase.
- **Oxygen.** Many patients will be prescribed oxygen by mask or nasal cannula (see p. 5) postoperatively, and some will require oxygen for a longer period. The number of litres of oxygen may be prescribed as a range (e.g. 4 to 6 L), and this is adjusted in response to the patient's oxygen saturation. The target oxygen saturation for the patient will be documented on the prescription chart.
- **Intravenous fluids.** It is important to ensure that IV fluids run at the prescribed rate and the cannula is inspected regularly using the visual infusion phlebitis (VIP) score. All input and output will be documented on a fluid balance chart.
- **Antibiotics.** Check the prescription chart for any additional medications (e.g. prophylactic antibiotics); depending on local policy a single dose is prescribed after the operation. As with all medicines, it is important to check for allergies prior to administration.
- **Wounds and drains.** Observe the wound site and any wound drainage and document the amount and type of drainage. Depending on the type of surgery, additional checks for example, if the operation is per vagina, record the blood loss by noting the number of sanitary pads. If the operation is transurethral, there will be continuous bladder irrigation.
- **Nasogastric tube.** This may be on free drainage or require manual aspiration. The amount and type of aspirate must be documented on the fluid balance chart.
- **Nil-by mouth.** All patients will be unable to eat and drink for a period of time. Instructions regarding when they can commence oral fluids will be part of the operation notes. If the surgery has involved the bowel, it will be necessary to wait for bowel sounds to return before the patient can start drinking. Inspect the mouth and provide regular mouth care/mouthwashes while the patient is unable to take oral fluids.
- **Pain Assessment using a Pain Assessment Tool.** The effectiveness of the pain management system used, e.g., patient-controlled analgesia (PCA) and any side-effects.
- **Postoperative nausea and vomiting (PONV).** PONV and this should be assessed when assessing pain. Many patients report that PONV is one of the most distressing aspects of

their hospital stay. Prophylaxis is often prescribed for patients at moderate to high risk for PONV (Anaesthesia UK, 2021).

- **Urine output.** If the patient is catheterised, it is important to closely monitor the urine output. An output of less than 0.5 mL/ kg per hour should be reported. If the patient is not catheterised, it is important to document when the patient first passes urine.
- **Temperature.** A patient may have a low temperature following surgery and so need to be slowly warmed. It is important to continue to monitor the patient's temperature as a raised temperature may be the first indication of an infection.
- **Blood glucose level.** If the patient has diabetes, they may be prescribed an insulin infusion that is titrated according to their blood glucose level. A variable dose regimen (sliding scale) will be prescribed.
- **Complications of reduced mobility.** Most patients will be able to mobilise very soon after their operation, but those with reduced mobility require re-assessment for pressure ulcer risk using a recognised assessment tool (e.g. Waterlow) and the risk of venous-thromboembolism risk. Inspect the patent's anti-embolism stockings to ensure that they are applied correctly.

Peri-Operative Care for People With Dementia

Increasing numbers of patients with dementia in the United Kingdom means more patients with cognitive impairment will require surgical care. Dementia is characterised by memory loss, impaired understanding of the perception of events and reduced communication skills (Mahoney, 2018). Patients with dementia are at increased risk of comorbidities, for example, cardiovascular disease and chronic obstructive airways disease (COPD) (Alcorn and Foo, 2017). This poses several challenges for nursing staff when providing peri-operative care to this vulnerable group of individuals.

KEY FACTS

- Few national consensus guidelines exist specifically for the peri-operative environment (Mahoney, 2018).
- An individualised approach to peri-operative care is required due to the varying degrees of cognitive impairment.

NURSING CONSIDERATIONS

Patients with dementia may be unable to comprehend their situation, may be frightened or show extreme behaviours. Therefore, it is recommended more time to prepare them for the anaesthesia and use a 'less-hurried' approach throughout the peri-operative pathway. Practitioners should understand how individuals with dementia may respond and information should be gathered from family and carers.

Dementia patients receiving a general anaesthetic may be at greater risk of postoperative cognitive decline. Therefore, careful assessment and consideration on the most appropriate anaesthesia to use should be considered (e.g. regional anaesthesia may be more appropriate). Other medical factors include frailty, poor nutritional state and comorbidities.

Practical considerations include:

- Gaining consent for surgery and associated procedures.
- Gaining and maintaining intravenous (IV) access.
- Patient being appropriately fasted before surgery.

- Postoperative delirium.
- Pain interpretation and management.
- Increased anxiety.

Nursing interventions should include:

- Communication amongst team members in terms of approach, anaesthesia and the requirement for increased time in preparing the patient for their procedure.
- Communication with the patient and their significant others (as appropriate).
- Observation of non-verbal communication in patients but also an awareness of your non-verbal communication.
- Avoid talking over the patient.
- Try to convey a sense of warmth, compassion and acceptance.
- Be aware a patient may struggle to find the right words when asked to reply to complex questions or 'quick-fire' ones.

References

Alcorn, S., Foo, I., 2017. Perioperative management of patients with dementia. BJA Educ. 17 (3), 94–98.

American Society of Anaesthesiologists, 2014. ASA Physical Status Classification System. https://www.asahq.org/standards-and-guidelines/asa-physical-status-classification-system.

Anaesthesia UK, 2021. Nausea and Vomiting. https://www.frca.co.uk/SectionContents.aspx?sectionid=113.

Department of Health, 2009. Reference Guide to Consent for Examination of Treatment, second ed. www.dh.gov.ukpublications.

Dougherty, L., Lister, S., West-Oram, A. (Eds.), 2015. Perioperative care. In The Royal Marsden Manual of Clinical Nursing Procedures: Student Edition. ninth ed. Wiley.

Johnstone J (2020) How to provide preoperative care to patients. Nursing Standard. doi: 10.7748/ns.2020.e11657

Peate I. (2016). Chapter 49: Pre-operative care. In Peate I. (2016). Medical-Surgical Nursing at a Glance. Wiley Blackwell.

Mahoney C. (2018). Peri-operative care for people with dementia: challenges and solutions. Nurs. Times. 114. 11. 53–56

NHS Improvement, 2018. Recommendations From the National Patient Safety Agency Alerts That Remain Relevant to the Never Events List 2018. https://improvement.nhs.uk/documents/2267/Recommendations_from_NPSA_alerts_that_remain_relevant_to_NEs_FINAL.pdf.

National Institute for health and Care Excellence [NICE], 2016. Routine preoperative tests for elective surgery. NICE guideline [NG45]. https://www.nice.org.uk/guidance/ng45/chapter/Recommendations#table-3-major-or-complex-surgery.

National Institute for health and Care Excellence [NICE], 2018. Venous thromboembolism in over 16s: reducing the risk of hospital-acquired deep vein thrombosis or pulmonary embolism. NICE guideline [NG89]. https://www.nice.org.uk/guidance/ng89/chapter/Recommendations#risk-assessment.

Royal College of Surgeons, 2018. Consent. https://www.rcseng.ac.uk/standards-and-research/gsp/domain-3/3-5-1-consent/.

Royal College of Anaesthetists, 2019. Guidelines for the Provision of Anaesthetic Services for Postoperative Care 2019. https://www.rcoa.ac.uk/gpas/chapter-4.

Royal College of Surgeons, 2019. Types of Surgery. https://www.rcseng.ac.uk/patient-care/having-surgery/types-of-surgery/.

World Health Organization, 2009. Safe Surgery Checklist. https://www.who.int/patientsafety/safesurgery/checklist/en/.

CHAPTER 14

Medicines Management

Medicines Administration

Preserving safety is key to nursing practice (Nursing and Midwifery Council [NMC], 2018), and is of paramount importance when administering medication by any route (National Institute for Health and Care Excellence [NICE], 2015). Nurses need to recognise there is individual responsibility at the administrator and prescriber level (Royal College of Nursing [RCN], 2020), and organisational and institutional responsibility for ensuring medicine safety (Royal Pharmaceutical Society [RPS], 2019; RCN, 2019). Therefore, it is imperative that the nurse follows the safety measures applicable to the clinical area they are working in. These now reflect that the key rights of medication have expanded from the original five to a total of nine (RPS, 2019. Ogston-Tuck, 2014. Elliot & Liu, 2010) (Ogston-Tuck, 2014). These are:

1. **Right patient:** the patient's identity should be checked against their identification (ID) band and the prescription chart. You should also ask the patient to confirm their name and date of birth verbally where possible. In primary care, where patients will not have an ID band, alternative means of identification should be used such as a photo ID or a photograph.

2. **Right medicine:** check that the prescription is legible, signed by an authorised prescriber, and that it matches the label on the medication. You also need to ensure that you know why this medication is being given and that the patient has no known allergies to the medication. If a patient has a known allergy, they should wear a red allergy band, with all allergies documented in full on the paper or electronic Medication Administration Chart. The prescription should provide the generic name, rather than the manufacturer's brand name, to ensure that the administrator is aware of the medication they are giving (i.e. Co-amoxiclav, not Augmentin).

3. **Right dose:** check that the correct dosage has been prescribed for the route of administration. This will involve performing any calculations required to ensure the correct amount is administered (see p. 201). It is also imperative that the maximum daily dose is not exceeded in any 24-hour period.

4. **Right route:** check that the prescribed route is appropriate for the patient and that a suitable preparation for that route is available. If a liquid dose is preferred over oral tablets, this will need to be ordered with the packaging clearly indicating that it is for oral administration.

5. **Right time:** check that the medication is given at the prescribed time. It is also important to check if the medication has specific administration requirements such as those that are given before or after food.

6. **Right documentation:** it is imperative that the prescription chart is signed to state that the medication has been given. If for any reason the medication is not able to be administered, this must also be documented with the reason for non-administration clearly identified. The reasons for non-administration are usually provided on the chart, and these reasons should be adhered to. It is not sufficient to state that the patient was not available but to establish why that was and whether the medication could be given at an alternative time. This would involve a discussion with the prescriber.

7. Right action: ensure that the medication is given for the right reason such as paracetamol to reduce systemic body temperature. This requires an understanding of the pharmacodynamics of the medication and the rationale for administration. If this is unclear from reading the nursing notes, you will need to seek clarification from the prescriber.

8. Right form: to ensure safe administration the right form must be used, i.e., intravenous rather than oral, but it also refers to medications that cannot be crushed or altered in any way, such as enteric-coated drugs. This is both the obligation of the prescriber and the administrator of the medication.

9. Right response: this right has been added to ensure that the patient is re-assessed to check if the desired response has been achieved (i.e. an analgesic providing pain relief). If the desired effect is not produced, then this needs to be addressed.

KEY POINTS

- Medicine may only be administered by a registered healthcare professional. In some instances, medication administration can be delegated, but this will be clear within the patient's records.
- The administrator, usually the nurse, must have knowledge of the action, usual dose and side effects of the drugs being administered as well as knowledge of legislation and local policies relating to the administration of medicines (RPS, 2019; RCN, 2019).
- Local policy may require that two nurses check certain medicines before administration. Always ensure that you familiarise yourself with these policies.

EQUIPMENT

Medicines to be administered with the equipment appropriate to the route of administration.
Patient's Medication Administration Record
Drug reference book (e.g. British National Formulary [most up to date version either electronic or hard copy])
Alcohol hand gel
Personal Protective Equipment (PPE) as required.

PROCEDURE

1. Check the location of the patient before dispensing the medication. Medication may need to be delayed if the patient is having a procedure.
2. Check that the patient understands the reasons for medication administration and any special instructions (e.g. swallow whole, after food, with water).
3. Decontaminate hands any PPE that is required.
4. Ensure that the patient understands what the medication is and why they are receiving it to provide informed consent.
5. Ascertain whether the patient has any drug allergies. Document any additional on the drug chart.
6. Ensure that the patient is wearing the appropriate name band, where applicable, with the correct identifying information.
7. Check the prescription chart has the patient's full name and hospital number correctly written or inputted and read the prescription to ascertain which medications require administration.
8. Check the route that each medicine should be given. If there is more than one route (i.e. per oral (PO)/intravenous [IV] consider which would be most appropriate in this instance).

9. Check the prescription is dated, legible and signed by an authorised prescriber.
10. Check if it is the correct time to administer the medicine and that the patient has not already received it.
11. Check any special observations (e.g. blood pressure, heart rate) or requirements relating to the medication (e.g. before or after food).
12. Identify the correct medication by checking the medicine external and internal packaging against the prescription chart.
13. Check the expiration date of the medicine on both the external and internal packaging.
14. Calculate how much is needed to achieve the prescribed dose (e.g. how many tablets or how much of the ampoule is to be drawn up).
15. Repeat steps 2 to 7 for all medicines due.
16. Check the patient's identity—using the patient's name band, a photograph or verbally, against the prescription chart, according to local policy.
17. Administer the medicine as prescribed. **Never leave unattended medication at the bedside**—this is considered incomplete medication administration. There are multiple safety issues with such practice.
18. Dispose of any packaging and other waste appropriately.
19. Check the patient is comfortable and knows how to report any unwanted side effects of the medication.
20. Sign/initial the prescription chart according to local policy to indicate that the medicine has been administered. If the medication cannot be administered for any reason, this must also be documented and reported and escalated to the prescriber as appropriate.
21. Monitor the effects of the medication and document in the nursing records. Report any abnormal effects/side effects immediately.

Special Considerations

- Patients have the right to refuse medication and thus it is essential to fully provide and document information on why the patient is receiving the medication so that an informed decision can be made
- If the patient does not have capacity, it may be that a 'best interest' approach is used. Do not assume refusal to indicate a lack of capacity
- Polypharmacy is becoming increasingly common (NICE, 2015) and thus medication should be reviewed when people are admitted to hospital or use a primary care service to ensure optimisation

---

Non-Medical Prescribing

In the UK, non-medical prescribing developed in 1992 from a need to provide high quality, timely, care and make better use of the resources available (Weeks et al., 2016). Historically, there were reported delays in case management whilst the nurse, or other allied health professional, waited for a doctor to provide the prescription (Cope et al., 2016). The Cumberledge report highlighted that this limited the quality of care provided (Department of Health and Social Security, [DHSS] 1986) and thus non-medical prescribing was introduced.

Non-medical prescribing falls into three different categories:

- Independent prescribing—the prescriber is responsible for assessing the patient, diagnosing, and making clinical decisions and a management plan that may well include prescribing.
- Supplementary prescribing—this is when there is a partnership between a medical prescriber (doctor or dentist), a supplementary prescriber and the patient to implement an agreed clinical management plan. An example of this could be a nurse-run hypertension clinic.

▪ Community Nurse Prescribing—this allows the community nurse to prescribe from the nurse prescribing formulary that includes some medications, dressings, emollients and medical devices such as catheter care equipment.

Whilst the three categories suggest that independent prescribers can prescribe any medication for any condition, the prescriber must still act in accordance with their professional regulatory body and their competence (RPS, 2016). The Nursing and Midwifery code highlights that nurses can only manage and treat the patient, which includes prescribing, if they have sufficient knowledge of that person's health status and health needs (NMC, 2018). The Royal Pharmaceutical Society has provided a competency framework (2016) that can be used as a guide for all prescribers.

KEY POINTS

- As the prescriber, you are well placed to review patient's prescription and consider all medications prescribed
- Reviewing medications also involves asking about side effects, which may also highlight drug interactions, and working with the patient to minimise these and changing the medication where required
- When prescribing, you also need to consider who will be administering the medication and if they will act appropriately if adverse effects are noted; this is of importance when prescribing controlled drugs

PROCEDURE

1. Assess the patient: this involves a full holistic assessment of the patient's current health and social care needs and a review of the current medication plan and adherence.
2. Consider options: this involves consideration of both pharmacological and non-pharmacological options which may include no treatment. The benefits and risks of treatment should be fully considered, including the patient's ability to take medication or adhere to a treatment plan.
3. Reach a shared decision: this involves listening to the patient and considering their needs and preferences. All treatment must be explained fully and the patients understanding ascertained before commenced.
4. Prescribe: as the prescriber you are responsible for being up-to-date on local and national prescribing regulations as well as competent at using the prescribing system within the local area. It is expected that appropriate drug formulary's (i.e. the BNF) will be used to assist the prescribing process.
5. Provide information: as with providing clear details on the treatment plan, clear information about the prescription must be given to the patient. This involves ensuring that the patient understands what the medication is and why it is being prescribed. It is also imperative that you provide the patient with the opportunity to ask questions and voice any concerns they might have.
6. Monitor and review: as the prescriber, you have an obligation to review the clinical management plan and assess the effectiveness of treatment. A review date should be planned during the consultation.
7. Prescribe safely: this involves having a continued awareness of your own level of competency and consistency working within your scope of practice. This also involves reporting errors, including near misses, to promote and foster a safety culture.

8. Prescribe professionally: be aware of professional, legal, and ethical obligations in relation to prescribing. The prescribing should be for the patient benefit and based on their need rather than prescriber preference.

9. Improve prescribing practice: as with all healthcare roles this involves reflecting on your practice, updating your competency as required under local and national policy and requesting feedback from patients and colleagues.

10. Prescribe as part of a team: regardless of the type of prescriber, all prescribers need to ensure that the prescribing role benefits the team. This role may also involve supporting other prescribers and requesting support and supervision within your role.

Controlled Drugs

Controlled drugs are used in the clinical setting but must be used in accordance with The Misuse of Drugs Regulations (2001) that provides restrictions based on production, prescription, administration and documentation. As such, there are specific steps to follow when administering controlled medications that are required by law. Local policy may also request that other procedures are followed, and as such, the healthcare professional must be fully aware of relevant guidance and policy.

KEY POINTS

- Ensure knowledge of legislation and local policies relating to the administration of controlled drugs.
- Two registered healthcare professionals are usually required, and local policy must be followed.
- It is imperative to note if the patient has ever had any adverse effects to controlled drugs, such as opioid analgesia.
- In some instances, patients will need to be monitored by a competent professional, aware of what they are observing, after administration.

EQUIPMENT

Patient's prescription chart
Controlled drugs register
Alcohol hand gel
PPE as appropriate

PROCEDURE

1. Decontaminate hands. Additional protective clothing may be necessary if indicated by the patient's condition (see Chapter 2)
2. Explain the procedure, to gain informed consent and cooperation
3. Check the patient understands the reasons for having the medication
4. Consider whether prescribed dose is safe for the person based on factors such as age, weight, comorbidities
5. If local policy stipulates two healthcare professionals, one administer and one witness, they must both be involved in **all** stages of this procedure:
   i. Check the '9 rights' (Elliot and Liu, 2010) and follow the principles of administration as described on pages 195 to 196.

    ii. Open the controlled drugs cupboard and select the appropriate drug, checking that the quantity corresponds with that indicated in the controlled drugs register.

    iii. Check the quantity remaining and replace in the cupboard.

    iv. Complete controlled drug record in accordance with local policy, usually a minimum of patient's name, dose to be administered, time and stock remaining (NICE, 2016).

    v. Lock the cupboard.

    vi. Select/draw up the correct amount/volume of the drug, performing any calculations as required.

    vii. Approach the patient, with a witness as required, and administer the drug by the prescribed route.

6. Discard all waste appropriately.
7. Check the patient is comfortable and is aware of the effects and side effects of the drug.
8. Ensure that both administer and witness sign both the prescription chart and the controlled drugs register—noting any wastage.
9. Ensure the Controlled Drugs register is returned to the appropriate place.
10. Monitor the effects of the drug, escalate and then document any adverse effects.

Antimicrobial Stewardship

Antimicrobial resistance is becoming increasingly common and is recognised by the World Health Organization (2018) as a public health concern. This resistance occurs when microorganisms adapt following exposure to antimicrobials and become resistant to its effects, an example of which is methicillin-resistant Staphylococcus aureus, (MRSA). As such, the World Health Organization stated the urgent need for international and national strategies to control the inappropriate use of antimicrobials (WHO, 2018). In consequence, the National Institute for Health and Care Excellence responded by stating that antimicrobial stewardship be operationalised in all settings (2015a). Therefore, individual health care professionals at both the prescriber and administrator level must consider the utility of this medication in supporting ongoing health and well-being.

KEY POINTS

- Establish if the patient has had resistance to treatments previously
- Consider past medical history, does the patient have reoccurring infections
- Focus on holistic support looking at social, economic, physical and mental health factors

PRESCRIBER

- Consider the patient's individual health needs.
- Consider the health needs of the wider population.
- Prescribe the shortest and most effective course of treatment.
- Check the patient understands the dosage and consequences of not completing the course of treatment (NICE, 2015a).

CLINICAL STAFF

- Make sure you are aware of relevant infection control policies and can advise patients on how to prevent/reduce the risk of infection.
- Have an awareness of signs and symptoms of systemic infection and sepsis (Public Health England, 2019).

Storage of Medicines

In line with legal requirements and local policies, it is part of the nurse's role to ensure that medicines are safely stored. The following principles apply to all situations involving the storage and administration of medicines:

KEY POINTS

- In some situations, the patient may self-administer medication. Local policy, usually involving a risk assessment, must be followed in relation to access to locked medication cupboards. Whilst it may be decided that the patient can access this independently, the storage cupboard must not be accessible to others
- If medication cannot be administered because it has passed its expiration date or has been stored incorrectly (i.e., at an inappropriate temperature), it must be disposed of correctly. This may well involve contacting the local health care provider or pharmacy for guidance

PROCEDURE

1. In compliance with the Medicines Act (1968), all medicines, lotions, and reagents must be stored in locked cupboards. Drugs for emergency use (e.g. cardiac arrest) may be kept with the emergency equipment in a sealed container, and must be replaced immediately after use.
2. All medicines, including emergency drugs and intravenous fluids, must be stored in an environment that meets the manufacturers' recommendations (e.g. minimum or maximum temperature).
3. Contents of boxes of dose units' (e.g. intravenous fluids, sterile topical fluids and ampoules should not be emptied out of their original containers and stored loose as this has been identified as a contributory factor in medication errors [Keers et al., 2013]).
4. Medication cupboards, must be locked when not in use. If a drug trolley is used, this must also be locked and immobilised when not in use.
5. Controlled drugs must be kept separate from other medicines, and the keys to the controlled drugs cupboard kept separately from other drug keys. A controlled drugs register must also be kept and audited regularly in line with local policy and national guidance.
6. All medications must be date checked and rotated so they are used before their expiry date. Regular checks of stored medication must be made to ensure that stock rotation is effective. The stock list of medications kept in the clinical area is agreed by pharmacy staff and the senior nurse.
7. The security of medications is the responsibility of the nurse in charge of the clinical area. No unauthorised person must be allowed access to the keys (refer to local policy regarding who has authorised access to the keys).

Drug Calculations

It is sometimes necessary to perform drug calculations for accurate administration of prescribed medications. Whilst you must be able to perform simple drug calculations using the formulas provided in the following sections, it is acceptable to check your answers using a calculator.

KEY POINTS

- Where medication requires two registered healthcare professionals, to calculate the dose, perform the calculations separately and then compare answers. This provides an additional safety measure that is not present if you work together on the calculation
- If you feel that the calculation is correct but that the medication to be administered is either too much or too little, check the prescription within a drug formulary

PROCEDURE: CONVERTING FROM ONE UNIT OF MEASUREMENT TO ANOTHER

It is sometimes necessary to convert from one unit of measurement to another to ensure that the correct amount of medication is administered. To convert units, you need to know the following:

1. 1 kilogram (kg) = 1000 grams (g)
2. 1 gram (g) = 1000 milligrams (mg)
3. 1 milligram = 1000 micrograms (mcg)

To convert grams (g) to milligrams (mg) or milligrams (mg) to micrograms (mcg), you need to multiply by 1000. This is achieved by moving the decimal point three places to the right (e.g. 6.5 mg × 1000 = 6500 mcg).

To convert micrograms (mcg) into milligrams (mg) or milligrams (mg) to grams (g), you need to divide by 1000. This is achieved by moving the decimal point three places to the left (e.g., 2500 mcg = 2.5 mg).

PROCEDURE: PERCENTAGE CONCENTRATION AND RATIOS

Some drug concentration may be measured as a percentage (%) or weight to volume (w/v). The percentage equates to the number of grams (weight) per 100 millilitres (volume), and the percentage remains constant, irrespective of the size of the container. i.e.:

- 1% lignocaine means 1 g of lignocaine dissolved in every 100 mL (i.e.1000 mg per 100 mL or 10 mg per mL).
- 5% glucose means 5 g of glucose dissolved in every 100 mL (i.e. 5000 mg per 100 mL or 50 mg per mL).

Occasionally, drug concentrations are written as ratios. The ratio 1:1000 equates to 1 g per 1000 mL, and the ratio: 1:10,000 equates to 1 g per 10,000 mL, e.g. adrenaline (epinephrine) 1:1000 (1 g per 1000 mL):

= 1000 mg per 1000 mL

= 1 mg per mL

e.g. adrenaline (epinephrine) 1: 10,000 (1 g per 10,000 mL)

= 1000 mg per 10,000 mL

= 1 mg per 10 mL

= 0.1 mg per mL

PROCEDURE: CALCULATING THE NUMBER OF TABLETS REQUIRED

To calculate the correct number of tablets, consider what you want and what you have, presented here as dose prescribed and dose per measure:

$$\text{number of measures required (i.e. tablets)} = \frac{\text{dose prescribed}}{\text{dose pre measure}}$$

Your first action is to convert the amount required into the same units of measurement as the tablets, then use the formula.

For example, 1 g of paracetamol is prescribed. Paracetamol is available in 500 mg tablets so you what is prescribed, and thus what you want, is 1000 mg:

$$1g = 1000 \text{ mg}$$

$$\text{number of tablets} = \frac{1000 \text{ mg}}{500 \text{ mg}}$$

$$= 2 \text{ tablets to be given}$$

Convert 1 g = 1000 mg
1000/500 = 2
2 tablets required

PROCEDURE: CALCULATING THE VOLUME TO GIVE OR DRAW UP

To calculate the correct volume, use the following formula:

$$\text{volume to give} = \frac{\text{dose required}}{\text{dose available}} \times \text{volume available}$$

For example, 75 mg of pethidine is prescribed. Pethidine is dispensed in ampoules containing 100 mg in 2 mL

$$\text{volume to give} = \frac{75}{100} \times 2 = 1.5 \text{ ml}$$

PROCEDURE: CALCULATING INFUSION RATES

This is covered in 'managing safe infusion therapy and blood transfusions', 'regulating flow rate' (see chapter 12)

Oral Route

Where possible, oral administration route is preferred as it is non-invasive and thus unlikely to introduce infection, not usually painful and not administered via a route that compromises privacy and dignity. Regular medications are often given orally, however, there are safety aspects to consider, you will need to assess if the patient can tolerate oral medication.

KEY POINTS

- Patients cannot be forced to take medication, and if the patient consistently refuses medication, resulting in a detrimental impact to health, the healthcare professional must check that accurate and understandable information has been provided, and the patient has capacity to make informed choices. Any medications declined must be referred to the prescriber. If there is a query over mental capacity, then local policies must be followed.
- The covert administration of medication can only be if the patient has been assessed as lacking capacity to decide, and the multidisciplinary team has agreed it is in the best interests of the patient to provide the medication (RPS, 2019). A care plan, stipulating this, must be included in the patient's notes
- If the patient appears to unable to swallow, a swallow assessment must be completed and the prescriber consulted for alternative route consideration.

EQUIPMENT

- Medications to be administered
- Medicine pots for tablets and measuring for liquids as required, oral syringes, tablet cutter
- Prescription chart
- Drug reference book or electronic version (e.g. British National Formulary)

PROCEDURE

1. Ask/assist the patient to assume a position that allows easy swallowing.
2. Make sure the patient has appropriate fluid with which to take the medication.
3. Decontaminate hands. Additional protective clothing may be necessary if indicated by the patient's condition (see Chapter 2).
4. Check the '9 rights' (Elliot and Liu, 2010) and follow the principles of administration as described on pages 195 to 196.
5. Calculate the volume of liquid or number of tablets or capsules required to achieve the prescribed dose (see p. 201). Do not break tablets unless they are scored across the middle. Use the tablet cutter to cut these tablets. If unsure if the tablet can be cut check the reference guide and if still unsure check with the ward pharmacist.
6. Dispense the prescribed amount into a medicine pot. If not in a blister pack, shake the tablets/capsules into the top of the container before transferring to the medicine pot to avoid handling them. Liquid preparations may involve the use of a measuring medicine pot or be drawn up in an oral syringe for the accuracy of measurement. When using an oral syringe, you can transfer the solution to a medicine pot.
7. Repeat this procedure for all oral medicines that are due.
8. Ensure you continue to follow the nine rights (Elliot and Liu, 2010).
9. Dispose of any packaging, disposable medicine pots, single-use syringes or other single-use equipment in the appropriate clinical waste.
10. Document the medications administered according to local policy.
11. Clean used equipment as appropriate and according to local policy.
12. Once you have left the patient's surroundings, decontaminate hands.

Administration of Nose Drops/ Nasal Spray

Medication is administered via the nasal route in both the community and hospital settings (Bailey et al., 2017). This can include immediate delivery of analgesics and sedatives after trauma (Johansson et al., 2013) and management of long-term conditions such as allergic rhinitis, depression, and migraines (NICE, 2018).

Medication can be easily administered via this route when others may not be accessible, such as when attempting intravenous access is challenging (Tucker et al., 2018), and the rapid delivery time of between 5 to 15 minutes is also beneficial (NICE, 2018). Whilst this route has been traditionally used in paediatrics, it is now becoming increasingly common in the adult setting (Bailey et al., 2017) .

KEY POINTS

- Explain to the patient that they must not sniff whilst spraying, if they do the medication will pass through the nasal cavity into the mouth where it will be swallowed and thus ineffective
- If the patient is self-administering their medication, the nurse should check the patient is aware of the manufacturer's guidance and able to follow it.

EQUIPMENT

- Medication administration record or patient group directive
- Nose drops/nasal spray as prescribed
- Clean tissues
- PPE as appropriate

PROCEDURE

1. Explain the procedure to gain informed consent and cooperation.
2. For nose drops, ask the patient to lie down or sit in a chair where they can hyperextend their neck. A pillow under the shoulders is beneficial.
3. For nasal sprays, the patient should be sitting upright with the head tilted slightly forward with the chin resting on the chest.
4. Decontaminate hands. Additional protective clothing may be necessary if indicated by the patient's condition (see Chapter 2).
5. Check the '9 rights' (Elliot and Liu, 2010) and follow the principles of administration as described on pages 195 to 196. Note whether the drops/spray are to be instilled into one or both nostrils.
6. If required, ask the patient to clear their nostrils by either blowing their nose or wiping the inside of the nostrils with a moistened tissue.

For nose drops:

7. Ask the patient to blow their nose (if able and not contraindicated).
8. Ask the patient to hyperextend their neck.
9. Remove the cap from the nose drops container and place it on the end to avoid contamination.
10. Using the dropper, administer the correct number of drops into each nostril, taking care not to touch the nose with the dropper. Replace cap.
11. Ask the patient to remain in this position for at least 2 minutes to allow absorption of the medication.
12. Wipe away any excess medication with a tissue or other suitable disposable item.

For nasal spray:

13. Ask the patient to blow their nose (if not contraindicated).
14. Remove the cap from the spray.
15. Shake the spray if required by manufacturer's instructions.
16. Ask the patient to bed the head so that the chin rests on the chest (Bartle, 2017).
17. Insert the spray just inside the nostril.
18. Ask the patient to inhale at the same time as activating the spray.
19. Repeat in the other nostril if prescribed. Replace cap.
20. Ask the patient to refrain from blowing their nose for about 20 minutes and instruct them not to sniff too vigorously following administration.
21. Check the patient is comfortable.
22. Discard any used tissues into clinical waste.
23. Return the nose drops/ nasal spray to the appropriate storage area.
24. Decontaminate hands.
25. Document administration on the prescription chart in accordance with local policy.
26. Evaluate the effect and report any abnormalities.

Pulmonary/Respiratory Route: Inhaler, Nebuliser

Inhalers and nebulisers are used in both the acute and long-term management of respiratory conditions (NICE, 2017; NICE, 2017a; NICE, 2019a; O'Driscoll et al., 2017). With inhalers, the types of inhaler can be metered dose, breathe-actuated, or dry powder (BMA and RPS, 2020), choice of device is dependent on the person's ability to use and tolerate administration (Booth, 2016).

It is estimated that as much as 86% of people use their inhalers incorrectly (Lavorini et al., 2020), and this could be due to a lack of dexterity or poor technique. As such, it is recommended that a spacer is used to improve inhalation with metered devices, and this also has the additional benefit of reducing drug deposition that can lead to candidiasis (Lavorini et al., 2020).

Nebulisers are often used in immediate care or when inhalers are insufficient for management. These can be jet, usually seen in the clinical setting, as this requires compressed gas to break down the particles (Booth, 2016), in other settings a nebuliser box driven by air may be used.

KEY POINTS

- The nurse's role when medication is to be administered is to educate the patient to self-administer. This involves being aware of the correct technique for the specific device and supporting the patient to follow the manufacturer's guidance.
- Patients need to be provided with information on how to care for their equipment.

EQUIPMENT

- Appropriate inhaler, and spacer, if required or nebuliser mouthpiece or mask, nebuliser chamber, and prescribed medication
- Medication Administration Record
- PPE as appropriate

PROCEDURE

1. Explain the procedure, to gain cooperation and informed consent
2. Decontaminate hands. Additional protective clothing may be necessary if indicated by the patient's condition (see Chapter 2)
3. Check the '9 rights' (Elliot and Liu, 2010) and follow the principles of administration as described on pages 195 to 196. Check the inhaler or nebuliser against the Medication Administration Record.

Using metred dose or breathe-actuated inhaler (Fig. 14.1). Instruct the patient to:
4. Remove the cap and shake inhaler, usually 4 to 5 times.
5. Tell the patient to breathe out gently and make a seal around the mouthpiece. As they start to inhale, advise them to press the top of the canister to actuate the inhaler and breathe in slowly for 3 to 5 seconds.
6. Then hold their breath for a minimum of 10 seconds before exhaling gently.
7. Wait 30 seconds before taking another inhalation.

Using inhaler with volumatic spacer. Instruct the patient to:
8. Shake the inhaler and insert it into the end of the spacer.
9. Ask the patient to place their mouth around the mouthpiece of the spacer and press the canister once to release the drug into the spacer.
10. Ask them to breathe in and out slowly five times and then remove the spacer from their mouth. Note, the valve of the mouthpiece will move in and out as the patient breathes.
11. Wait 30 seconds before administering a second dose.

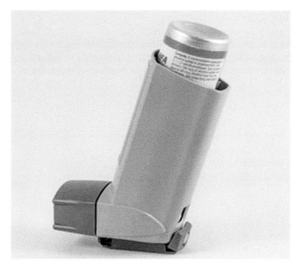

Fig. 14.1 Example pressurised metered-dose inhaler. (Kacmarek, R. M., Stoller, J, K., & Heuer, A. (2019). *Egan's Fundamentals of Respiratory Care*. Elsevier.)

Using dry powdered inhaler. Instruct the patient to:
12. Remove lid or cap.
13. Add dose as required.
14. Place mouthpiece into their mouth and make a firm seal.
15. Inhale deeply for 3 to 5 seconds.
16. Follow steps for a second dose, as required.
Using a Nebuliser:
17. Check that the liquid medication is sealed and in date.
18. Pour liquid into the nebuliser chamber.
19. Attach tubing to appropriate compressed gas, either oxygen or air, and to mouthpiece or face mask (if using a face mask ensure it is fitted correctly onto the patient).
20. Turn the flow rate up to 6 L/min to administer.
21. Observe the patient to ensure comfort and that no gas is escaping if using a mask.
22. If using a mouthpiece, provide correct instructions in accordance with the manufacturer's guidance.
With all methods:
23. Replace the inhaler cap on and return the inhaler into a locked cabinet or remove nebuliser equipment and dispose of equipment in clinical waste, if required.
24. Check the patient is comfortable.
25. Document effectiveness.

Administration of Ear Drops

Ears are an essential part of the sensory system and essential for both hearing and balance (Millwark, 2017). Therefore, ear health is important to well-being. The health of the ear can be affected by the buildup of cerebrum (ear wax) that can cause hearing loss, earache, tinnitus and vertigo (NICE, 2016a) as well as ear infections (Kilkenny, 2019). In many of these conditions, ear drops may be prescribed.

- Patients may be able to administer the medication themselves. If this is the case, observe the initial administration to check that the correct procedure is being followed.
- Ear drops are contraindicated when there is a perforated tympanic membrane (ear drum)

EQUIPMENT

- Medication administration chart
- Ear drops as prescribed
- Clean tissues or another appropriate disposable wipe

PROCEDURE

1. Explain the procedure, to gain informed consent and cooperation.
2. Explain the action of the ear drops and the expected outcome.
3. Decontaminate hands. Additional protective clothing may be necessary if indicated by the patient's condition (see Chapter 2).
4. Ask the patient to sit upright with their head tilted slightly away from the affected ear or to lie on their side with the affected ear uppermost.
5. Check the '9 rights' (Elliot and Liu, 2010) and follow the principles of administration as described on pages 195 to 196. Check the ear drops against the Medication Administration Chart, noting which ear is to have the drops instilled.
6. Check the patient is comfortable and can tolerate the position for the required timespan.
7. Remove the cap from the ear drops container and place on the end to avoid contamination.
8. Gently pull the pinna of the ear upwards and backwards (Fig. 14.2).

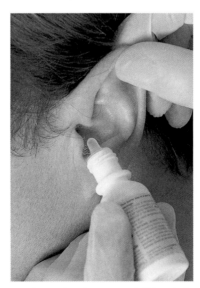

Fig. 14.2 Administration of prescribed drops into the ear canal. (Crisp, J., Douglas, C., Rebeiro, G., Sharma, S.K. & Waters, D. (2021). *Potter & Perry's Fundamentals of Nursing*, South Asia Edition. Elsevier Inc.)

9. Squeeze the bottle or dropper to dispense the prescribed number of drops into the ear, taking care not to touch the skin with the dropper.
10. Release the pinna.
11. Replace the cap.
12. Instruct the patient to remain in this position for 1 to 2 minutes to allow the drops to reach the eardrum.
13. When the patient is sitting upright, use the tissue to wipe away any excess fluid from the outer ear.
14. If prescribed, repeat the process in the other ear after 5 to 10 minutes.
15. Check the patient is comfortable.
16. Dispose of used tissues or other disposable wipes in clinical waste.
17. Return the nose drops/ nasal spray to the appropriate storage area.
18. Decontaminate hands.
19. Record administration on the Medication Administration Record.
20. Evaluate the effect of the ear drops and report any abnormalities in the nursing notes.

Administration of Eye Drops or Ointment

Eyes are an essential part of sensory system and thus eye health is essential for both physical and mental well-being. Both acute and chronic eye conditions, may require eye drops or ointments, these include corneal injury, glaucoma, and dry eye syndrome (NICE, 2017, 2017a, 2019b).

KEY POINTS

- Patients may well be able to administer the medication themselves. If this is the case observe the initial administration to check that the correct procedure is being followed.
- If there are signs of allergy do not administer the medication and alert the prescriber (Shaw, 2016)
- Remove contact lenses before administration

EQUIPMENT

- Medication administration record
- Eye drops and/or ointment as prescribed
- Low-linting gauze

PROCEDURE

1. Explain the procedure to gain informed consent and cooperation.
2. Instruct the patient to tilt their head backwards and look up or lie down, as able.
3. Explain that vision may be blurred for a short whilst after administration of the drops/ ointment.
4. Decontaminate hands. Additional protective clothing may be necessary if indicated by the patient's condition (see Chapter 2).
5. Check the '9 rights' (Elliot and Liu, 2010) and follow the principles of administration as described on pages 195–196. Check the eye drops against the Medication Administration Record, noting which eye is to have the drops/ointment instilled.

Eye drops:

6. Shake the bottle and remove the cap from the container, placing it on the end, or a pre-cleaned surface, to avoid contamination.

7. Using the low-linting gauze, gently pull the lower lid downwards to form a small pocket for the drops/ointment, usually with your non-dominant hand.

8. Hold the dispenser between your thumb and middle finger about 2 cm from the patient's eye, usually with your dominant hand.

9. Ask the patient to tilt head backwards and look up.

10. Press the bottom of the bottle with your forefinger to dispense the prescribed number of drops.

11. Ask the patient to close (but not squeeze) the eye for about 60 seconds to disperse the medication.

12. Repeat for the other eye if prescribed (see Fig. 14.3).

Eye ointment:

13. Remove the cap from the container and place it on the end, or a pre-cleaned surface, to avoid contamination.

14. Using low-linting gauze, gently pull the lower lid downwards.

15. Squeeze the tube gently until a small amount (approximately 1 to 2 cm) of ointment forms a 'ribbon'. Apply the ribbon inside the lid margin, from the inner to outer aspect of the eye. Do not touch any part of the eye with the tube.

16. Ask the patient to close (but not squeeze) their eyes to disperse the medication. They should keep their eyes closed for approximately 60 seconds.

17. Wipe away any excess medication that runs down the cheek with a clean tissue.

18. Repeat for the other eye if required.

19. Replace the cap of eye drops/ointment.

20. If more than one medication is required, repeat the process after 2 to 3 minutes.

Both methods:

21. Check the patient is comfortable and that vision has returned to normal.

22. Dispose of used gauze in clinical waste.

23. Return the eye drops/ointment to the appropriate storage area.

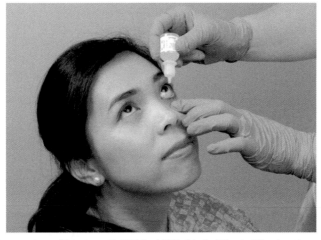

Fig. 14.3 Instilling eye drops. (Stromberg, H. (2021). *deWit's Medical-Surgical Nursing: Concepts & Practice*, 4th ed. Elsevier Inc.)

24. Decontaminate hands.
25. Document administration on the Medication Administration Record.
26. Evaluate the effect of the drops/ointment in the nursing records and report any abnormalities.

Topical Application

Topical medication application commonly refers to creams and ointments applied to the skin such as corticosteroids for eczema and contact dermatitis (BMA and RPS, 2020) but also refers to transdermal patches, commonly used for pain management in long-term conditions (NICE, 2019c), eyes and ear drops, and wound dressings. As eyes and ear drop administration have been described on p. 208 and 209 and wound care in chapter 15, this section focuses on skin applications, including transdermal patches.

KEY POINTS

- If a patient presents with an opioid analgesic patch on admission, notify the prescribing team to ensure that appropriate analgesia is continued.
- In the in-patient setting, nicotine replacement therapy needs to be considered for smokers and this may well include a patch.
- Site of administration should be alternated every time a patch is changed, in accordance with manufacturer's instructions.
- Do not administer a transdermal patch if signs of inflammation (i.e. redness, swelling, heat).

EQUIPMENT

- Take appropriate measures to ensure privacy and dignity (i.e. (do not disturb) clip on a curtain or sign on a door)
- Medication Administration Record
- Cream, ointment, lotion, or topical patch as prescribed
- Nonsterile gloves and sterile gauze to apply cream/lotion/ointment

PROCEDURE

1. Explain the procedure to gain cooperation and informed consent.
2. In many instances' patients will apply the cream, ointment or patch themselves. The nurse should thus ensure that they are applying it correctly.
3. Decontaminate hands. Where required, wear a single-use disposable plastic apron. Additional protective clothing may be necessary if indicated by the patient's condition (see Chapter 2).
4. Check the '9 rights' (Elliot and Liu, 2010) and follow the principles of administration as described on pages 195–196. Check the lotion/ointment/patch against the prescription.
5. Locate the appropriate part of the body and assess the skin.
Topical Patch:
6. Remove backing and apply the patch to clean, dry skin. Ensure that you are following the manufacturer's instructions.
Topical cream, ointment, or lotion:
7. Put on gloves and rub in with a piece of low-linting sterile gauze. Your gloves will protect you from absorption of the active ingredients.

All methods:
8. Check the patient is comfortable.
9. Remove apron and gloves and discard, with the used gauze, in clinical waste.
10. Decontaminate hands.
11. Document both the site of administration and the condition of the skin in accordance with local policy.

Vaginal Preparations

Per vaginum topical application and pessaries are usually prescribed for vaginal dryness, commonly oestrogen for post-menopausal women (NICE, 2015b) and candidiasis infections (NICE, 2017b). As such, the prescriber needs to consider when this route would be most appropriate, and the healthcare professional administering the medication must be able to effectively administer and where appropriate educate and support the patient to self-administer.

KEY POINTS

- Note the prescription time. It is best to administer vaginal medications at night where the patient will remain recumbent for several hours.
- Be aware of side effects. Some medications may cause temporary stinging, but prolonged discomfort is suggestive of a reaction and will warrant removal of cream or ointment

---

EQUIPMENT

Maintain privacy and dignity by closing curtains, providing screens, or closing the door.
   A (do not disturb) clip or sign can also be used
Medication Administration Record
Equipment tray
Cream or pessary as prescribed
Vaginal applicator
Low-linting gauze swabs
Protective pad as required
Disposable clinical waste bag

PROCEDURE

1. Explain the procedure, to gain cooperation and informed consent.
2. Wherever possible, the woman should be assisted as necessary to administer the cream or pessary herself. If this is not possible, ask/assist her to lie on her back with her heels together, knees bent and legs apart.
3. Decontaminate hands. Put on nonsterile gloves and a single-use disposable apron. Additional protective clothing may be necessary if indicated by the patient's condition (see Chapter 2).
4. Check the '9 rights' (Elliot and Liu, 2010) and follow the principles of administration as described on pages 195–196. Check the pessary/cream/ointment/other against the Medication Administration Record.

When administering a pessary or cream into the vagina:

5. Remove the pessary from the packaging and insert into the applicator. If using a vaginal cream, this is usually pre-loaded in the applicator. Place in equipment tray.
6. Raise the bed to a safe working height to avoid stooping. Advise the patient of this before doing so.
7. Place an absorbent pad under the patient's buttocks.
8. Ask patient to bend knees, bring feet together and then relax her knees. Help into position as necessary.
9. Expose the genital area and retract the labia to expose the vagina. Gently insert the applicator into the vagina as far as is comfortable.
10. Holding the applicator, press the plunger to release the pessary or cream high in the vagina.
11. Remove the applicator and place in the tray. Wipe away any traces of cream and remove the absorbent pad. Discard all waste into the clinical waste bag.

Application of topical cream/ointment:

12. Follow steps 2 to 5 as outlined above.
13. Apply in accordance with the manufacturer's instructions and prescription.

Both methods:

14. Offer the patient a liner or pad to protect underwear. Replace bedclothes.
15. Remove gloves and place in a clinical waste bag.
16. Check the patient is comfortable and lower the bed to a safe height. Ask the patient to remain recumbent for as long as they are able, up to 30 minutes.
17. Remove apron and decontaminate hands.
18. Document administration according to local policy.
19. Evaluate the effect of medication and document any adverse reactions in nursing records.

Rectal Route: Administration of Suppositories

Medications are given rectally for numerous reasons that include enemas, usually for constipation (Peate, 2014), suppositories or topical application for acute episodes of haemorrhoids (NICE, 2016b), but also for the treatment of seizures (NICE, 2020) and it can also be considered as an alternative route when the oral route is not appropriate. As such, the prescriber needs to consider when this route would be most appropriate, and the healthcare professional administering the medication must be able to effectively administer and where appropriate educate and support the patient to self-administer.

KEY POINTS

- Be aware that the patient may prefer a different person to administer the rectal medication, and this could be due to cultural, personal, or religious reasons. In all instances, the patient's wishes should be respected (NMC, 2018).

EQUIPMENT

Draw the curtains, screen, or door closed and apply a (do not disturb) sign where possible to ensure dignity, privacy, and comfort

Medication Administration Record

Suppositories as prescribed
Equipment tray
Lubricant
Small clinical waste bag
Gauze swabs

PROCEDURE

1. Explain the procedure, to gain informed consent and cooperation.
2. Decontaminate hands. Put on single-use disposable gloves and apron. Additional protective clothing may be necessary if indicated by the patient's condition (see Chapter 2).
3. Depending on the reason and type of medication, the bowels should be opened prior to administration if possible.
4. A rectal examination to assess whether faecal matter is present may be performed by a competent healthcare professional prior to administration of suppositories designed to relieve constipation.
5. Ask/assist patient to remove clothing below the waist, and lie in the left lateral position.
6. Place an absorbent pad under the buttocks.
7. Check the '9 rights' (Elliot and Liu, 2010) and follow the principles of administration as described on pages 195–196. Check the suppository against the Medication Administration Record.

Suppository administration:

8. Remove all packaging around the suppository.
9. Squeeze some lubricant onto a piece of gauze and lubricate the blunt end of the suppository.
10. Raise the bed to a safe working height to avoid stooping and advise the patient of this.
11. Pull back the bedclothes and ask the patient to lie in the left lateral position with knees drawn up.
12. With your left hand, part the patient's buttocks and visualise the anus, noting any haemorrhoids or skin tags that may make insertion difficult.
13. Warn the patient that they will feel the suppository being inserted into the rectum.
14. Ask the patient to relax; encouraging deep breathing may help.
15. Gently insert the suppository into the anal canal blunt end first, using the index finger of your right hand.
16. Repeat the process if more than one suppository is required.
17. Wipe away excess traces of lubricant from the anal area and remove gloves.
18. If it is an evacuant suppository (e.g. glycerine or bisacodyl), leave the patient in a comfortable position with a call bell at hand. To be effective, the suppositories need to remain in position for at least 15 minutes (Peate, 2014) and patients should be discouraged from opening their bowels before this time.

Application of topical cream/ointment:

19. Follow steps 2 to 5 as outlined above.
20. Apply in accordance with the manufacturer's instructions and prescription.

Both Methods:

21. Replace bedclothes and lower the bed.
22. Place all used equipment, gloves and apron in clinical waste and wash decontaminate hands.
23. Document administration of the suppository as per local policy.
24. Document the effect of the suppository and report any adverse effects.

Subcutaneous Injection

Injections administered via the subcutaneous route (SC) are injected into the fatty layer underneath the epidermis and dermis. Examples of medications that are commonly administered via this route are insulin and low molecular weight heparins. Fluids can also be infused via the subcutaneous route for hydration purposes.

These subcutaneous injections provide a slow, sustained release of medication and are used when the medication is not irritant, and the total volume injected to be injected does not exceed (Shepherd, 2018). Both prescriber and administrator need to check that the most appropriate route for medication efficacy is being used.

There are several sites suitable for the administration of subcutaneous injections (Fig. 14.4). For a patient receiving regular, daily, injections, the sites will need to be rotated to prevent potential tissue damage (Ogston-Tuck, 2014). When administering via this route, you will require a 23G (blue) or 25G (orange) with a length of 4 to 6 mm or an insulin needle for SC injections (Shepherd, 2018). These need to be short enough so they do not reach the muscle.

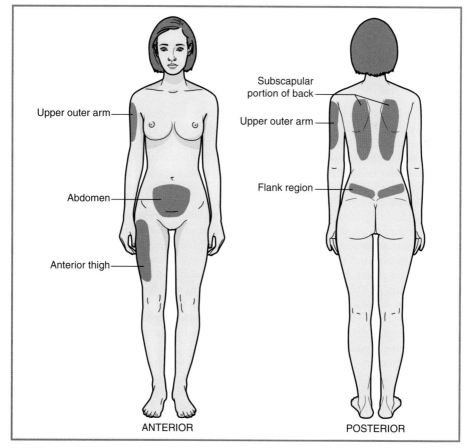

Fig. 14.4 Common sites for subcutaneous injection. (Niedzwiecki, B., Pepper, J., & Weaver, P. A. (2020). *Kinn's The Clinical Medical Assistant: An Applied Learning Approach*, 14th ed. Elsevier.)

KEY POINTS

- The patient may require the skin to be cleaned and request that this is done with an alcohol-impregnated swab. It is the healthcare professional's role to advise that this is no longer supported as evidence suggests that this can cause the skin to harden over time this will be specifically relevant to those receiving daily injections.
- There may be some situations where a 90-degree angle is used, but this is highly unusual and would only occur if a patient were extremely underweight. A clinical decision on the utility of the medication would need to be considered in this instance.

EQUIPMENT

- Patient's medication administration chart
- Prescribed medication (this is often a pre-filled syringe with a needle)
- Equipment tray, cleaned with a hard surface wipe
- Syringe of appropriate size (0.5 to 2 mL) as required
- Blue (23G) or orange (25G) sterile needle as required
- Draw the curtains, screen, or door closed and apply a do not disturb sign where possible to ensure dignity, privacy, and comfort
- Non-linting gauze
- Sharps container

PROCEDURE

1. Explain the procedure to gain informed consent and cooperation.
2. Ask/assist the patient to choose the site of injection.
3. Decontaminate hands.
4. A single-use disposable apron should be worn and potentially nonsterile latex-free gloves, depending on local policy.
5. Protective clothing may also be necessary if indicated by the patient's condition (see Chapter 2).
6. Check the '9 rights' (Elliot and Liu, 2010) and follow the principles of administration as described on pages 195–196. Check the medication against the prescription.
7. If using a pre-filled syringe, do not expel the air bubble, as this is designed to remain in the syringe, next to the piston. When the small amount of drug is given, the air fills the needle hub/nozzle of the syringe and needle, ensuring that all fluid has been expelled from the syringe. This prevents the drug from tracking back to the surface as the needle is withdrawn, which can cause skin irritation and discomfort (Ogston-Tuck, 2014).
8. If drawing up the medication, open the syringe packaging at the plunger end and remove the syringe, check that the packaging is intact, and in date. Check that the plunger will move freely inside the barrel.
9. Taking care not to touch the nozzle end, hold the syringe in one hand and open the needle packaging at the hilt (coloured) end (ideally a drawing up needle should be used here), check that the packaging is both intact and in date. Attach the needle firmly to the syringe and loosen, but do not remove, the needle cover (sheath). Place in the cleaned equipment tray.
10. If a glass ampoule of liquid is being used, ensure that all the contents are in the bottom of the ampoule, then break off the top using a clinical wipe or another appropriate item, to protect your fingers. If a plastic ampoule is being used, break off the top, taking care not to touch the top of the ampoule with your fingers.

11. Pick up the syringe and needle, allowing the loosened needle cover to slide off into the tray or receiver.
12. If using an ampoule, carefully insert the needle into the solution, taking care not to allow it to scrape against the bottom of the ampoule.
13. Draw back on the plunger, using your thumb and middle finger on the plunger with your first finger against the flange of the syringe until the required amount is in the syringe.
14. If the medicine is in powder form, draw up the diluent, then clean the rubber stopper with an alcohol-impregnated wipe for 30 seconds and leave to dry for 30 seconds (Loveday et al., 2014) and inject the appropriate amount of diluent into the ampoule/vial. Mix thoroughly by gently agitating the ampoule/vial until the powder has dissolved.
15. Now drawing up the same amount of air as liquid solution is required. This will produce a negative pressure ensuring easy withdrawal of the solution.
16. Then holding the ampoule/vial upside down at eye level, pull back the plunger to draw the liquid into the syringe. Make sure that the needle remains below the surface of the liquid to prevent any air from being drawn into the syringe.
17. Replace the ampoule back into the equipment tray and change to the appropriately sized needle using a non-touch technique. If using gloves, these will need to be removed, and hand hygiene performed, before donning a new set of disposable latex-free gloves.
18. Hold the syringe upright at eye level and encourage any air to rise to the top of the syringe. Gently tap the barrel of the syringe if necessary to make air bubbles rise to the top. Then, expel the air by gently pressing the plunger until droplets of liquid are seen at the top of the needle.
19. Now, approach the patient with the equipment tray and prescription chart. If in the secondary care setting, you may well need to raise the bed to a safe working height to avoid stooping.
20. Select the site of administration and ask/assist the patient to adopt a suitable position, if necessary, and expose the chosen injection site.
21. Clean the skin using soap and water if visible soiled (WHO, 2010).
22. Pinch up the skin using the thumb and first finger of your non-dominant hand and insert the short needle into the subcutaneous tissue at an angle of 90 degrees (Fig. 14.5).
23. Keeping the skin pinched, inject the solution slowly. On completion, pause briefly, up to 10 seconds, before withdrawing the needle to prevent the seeping into the dermis (Fig. 14.6).

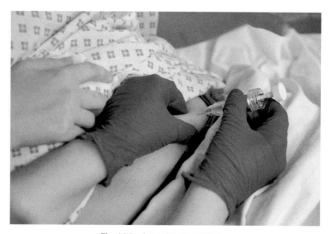

Fig. 14.5 Inserting the needle.

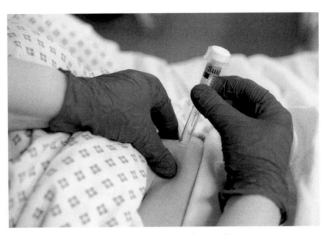

Fig. 14.6   Withdrawing the needle.

24. Do not massage the site as this affects the absorption of the drug and increases the risk of capillary damaging and bruising (Shepherd, 2018).
25. If required, use the gauze to wipe away any blood.
26. Dispose of the syringe and needle into the sharp's container immediately. Never re-sheath the needle.
27. Lower the bed. Check the patient is comfortable and is aware of the effects and side effects of the medication. Advise that there may well be local irritation at the injection site but that this is temporary.
28. Dispose of any waste, gloves, and apron in the clinical waste.
29. Decontaminate hands.
30. Sign the prescription chart as per local policy to indicate that the medication has been administered. Document the site of injection as well as any abnormalities or complications with the procedure.
31. Store medications according to the manufacturer's guidance. Some medications (e.g. insulin) must be kept in the refrigerator.

Intramuscular Injection

Intramuscular (IM) injections are used when rapid absorption of medication is required as they deliver medication into the well-perfused muscle beneath the subcutaneous tissue. The onset of action usually occurs within 10 to 15 minutes after the injection so could be given for anti-emetics and analgesics when there is a need for swift management and peripheral access is challenging.

Unlike the subcutaneous route, intramuscular injections allow for a larger volume of fluid, up to 5 mL in adults (Ogston-Tuck, 2014). Key sites for intramuscular injection in adults are:

- Ventrogluteal site (Fig. 14.7)
- Deltoid site (see Fig. 14.7)
- Vastus lateralis site (see Fig. 14.7)
- Rectus femoris site

All intramuscular injections should be given at a 90-degree angle so that the needle reaches the muscle and to minimise pain (Ogston-Tuck, 2014). Needle gauge and length are essential factors to consider when giving injections via this route to ensure that delivery is given into the

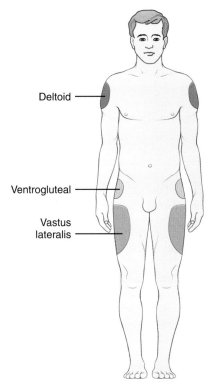

Fig. 14.7 The deltoid, ventrogluteal and vastus lateralis are the most common intramuscular injection sites. (Dehn, R. & Asprey, D. (2021). *Essential Clinical Procedures*, 4th ed. Elsevier Inc.)

muscle (Greenway, 2014). As such, it is essential that each patient should be assessed individually before the procedure to enable accurate selection of needle length.

KEY POINTS

- If the patient is undernourished, (cachexic), a different needle length and gauge may be used. In rare instances, the angle of injection may be reduced to 45 degrees
- Make sure that you follow local drug policy, and some medications will require two staff to check the prescription and observe the administration
- Ensure that the z-track technique is used; not doing so poses the risk of the vesicant or irritant to seep back into the subcutaneous tissue and cause pain

EQUIPMENT

- Patient's medication administration record
- Prescribed medicine and diluent, if required
- Cleaned equipment tray
- Sterile syringe of appropriate size (2 to 5 mL)
- Sterile needle-usually green (21G) for adult patients
- Alcohol-impregnated swab

- Low-linting gauze
- Sharps container

PROCEDURE

1. Explain the procedure, to gain informed consent and cooperation.
2. Decontaminate hands. A single-use disposable apron and nonsterile gloves should be worn. Protective clothing may also be necessary if indicated by the patient's condition (see Chapter 2).
3. Check the '9 rights' (Elliot and Liu, 2010) and follow the principles of administration as described on pages 195–196. Check the medication against the prescription.
4. Follow steps 3 to 16 of subcutaneous injection (see p. 216).
5. Use the z-track track to pull the subcutaneous tissue away from the muscle.
6. Hold the syringe like a dart in your dominant hand, advise the patient that you will be administering the medication and insert the needle swiftly and firmly at an angle of 90 degrees to the skin.
7. Depress the plunger steadily and slowly, administering the liquid in 10 seconds or less, until the syringe is empty.
8. Quickly and smoothly withdraw the needle from the skin and press firmly on the site with the gauze until any bleeding ceases.
9. Do not resheathe the needle. Discard it, still attached to the syringe, into the sharp's container.
10. Assist the patient into a comfortable position and replace the bed clothes. Lower the bed to a safe height.
11. Dispose of any waste, gloves and aprons in the clinical waste.
12. Decontaminate hands.
13. Document administration according to local policy.
14. Check for the desired effect and for any side effects, especially if administering an analgesic or anti-emetic. Document and report any complications or adverse reactions.

References

Bailey, A.M., Baum, R.A., Horn, K., et al., 2017. Review of intranasally administered medications for use in the Emergency Department. J. Emerg. Med. 53 (1), 38–48.

Bartle, J., 2017. How to use a corticosteroid nasal spray. Nurs. Stand. 31 (52), 41–43.

Booth, A., 2016. Nebulised therapy in respiratory disease management: best practice. Nurse Prescribing. 14 (12), 586–592.

British Medical Association & Royal Pharmaceutical Press, 2020. British National Formulary (BNF) 79. Pharmaceutical Press, London.

Cope, L.C., Abuzour, A.S., Tully, M.P., 2016. Non-medical prescribing: where are we now? Ther. Adv. Drug Saf. 7 (4), 165–172.

Department of Health and Social Security, 1986. Neighbourhood nursing: a focus for care. Her Majesty's Stationary Office, London.

Elliot, M., Liu, Y., 2010. The nine rights of medication administration: an overview. Br. J. Nurs. 19 (5), 300–305.

Greenway, K., 2014. Rituals in nursing: intramuscular injection. J. Clin. Nurs. 23 (24), 3583–3588.

Johansson, J., Sjöberg, J., Nordgren, M., et al., 2013. Prehospital analgesia using nasal administration of S-ketamine—a case series. Scand. J. Trauma Resusc. Emerg. Med. 21 (38), 1–5.

Keers, R.N., Williams, S.D., Cooke, J., et al., 2013. Causes of medication administration errors in hospitals: a systematic review of quantitative and qualitative evidence. Drug Saf. 36 (11), 1045–1067.

Kilkenny, N. (2019) The nurse's role in ear care: undertaking hearing assessment and ear cleaning. Br. J. Nurs. 28 (5), 281–283.

Lavorini, F., Barreto, C., van Boven, J.F.M., et al., 2020. Spacer & valved holding chambers—the risk of switching to different chambers. J. Allergy Clin. Immunol. 8 (5), 1569–1573.

Loveday, H., Wilson, J.A., Pratt, R.J., et al., 2014. National Evidence-Based Guidelines for Preventing Healthcare-Associated Infections in NHS Hospitals in England. J. Hosp. Infec. 86S1 (2014), S1–S70.

Gov.uk. (1968). Medicines Act, 1968. Chapter 67. https://www.legislation.gov.uk/ukpga/1968/67

Millwark, K., 2017. Ear care: an update for nurses (part 1). Pract. Nurs. 28 (4), 154–160.

National Institute for Health and Care Excellence, 2014. CG179 Pressure Ulcers: Prevention and Management. National Institute for Health and Care Excellence, London.

National Institute for Health and Care Excellence, 2015. Medicine Optimisation. National Institute for Health and Care Excellence, London.

National Institute for Health and Care Excellence, 2015a. NG15 Antimicrobial Stewardship: Systems and Processes for Effective Anti-microbial Use. National Institute for Health and Care Excellence, London.

National Institute for Health and Care Excellence, 2015b. Menopause: Diagnosis and Management. National Institute for Health and Care Excellence, London.

National Institute for Health and Care Excellence, 2016. NG46 Controlled Drugs: Safe Use and Management. National Institute for Health and Care Excellence, London.

National Institute for Health and Care Excellence, 2016a. NICE Clinical Knowledge Summaries: Earwax. https://cks.nice.org.uk/earwax#!scenario

National Institute for Health and Care Excellence,2016b. NICE Clinical Knowledge Summaries: Haemorrhoids. https://cks.nice.org.uk/haemorrhoids#!scenario

National Institute for Health and Care Excellence, 2017. Asthma: Diagnosis, Monitoring and Chronic Asthma Management. National Institute for Health and Care Excellence, London.

National Institute for Health and Care Excellence, 2017a. NICE Clinical Knowledge Summaries: Corneal Superficial Injury. https://cks.nice.org.uk/corneal-superficial-injury#!scenario

National Institute for Health and Care Excellence, 2017b. NICE Clinical Knowledge Summaries: Candida Female Genital: Uncomplicated Infection. https://cks.nice.org.uk/candida-female-genital

National Institute for Health and Care Excellence, 2018. NICE Clinical Knowledge Summaries: Allergic Rhinitis. https://cks.nice.org.uk/allergic-rhinitis#!scenario

National Institute for Health and Care Excellence, 2015. NG15 Antimicrobial Stewardship: Systems and Processes for Effective Antimicrobial Medicine Use. https://www.nice.org.uk/guidance/ng15/resources/antimicrobial-stewardship-systems-and-processes-for-effective-antimicrobial-medicine-use-pdf-1837273110469

National Institute for Health and Care Excellence, 2019a. Chronic Obstructive Pulmonary Disease in Over 16s: Diagnosis and Management. National Institute for Health and Care Excellence, London.

National Institute for Health and Care Excellence, 2019b. NICE Clinical Knowledge Summaries: Glaucoma. https://cks.nice.org.uk/glaucoma#!scenario.

National Institute for Health and Care Excellence, 2019c. Key Therapeutic Topic KTT21: Medicines Optimisation in Chronic Pain. National Institute for Health and Care Excellence, London.

National Institute for Health and Care Excellence, 2020, Treating Prolonged or Repeated Seizures and Status Epilepticus. National Institute for Health and Care Excellence, London.

Nursing and Midwifery Council, 2018. The Code: Professional Standards of Practice and Behaviour for Nurses and Midwives. Nursing & Midwifery Council, London.

O'Driscoll, B.R., Howard, L., Earis, J., et al., 2017. BTS Guideline for oxygen for oxygen use in adults in healthcare and emergency settings. Thorax. 72 (1), i1–i88.

Ogston-Tuck, S., 2014. Intramuscular injection technique: an evidence based approach, Nurs. Stand. 29 (4), 52–59.

Peate, I., 2014. How to administer an enema. Nurs. Stand. 30 (4), 34–36

Public Health England, 2019. Antimicrobial Resistance (AMR): Applying All Our Health. https://www.gov.uk/government/publications/antimicrobial-resistance-amr-applying-all-our-health/antimicrobial-resistance-amr-applying-all-our-health.

Royal College of Nursing, 2020. Medicines Management: An Overview for Nursing. Royal College of Nursing, London.

Royal Pharmaceutical Society, 2016. A Competency Framework for all Prescribers. Royal Pharmaceutical Society, London.

Royal Pharmaceutical Society, 2019. Professional Guidance on the Administration of Medications in Healthcare Settings. Royal Pharmaceutical Society, London.

Royal Pharmaceutical Society and Royal College of Nursing, 2019. Professional Guidance on the Administration of Medicines in Healthcare Settings. Royal Pharmaceutical Society, London.

Shaw, M., 2016. How to administer eye drops and ointments. Nurs. Stand. 30 (39), 34–6.

Shepherd, E., 2018. Injection technique 1: administering drugs via the intramuscular route. Nurs. Times. 114 (8), 23–25.

Tucker, C., Tucker, L., Brown, K., 2018. The intranasal route as an alternative method of medication administration. Crit. Care Nurse. 38 (5), 26–31. doi:10.4037/ccn2018836. PMID: 30275061.

Weeks, G., George, J., Maclure, K., et al., 2016. Non-medical prescribing for acute and chronic disease management in primary and secondary care (review). The Cochrane Database of Systematic Reviews Collaboration. Wiley, Chichester.

World Health Organization, 2010. WHO Best Practices for Injections and Related Procedures Toolkit. World Health Organization, Geneva.

World Health Organization, 2018. Antimicrobial Resistance. https://www.who.int/en/news-room/fact-sheets/detail/antimicrobial-resistance.

CHAPTER 15

Wound Care

Wound Assessment

The purpose of wound assessment is to gather and document information about the wound and surrounding skin, to ascertain whether the wound is healing, unchanged or deteriorating. A thorough assessment enables nurses to select the most appropriate type of wound dressing. There are a variety of wound assessment tools which provide a systematic approach and provide prompts, around key parameters to determine the condition of the wound (Peate and Glencross, 2015). An assessment tool should also identify factors that may adversely affect a person's ability to heal effectively, such as poor nutrition and poor circulation. Once the wound assessment is completed, an appropriate plan of care must be written with specific objectives to guide the management of the wound.

WOUND ASSESSMENT TOOLS

Most wound assessment tools incorporate consideration of factors known to influence wound healing:

1. Cause and type of wound—it is essential to identify and record the cause of the wound, when and how the wound occurred. Acute wounds may be described as traumatic caused by injury (including burns), or surgical intervention. Acute wounds usually heal quickly and without complication, provided that infection does not occur (Carlin, 2022). Chronic (or older) wounds may be caused by ischaemia (reduced blood supply) or pressure (such as a pressure ulcer), therefore, may take longer to heal. Pressure ulcers must be graded to determine their severity (see p. 288), and leg ulcers require specialised assessment by experienced practitioners (Munro & Beck, 2021. NMC, 2018).

2. Wound location—the location of the wound may have implications for the patient and influence the choice of dressing. For example, a sacral pressure ulcer may become contaminated with urine or faeces, the wound may be difficult to dress and the patient may feel uncomfortable if the dressing is too big. A deep laceration on a patient's hand may restrict their ability to work; a longer-lasting water-resistant dressing may be more appropriate.

3. Wound measurement—measurements of the size of the wound are recorded at the initial assessment and then usually weekly using the same tool. The simplest method is to use a disposable tape measure to record the length and width of the wound. The most accurate method is to trace around the wound margins using a transparent acetate sheet with a grid matrix; the surface area can then be calculated by counting the number of grid squares within the outline. Photography can be used to produce a figure of the wound with a transparent grid overlay, or with a ruler placed alongside the wound to show the size. The patient's confidentiality, privacy and dignity must be considered at all times, and photography must be used in accordance with local policy and the patient's informed consent.

4. Wound margins—when assessing a wound, it is essential to review the wound edges (margins). In the initial stages of a wound formation, the edges will usually be red and slightly raised due to the inflammatory response of the healing process. After 48 to 72 hours this should have settled, and the wound margins will start to appear paler as healing progresses. Finally, tissue migrates from the edges across the wound in the process of epithelialisation (see below). If wound edges appear red and raised in the later stages of wound healing (>72 hours from the wound forming), this may indicate a wound infection.

5. The appearance of the tissue type in the wound bed—there are five tissue types found in the wound bed, which indicate the stage of healing. These can be described by colour or descriptors.
   - Red—granulation tissue: this indicates a healing wound.
   - Pink/pale purple—epithelisation: this indicates the later stages of wound healing as new protein cells help to complete the wound repair.
   - Green—infected: indicates the presence of an infection.
   - Yellow—sloughy: this is devitalised tissue that may need a special dressing designed to lift it from the wound bed.
   - Black—necrotic: this is dead or ischaemic tissue that usually requires surgical removal.

Wounds may present with more than one tissue type. When a wound presents with a combination of tissue types, each must be documented with an estimated percentage. For example, 70% granulation, 10% slough and 20% epithelialisation

6. Presence of exudate—this refers to the type of exudate (colour, appearance and viscosity) and volume of exudate. Colour, appearance and viscosity can be assessed by inspecting the dressing when it is removed. However, assessing the volume of exudate is subjective and should be documented using descriptors such as minimal, moderate or large. A useful measurement entails recording the number of dressing changes, to determine if these have become more or less frequent. This is important as increasing exudate together with pain may indicate infection.

7. Odour—the presence of a an odour may indicate increasing infection. Heavily infected wounds can cause an offensive odour that can be detected before and after the wound dressing. Patients may feel embarrassed and uncomfortable in front of other people. Specialist dressings including activated charcoal dressings can help absorb odour.

8. Condition of the surrounding skin—it is important to assess and document the condition of the surrounding skin as this will provide information about the patent's general health status, and changes should alert the nurse to any changes. For example: dry, flaky and itchy skin may indicate eczema; dry and scaly skin may indicate dehydration; redness may be a sign of inflammation or injury (often present in the first 48 hours following an acute wound); or skin may appear white and spongy due to maceration (where the skin has become 'soggy'). It is good practice to determine the skin temperature by feeling the skin with the back of the hand.

9. Pain—the presence of pain will affect the comfort and wellbeing of the patient and is also likely to indicate a potential infection. As pain is unique to the individual, it is important to incorporate a pain assessment to determine the severity of the pain and any related issues.

10. Wound healing is complex—there are intrinsic factors such as age, malnutrition, dehydration, smoking, poor circulation, the patient's medical condition; and extrinsic factors, such as sustained pressure, medication, infection, poor surgical technique, poor wound management and the patient's environment. Psychological factors relating to body image, anxiety and grief may also affect the person's (Hussey & Young, 2020) response to a complex wound.

Performing a Wound Dressing Change

When carrying out a wound dressing change, the procedure should be performed using an aseptic non-touch technique (see below) (Denton and Hallan, 2020). Prior to the procedure the nurse must check the wound care plan and the current dressing to determine what type is being used and whether it has been adequate (e.g. whether more padding to absorb exudate is needed). The wound care plan should be followed which involves assessing the wound, noting any changes, and potentially changing the type of dressing depending on how the wound is healing. All healthcare professionals undertaking wound dressing changes must be competent in all elements of wound dressing technique and ANTT.

> **KEY FACTS**
>
> - The type of dressing pack will vary according to availability, individual preference and the type of wound.
> - Correct use of ANTT and prevention of infection can help to reduce the requirement for antimicrobial prescribing (page 5).

EQUIPMENT

Dressing trolley or other suitable surfaces

Dressing pack, a syringe (for irrigating the wound), cleansing solution and new dressing according to the wound care plan/local policy

Other equipment (e.g. scissors) as required

Alcohol hand-rub or handwashing facilities

Draw screens around the bed for privacy and ensure adequate light. Clear the bed area, close windows, turn off fans, and all other necessary actions to ensure that there is not a draft and the temperature is adequate.

PROCEDURE

1. Check wound care plan to determine the type of dressing required, frequency of change, and other key elements.
2. Decontaminate hands.
3. An apron should be worn. Additional protective clothing may be necessary if indicated by the patient's condition (see Chapter 2).
4. Explain the procedure to gain consent and cooperation. Do not leave the patient unattended on a raised bed.
5. Check patient comfort (e.g. convenience, position, need for the toilet).
6. Assess the wound dressing.
7. Administer analgesics as appropriate and allow time to take effect.
8. Adjust bedclothes to permit easy access to the wound but maintain warmth and dignity.
9. Clean the trolley or another appropriate surface according to local policy. (Loveday et al., 2014). If antimicrobial wipes impregnated with alcohol are indicated in the policy, those designed for hard surfaces (not skin wipes) must be used and allowed to dry thoroughly.
10. Gather the equipment, check that the equipment is intact, and thus sterile, and in date of all equipment and solutions. Place these on the bottom of the trolley or somewhere convenient (Fig. 15.1).

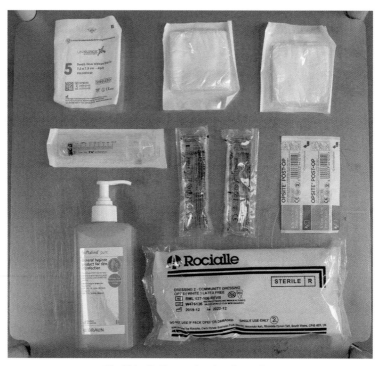

Fig. 15.1   Setting up the dressing trolley.

11. If scissors are needed to cut non-sterile tape, wash your scissors, dry thoroughly, clean with an alcohol-impregnated swab and place on the bottom of the trolley. If sterile scissors are needed (e.g. to cut a sterile dressing), these are usually packed separately.

12. Take the trolley to the bed area. Adjust the bed to a safe working height to avoid stooping. In some clinical areas, dressings are performed in a clean treatment room rather than at the bedside, to reduce the risk of cross-infection.

13. Remove the dressing pack from its outer packaging; place it on the clean trolley/surface.

14. Using your fingertips and touching the edges of the paper only, open the pack and lay it flat to create a sterile field (Figs. 15.2 and 15.3).

15. Carefully pick up the edge of the waste bag and place it at one corner of the sterile field. Some practitioners put their hand inside the clinical waste bag and use it as a 'glove' to arrange the sterile equipment on the trolley. The waste bag should be positioned so that used swabs can be discarded without passing over the sterile field.

16. Touching only the corner of the pack carefully move the gloves to the edge of the sterile field.

17. Taking care not to contaminate the sterile field, carefully pour the cleansing solution into the tray (Fig. 15.4). Open the dressing, syringe, and all other equipment detailed in the wound care plan, onto the sterile field.

18. Adjust bedclothes to expose the wound, then loosen the existing dressing, but do not remove it.

19. Decontaminate hands.

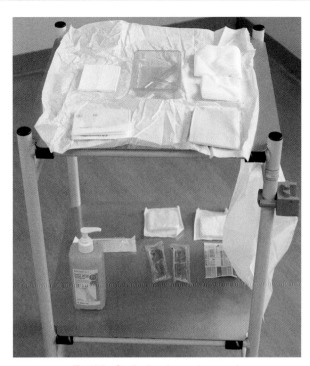

Fig. 15.2   Sterile dressing pack opened.

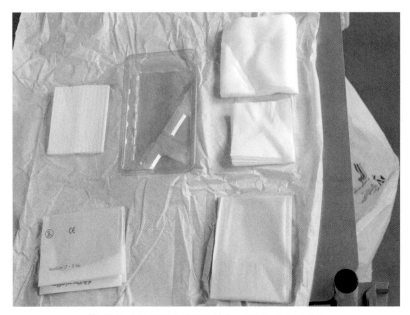

Fig. 15.3   Arranging contents of dressing pack on trolley.

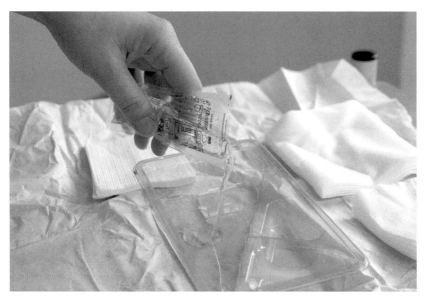

Fig. 15.4 Pouring cleaning solution into sterile tray.

20. Depending on local policy, either use unsterile gloves or open the yellow waste bag and put your hand inside so that the bag acts as a glove. Use this to remove the soiled dressing.

21. Inspect the dressing to determine the type and amount of exudate.

22. Taking care not to touch the outside of the gloves, put on the sterile gloves (see p. 2).

23. Fold the dressing towel over your fingertips to avoid contamination with the bedclothes or skin, and place close to the wound, if required.

24. Use a gauze swab dipped in cleansing solution to clean around the wound to remove blood, slough or exudate. Gauze should not be used to clean inside the wound as this has been shown to damage the delicate granulating tissue of a healing wound. In some clinical settings, the solution is warmed to prevent cooling and vasoconstriction at the wound site.

25. A syringe (usually 20 mL unless the wound is very large) should be used to gently irrigate any wound that needs cleaning (Figs. 15.5 and 15.6). Irrigation removes cellular debris, surface bacteria, wound exudate, dressing residue and residual topical agents (Fry, 2017)

26. To irrigate a wound, use a syringe primed with a solution in one hand and a gauze swab on the skin below the wound in the other. Making sure that neither the syringe nor gauze come into contact with the wound, allow the solution to flow into the wound, collecting the solution in the gauze swab held below the wound.

27. Use fresh gauze swabs to dry around the wound (not the wound itself), using each swab once only from the centre to the edges (Fig. 15.7). If there is any infection, swab from clean towards infected areas.

28. Gently apply the new dressing, making sure it is secure (Figs. 15.8 and 15.9).

29. Place any sharps (e.g. stitch cutters) in a sharps bin. Wrap all used disposable items in the sterile field and place in the waste bag. Remove gloves and discard in the waste bag. This should then be sealed/tied and placed in the clinical waste.

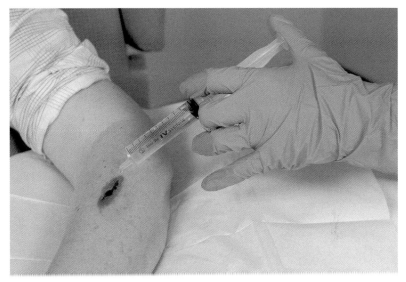

Fig. 15.5 Irrigating the wound.

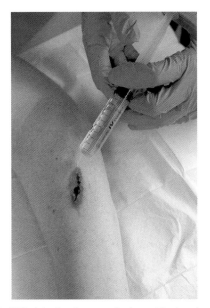

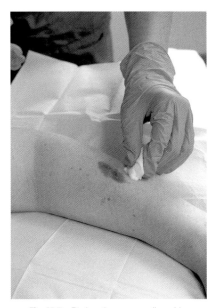

Fig. 15.6 Irrigating the wound using a 10 mL syringe.   **Fig. 15.7** Drying the surrounding skin.

30. Replace the bedclothes and assist the patient as necessary into a comfortable position. Readjust the bed to a safe height.
31. Remove apron, discard in the clinical waste and decontaminate hands.
32. Return any unused items to the stock cupboard. Clean the trolley according to local policy.
33. Document the dressing change and condition of the wound. Report any abnormalities.

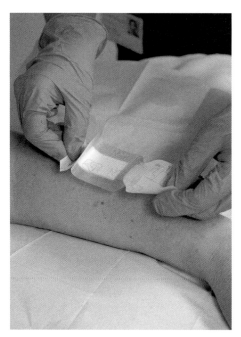

Fig. 15.8 Applying sterile dressing.

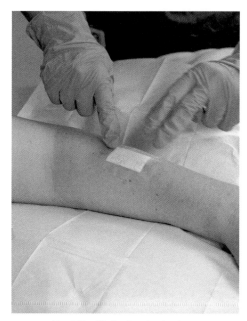

Fig. 15.9 Sterile dressing in place.

Removal of Skin Closure: Sutures / Staples

RATIONALE

The type of surgery will determine the type of skin closure used. The removal of sutures or staples should not be painful, although the patient may anticipate pain or discomfort. Explanation and careful positioning may alleviate this.

KEY POINTS

- If the wound is longer than 15 cm, or if the incision is in a place where there may be a strain on the skin and underlying tissues, it is better to remove alternate sutures/staples, starting with the second one along. This allows you to check that the wound does not begin to open at any point before the rest are removed. If the wound begins to open (dehisce), the remaining sutures/staples may be left until the following day and reassessed. In some instances, the number of sutures/staples removed needs to be documented. With continuous sutures and if the wound begins to gape stop, and do not remove any more.
- When removing sutures, only make one cut until you can determine where the loose end is and it is visible. Cut the suture as close to the skin as possible. The part of the suture that has been lying on the skin must not be pulled under the skin during removal as this will introduce microorganisms into the skin.
- Skin-closure strips are used to pull the edges of the wound together to promote healing. Starting at the centre of the wound, attach the strip to the skin on one side of the wound. Making sure that the skin edges are aligned without creating excessive tension, lay it over the wound and attach it to the skin on the other side. The next and any subsequent strips should be attached first to alternate sides of the wound. This will apply even pressure to the wound edges.

EQUIPMENT

1. Dressing pack containing sterile gloves
2. Sterile scissors/stitch cutter and forceps or staple remover as appropriate
3. Alcohol hand-rub or handwashing facilities
4. Draw screens around the bed and ensure adequate light. Clear bed area, close windows, turn off the fan, etc.

PROCEDURE

1. Consult the wound care plan to determine when the sutures/staples are due for removal, the dressing type
2. Decontaminate hands. An apron should be worn.
3. Additional protective clothing may be necessary if indicated by the patient's condition (see Chapter 2)
4. Explain the procedure, to gain consent and cooperation
5. Check patient comfort (e.g. position, convenience, need for the toilet)
6. Administer analgesics if appropriate and allow time to take effect
7. Adjust the bedclothes to permit easy access to the wound but maintain warmth and dignity
8. Prepare the dressing trolley for an aseptic dressing (see p. 227)
9. Taking care to maintain sterility, open the stitch cutter and forceps or staple remover onto the sterile field.
10. Adjust any bedclothes to expose the wound then loosen the existing dressing but do not remove it.

11. Decontaminate your hands.

12. Open the sterile waste bag and put your hand inside so that the bag acts as a glove. Use this to remove and inspect the old dressing.

13. Turn the bag inside out so that the dressing is contained within it, and using the adhesive strip, attach the bag to the side of the trolley or other convenient place close to the wound

14. Taking care not to touch the outside of the gloves, put on the sterile gloves (see p. 10)

15. Inspect the wound for signs of healing. If the wound looks inflamed or there is any exudate (pus) present, advice should be sought from an experienced nurse. It may be necessary to remove just one or two sutures/staples to allow the pus to drain.

16. Do not clean the wound before removing the sutures/staples, as the cleansing solution may seep into the holes made by the sutures/staples when removed.

17. If the wound is longer than 15 cm, remove alternate sutures/staples and check that the wound is fully healed before removing the rest:

   ▪ Individual sutures—use the forceps to lift up the knot of the suture. In your other hand, hold the scissors or stitch cutter flat against the skin and slide it under the suture to cut it (Fig. 15.10). The place where you cut it is important; in order to prevent infection, the part of the suture that has been lying on the skin must not be drawn underneath the skin.

   ▪ Staples—a special instrument is used to remove staples (Fig. 15.11). This should be placed under the centre of the staple and squeezed hard. This bends the staple so that it comes out of the skin easily and does not have to be 'hooked' out. The staple can be steadied, if necessary, by holding it with forceps.

   ▪ Continuous suture—this means the incision is held together with one thread, which passes under and over the incision about every centimetre. There is a knot at each end. Use the forceps to lift the knot at one end and cut the first 'suture' at the end furthest from the knot. Lift the knot to remove the loose end from under the skin and cut close to the skin. Slide the forceps under the next stitch, raise it to remove the underlying thread and cut it close to the skin. Repeat this process with all the

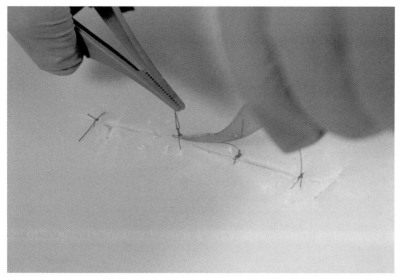

Fig. 15.10 Removing sutures using a stitch cutter.

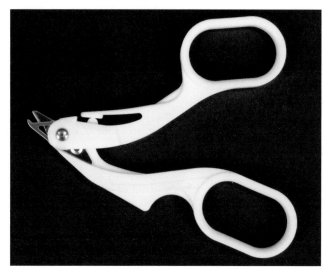

Fig 15.11 Staple remover.

others, making sure that the part that has been on the skin is not pulled underneath the skin. Never cut both ends of a suture or you will be unable to remove the hidden part underneath the skin.

- Subcutaneous suture—this is a continuous suture, but it is not visible above the skin. There is usually a bead at each end. Cut the thread holding one bead and gently pull the other until the whole thread is removed from under the skin.

18. Use a gauze swab dipped in the cleansing solution to clean and then dry around the wound if necessary (not the wound itself).
19. If there are any small areas where the skin edges are not completely healed together, skin-closure strips may be applied.
20. If appropriate, apply the new dressing.
21. Place any sharps (e.g. stitch cutters) in a sharps bin. Forceps, if not disposable, should be returned to the sterile supplies department for decontamination.
22. Wrap all non-sharp disposable items in the sterile field and place in the waste bag. Remove gloves, discard into the clinical waste bag and tie securely.
23. Replace the bedclothes and assist the patient as necessary into a comfortable position. Readjust the bed to a safe height.
24. Remove apron, discard in the clinical waste bag and decontaminate hands.
25. Return any unused items to the stock cupboard. Clean the trolley according to local policy.
26. Document the care given and the condition of the wound. Report any difficulties with the procedure, changes or abnormalities.

Wound Drainage

PRINCIPLES

Open System

This refers to a hollow or corrugated tube, that are occasionally used. These are situated in the wound to promote drainage (Fig. 15.12). If there is a large amount of drainage, the end

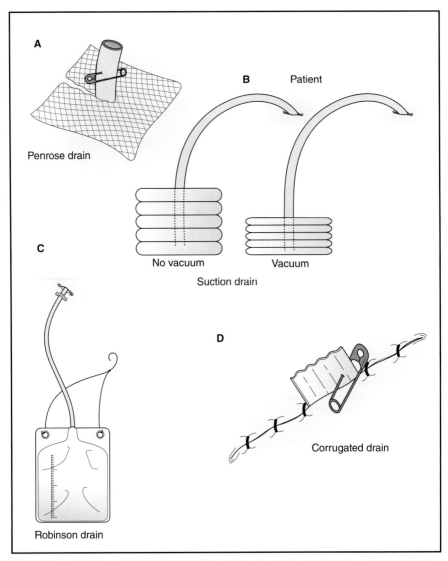

Fig. 15.12 Types of drain available. (Nicol, M., Bavin, C., Cronin, P., Rawlings-Anderson, K., Cole, E., & Hunter, J. (2008). *Essential Nursing Skills*, 3rd ed. Elsevier Ltd.)

of the drain may be inserted into a stoma bag (see p. 282). This is designed to keep the wound area free from drainage, and thus reduce the risk of infection, and to prevent damage to the skin.

Closed System

This refers to a system whereby the drain is attached to tubing and a bag for the collection of drainage. This means that the system is 'closed' and thus, the risk of infection is greatly reduced. Closed systems may incorporate a vacuum to encourage active drainage (Fig. 15.13).

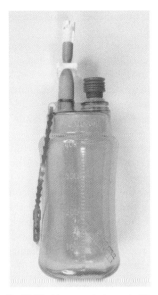

Fig. 15.13   Vacuum drainage bottle.

- The bag or bottle should be supported by an attachment to the bed or patient's clothing to prevent pulling, kinking, blockage and accidental dislodgement of the drain.
- Asepsis must be maintained when changing the bag or bottle.

CHANGING A VACUUM DRAINAGE BOTTLE

The presence of a vacuum is usually indicated by the small concertina of plastic folds at the top of the bottle; when the vacuum is no longer present, the concertina effect is lost (see Fig. 15.13). If only a small amount of drainage is expected, a small concertina container may be used. This is squeezed flat to create a vacuum, and then the stopper is replaced to maintain the vacuum. The used bottle, once clamped, should be discarded into the clinical waste bag. It should not be emptied because of the risk of splashing and contact with blood.

EQUIPMENT

New sterile vacuum drainage bottle (check that a vacuum is present)
Orange/Yellow clinical waste bag

PROCEDURE

1. Decontaminate hands.
2. Put on an apron and clean gloves.
3. If there is a danger of splashing, goggles should be worn.
4. Explain the procedure, to gain informed and cooperation.
5. Adjust the bed to a safe working height. Take care not to dislodge the drain.

6. Detach the drainage bottle from the bed, taking care not to let the bottle slip or the drainage tube may be pulled out.

7. With the clamps that are provided as part of the system, clamp off both the drainage tube (above the connection to the bottle) and the bottle.

Bottle system

8. Carefully remove the drainage tube from the 'old' bottle, taking care not to touch the last 2 to 3 cm to keep it sterile.

9. Note the volume of drainage, then discard the bottle with its contents into the clinical waste bag

10. Using an aseptic non-touch technique connect the tubing firmly into the new bottle and release the vacuum clamp (see Fig. 15.13). Release the clamp on the drainage tubing.

Small concertina system

11. If it is necessary to empty the drainage and replace the vacuum container, detach the container, empty into a jug taking care to avoid splashing

12. Squeeze the container flat, push the tubing firmly back into the container and release the clamp on the drainage tubing

13. If drainage is no longer required, remove the drainage tubing and insert the stopper. Discard into the clinical waste system.

14. Secure the container to the bed or patient's clothing to prevent pulling. Check the vacuum is present.

Both methods

15. Remove gloves, discard into the clinical waste bag and close securely.

16. Check the patient is comfortable, and the drain is not pulling. Adjust the bed to a safe height.

17. Dispose of equipment and clinical waste appropriately.

18. Remove apron, discard in the clinical waste and decontaminate hands.

19. Document the amount and type of drainage according to local policy.

Removal of Wound Drain

KEY POINTS

- Clamping the tubing prevents suction during removal, which may be painful for the patient.
- If the drain site appears inflamed or purulent, a swab for culture and sensitivity should be taken.
- Check that the entire drain has been removed. If the drain cannot easily be removed, leave it in position and report it to the nurse in charge.

EQUIPMENT

As for the aseptic dressing technique (see p. 5) plus:
Sterile stitch cutter or sterile scissors
Sterile disposable forceps
Sterile dressing towel

PROCEDURE

1. Decontaminate hands.
2. Put on apron.
3. Additional protective clothing may be necessary if indicated by the patient's condition (see Chapter 2).

4. Explain the procedure, to gain consent and cooperation.
5. Prepare the patient, bed area and equipment as described for the aseptic dressing technique.
6. Note the amount of drainage. If the drain has a vacuum bottle attached, clamp the tubing with the clamp provided to prevent suction during removal of the drain.
7. Put on sterile gloves and clean the site, if necessary, so that the knot of the suture holding the drain in place is visible and accessible. Place the sterile towel under the tubing.
8. Lift up the knot of the suture with the sterile forceps, and using the stitch cutter, cut the suture close to the skin, and remove the suture (see p. 231).
9. Fold a gauze swab several times to create an absorbent pad and hold this over the site.
10. Warn the patient to expect a pulling sensation, gently remove the drain onto the sterile towel. Use counter-pressure on the skin with the other hand if resistance is felt.
11. Maintain pressure over the site until bleeding/drainage is minimal. Cover the site with a sterile dressing.
12. Detach the bottle from the bed/clothing. Wrap the bottle and the tubing in the sterile towel and discard into the clinical waste bag.
13. Place any sharps (e.g. stitch cutter) in the sharps bin. Scissors, if not disposable, should be returned to the sterile supplies department for decontamination. Remove gloves and discard with dressing pack into the clinical waste bag and close securely.
14. Check the patient is comfortable and readjust the bed height.
15. Remove apron and decontaminate hands.
16. Document the time and date of removal, the amount and type of drainage, and the condition of the wound.

Topical Negative Pressure

Topical negative pressure (TNP) wound therapy (also known as vacuum-assisted closure therapy) is increasingly being used to promote and accelerate the closure of wounds. TNP wound therapy provides a uniform negative pressure to the wound bed to stimulate blood flow and generate the formation of granulation tissue (Norman et al., 2022). TNP therapy also draws off excess exudate to promote an optimum moist wound bed environment, reduces the number of bacteria (bacterial load) from the wound bed, removes odour, and reduces oedema from the surrounding tissues (Peate and Glencross, 2015). At the same time, the negative pressure draws the wound edges together to encourage wound contraction.

A range of different devices are available from several manufacturers, and detailed information on each device, its application, and relevant materials will be found in the manufacturer's instruction manual. Inappropriate or wrongly applied TNP wound therapy can harm the patient, and it is the nurse's responsibility to ensure they are familiar with the device to maintain safety. Help and support are available in many clinical settings from the Tissue Viability Specialist. Nurses can also contact the manufacturer's representative for advice, training and education.

TNP wound therapy can be applied to wounds that are slow to heal, have excessive wound fluid (exudate), or wound cavities. TNP wound therapy has been found to be effective for patients with acute or traumatic wounds (e.g. dehisced surgical wounds, flaps, skin grafts, and partial thickness burns), and chronic wounds (e.g. pressure ulcers, diabetic ulcers and venous leg ulcers). Not all wounds will benefit from TNP wound therapy; it may have a detrimental effect on patients with fistulae, malignancy, presence of necrotic tissue, and osteomyelitis (Huang et al., 2014; Kaufman-Rivi et al., 2013).

The equipment used to apply TNP wound therapy generally consists of a wound contact dressing (e.g. gauze material or foam), drainage tubes, and a wound drainage collection canister, which is attached to the powered vacuum pump. A transparent film dressing is used to cover the contact dressing to ensure a tight seal around the edges of the wound. It is important to refer to the manufacturer's instructions for the device being used.

As with all wound management, an initial wound assessment must be undertaken before TNP wound therapy is applied. It is also crucial to assess its effectiveness each time the dressing is changed. Dressings are usually changed every 48 to 72 hours using an aseptic technique. If the wound is infected the dressing may need to be changed every 12 to 24 hours (Wu et al., 2022). Document the assessment of the wound following local policy. This should include any concerns about the condition of the wound or treatment, the amount of drainage in the canister when the TNP wound therapy dressing was changed and the pressure setting.

When the vacuum pump is switched on with the prescribed pressure, the TNP wound therapy dressing contracts and becomes hard as the air pressure beneath the dressing is removed. When setting the prescribed negative pressure, always take advice from the manufacturer's recommendations to ensure the correct pressure is used. If the pressure is incorrect, the patient may experience pain and bruising at the wound bed, which will adversely affect the healing process. The negative pressure may need to be increased slowly to reach the required level according to the patient's tolerance and comfort. The device can be programmed to apply continuous or intermittent negative pressure.

The device must be regularly monitored and check it is working correctly depending on local policy. Always check the manufacturer's instructions about the alarms, which may be visual or audible. For example, alarms may be triggered when the canister is full, the drainage tubes are blocked or kinked, the transparent film dressing is leaking, or the battery life is low. Portable devices need the batteries recharged as required; static devices must be connected to the wall socket but usually have a backup battery for short-term use, therefore, regular checks must be made to confirm the battery is charging.

Some patients may be unable to tolerate TNP due to pain, and intermittent therapy cycling may affect the patient's sleep (Shreiber, 2016). Consequently, a comprehensive pain assessment and plan should be developed in collaboration with the patient (Peate and Glencross, 2015).

References

Carlin AS (2022) Essentials of wound care: assessing and managing impaired skin integrity. Nursing Standard. doi: 10.7748/ns.2022.e11964

Denton, A., Hallam, C., 2020. Principles of asepsis 1: the rationale for using aseptic technique. Nurs. Times [online]. 116, 38–41.

Fry, D.E., 2017. Pressure irrigation of surgical incisions and traumatic wounds. Surg. Infect. 18 (4), 424–430. doi:10.1089/sur.2016.252.

Huang, C., Leavitt, T, Bayer, L.R., et al., 2014. Effect of negative pressure wound therapy on wound healing. Curr. Probl. Surg. 51 (7), 301–331.

Hussey G. Young T. (2020). The impact of psychological factors on wound healing. Wounds Internationa. 11. 4. 58–62

Kaufman-Rivi, D., Hazlett, A.C., Hardy, M.A., et al., 2013. Provider experiences with negative-pressure wound therapy systems. Adv. Skin Wound Care. 26 (7), 311–318.

Loveday, H.P., et al., 2014. National evidence-based guidelines for preventing healthcare associated infections in NHS hospitals. J. Hosp. Infect. 8651, S1–S70.

Munro JA, Beck AD. (2021) The Effect of UK Nursing Policy on Higher Education Wound Care Provision and Practice: A Critical Discourse Analysis. Policy Polit Nurs Pract. 22(2):134–145. doi: 10.1177/1527154421994069. Epub 2021 Mar 11. PMID: 33706598; PMCID: PMC8056706.

Norman G, Shi C, Goh EL, Murphy EM, Reid A, Chiverton L, Stankiewicz M, Dumville JC. (2022). Negative pressure wound therapy for surgical wounds healing by primary closure. Cochrane Database Syst Rev. 26;4(4):CD009261. doi: 10.1002/14651858.CD009261.pub7. PMID: 35471497; PMCID: PMC9040710.

Nursing and Midwifery Council. (2018) The Code. www.nmc.org.uk

Peate, I., Glencross, W., 2015. Wound Care at a Glance. John Wiley & Sons, Incorporated.

Schreiber, M.L., 2016. Negative pressure wound therapy. Med. Surg. Nurs. 25 (6).

Wu L. Wen B. Xu Z. Lin K. (2022). Research progress on negative pressure wound therapy with instillation in the treatment of orthopaedic wounds. International Wound Journal. 19. 6. 1449–1445

CHAPTER 16

Patient Hygiene

Assisting With a Bath or Shower

Personal care and hygiene are individual for each patient, with showering and bathing being fundamental aspect of nursing care (Nursing and Midwifery Council (NMC), 2018a). Nurses are required to 'demonstrate knowledge, skills and ability to act as a role model for others in providing evidence-based, person-centred nursing care to meet people's needs related to...hygiene' (NMC, 2018b, p. 17). Nurses must discuss the patient's preference for a bath or a shower, assess how much the patient is able to do for themselves and how much assistance may be required. If a shower is not available, some patients may prefer to use running water while sitting in an empty bath.

KEY POINTS

- Some hospitals require patients to use antiseptic cleansing solution rather than soap, as prophylaxis against methicillin-resistant Staphylococcus aureus (MRSA).
- The hands can usually tolerate higher temperatures than the rest of the body. The elbow is more sensitive and will minimise the risk of the water being too hot. The safest option is to use a bath thermometer.
- If leaving patients to wash themselves make sure they have access to a call bell for assistance.

EQUIPMENT

- Shower gel or antiseptic cleansing agent, according to local policy
- Flannel/sponge and towels
- Brush and/or comb
- Toothbrush, toothpaste and denture pot if appropriate
- Shampoo (if required)
- Clean clothing
- Toiletries, make-up, etc., according to individual preference
- Shower stool or plastic chair
- Hoist and/or other aids to mobility as required

PROCEDURE

1. Explain the procedure to gain consent and cooperation. Ascertain whether the patient wishes to use the toilet before taking them to the bathroom.
2. Put on plastic apron and any additional protective clothing as necessary.
3. Check that the bathroom is available and that the bath/shower is clean.
4. Run the bath water/check shower is working.
5. Help the patient to collect together clothes and toiletries.

6. Assist the patient to the bathroom and make sure that access by others is restricted, to ensure privacy.
7. For bathing: use a bath thermometer to check the temperature of the water. The temperature should be less than 40°C.
8. Assist the patient with undressing, maintaining dignity by covering them with a towel.
9. Observe the condition of the patient's skin, especially at the pressure points, such as heels and sacrum. Note and record any signs of inflammation, bruising, discoloration or rash, and the integrity of the skin and its hydration, whether dry, clammy or sweaty, etc.
10. For bathing: assist the patient to get into the bath. A mechanical hoist is likely to be required for immobile patients.
11. For showering: assist the patient to sit on the shower stool or chair and adjust the water flow to the correct temperature.
12. Assist the patient to wash. Encourage patients to do as much as they can themselves.
13. If required, assist the patient to wash their hair, using the flannel as an eye-guard to avoid getting shampoo in the eyes.
14. Assist the patient out of the bath or shower, using a hoist if required. Cover the patient with a towel as soon as possible, to provide warmth and maintain dignity.
15. Help the patient to: dry themselves; apply toiletries as requested; dress in chosen clothing; brush or comb their hair; clean their teeth or dentures as appropriate.
16. Assist the patient to return to bed, chair or day room, using a mechanical hoist if required. Check the patient is comfortable.
17. Return/replace towels and toiletries as appropriate.
18. Clean the bath or shower and then decontaminate hands.
19. Document the care noting how much assistance the patient required, the state of their skin and pressure areas and the patient's general condition. Report any significant changes.

Bed Bath

Assisting a patient with a bed bath provides an opportunity to carry out a holistic assessment, as it allows time to discuss any concerns they may have while assessing the physical (such as checking skin integrity) and psychological status of the individual. (Lawton and Shepherd, 2019a). Nurses must discuss and assess hygiene needs with patients; in order to develop an individual care plan, for example, some patients may prefer to bathe in the evening as it helps them to settle, others may prefer to bathe in the morning while others will wish to bathe morning and evening. In addition to assisting with a patient's hygiene needs, urethral catheter care, mouth and denture care, foot care and eye care should be addressed.

KEY POINTS

- A bed bath is not as effective as showering or bathing and should only be undertaken when there is no alternative (Dougherty and Lister, 2015). Patients should be encouraged to do as much as possible to promote independence and self-esteem.
- Some hospitals require patients to use an antiseptic cleansing solution instead of soap as part of their infection control policy. Patients may prefer not to use soap on their face and, if they have any skin conditions, may use an emulsifying ointment in the water instead of soap. Increasingly, disposable wipes impregnated with a cleansing solution are used.
- The back is left until last so that it can be washed and the clean sheet inserted at the same time, to prevent unnecessary movement for the patient. One nurse can often manage until this point but will need assistance to roll the patient and make the bed with clean linen.

- The use of non-sterile gloves is not required routinely for washing and dressing patients (World Health Organization, 2009). However, nurses should wear gloves when there is a risk of exposure to blood and body fluids (Royal College of Nursing, 2018), and evidence suggests that patients may prefer nurses to wear gloves to provide intimate care (Loveday et al., 2014).

EQUIPMENT

- Cleansing wipes or antiseptic cleansing agent
- Disposable wash cloths
- Two towels
- Toiletries, make-up, etc., according to individual preference
- Brush and/or comb
- Toothbrush and toothpaste, tumbler of water and bowl/receiver
- Bowl of water (hand hot)
- Clean night clothes
- Trolley or suitable work surface
- Linen bag and bags for fouled or infected linen if required
- Clean bed linen
- Clinical waste bag

PROCEDURE

1. Discuss the procedure to gain cooperation and consent.
2. Ascertain if the patient wishes to use a bedpan/urinal or commode prior to their bed bath.
3. Ask if the patient has any pain, administer appropriate analgesia and allow it to take effect before starting the bed bath.
4. The patient requiring a bed bath will need assistance, however they should be encouraged to try to help.
5. Maintain privacy, warmth and dignity.
6. Put on plastic apron and gloves, if necessary, plus any additional protective clothing required.
7. Assist the patient into a comfortable position. Clear space at bedside for bowl of water and toiletries. Adjust bed to a suitable working height.
8. Assist the patient to remove any night clothes, ensuring the patient is covered with a sheet or blanket to maintain warmth and dignity.
9. Ask if the patient would like soap on the cloth to wash their face. Assist the patient with washing the face, ears and neck. If soap is used, rinse well and dry thoroughly.
10. Wash, rinse and dry the body in a logical order, exposing only the part of the body to be washed. The suggested order is arms, chest, abdomen, genital area, legs and feet and then back; however, this should be discussed with the patient to ascertain any preferences. Change the water as it cools or becomes dirty. If two nurses are present, one should wash and rinse while the other dries the body and applies toiletries as requested (e.g. talc, deodorant or body cream). This reduces the amount of time the body is exposed.
11. As the patient is washed, observe the condition of the skin. Document any signs of inflammation, bruising, discoloration or rash, including the skin integrity and hydration (e.g. whether dry, clammy or sweaty).

12. Put on gloves and assist the patient to wash, rinse and dry the genital area using a disposable cloth. Remember to wash from the front of the perineal area to the back. In males, ensure that the foreskin is repositioned after washing, and dry underneath it. If a urinary catheter is in place, wash carefully around the urethral meatus and catheter tubing, moving away from the meatus, and dry carefully. Change the water after washing the genital area.

13. Once the back and genital areas are washed, the bottom sheet can be changed. This will require two nurses. To change the bottom sheet, loosen the sheet and roll it into the centre of the bed, as far as possible under the patient. Open out the clean sheet lengthwise and, leaving a sufficient amount to tuck in, roll the rest into the centre of the bed. Secure the corners and tuck in the middle to anchor the sheet. Holding the top sheet to ensure the patient is covered, ask the patient to roll over to the opposite edge of the bed. The old sheet may now be removed and put in the laundry bag, the clean sheet pulled through and tucked in.

14. Assist the patient to put on night clothes.

15. Remake the bed.

16. Assist the patient to clean teeth or dentures. If the patient is going to sit out of bed after the bed bath, it is often easier to clean the teeth when sitting in a chair.

17. Assist the patient to brush or comb hair and to clean and file nails if necessary.

18. Lower bed.

19. Ensure the patient is left comfortable and has belongings within easy reach.

20. Wash and dry the bowl. Rinse out the flannel if this has been used and leave to dry. Discard any disposable wipes used into the clinical waste. Return the linen bag to its collection point.

21. Remove apron and decontaminate hands.

22. Record the procedure in the nursing documentation, noting how much the patient could do without assistance and the condition of the skin, eyes, mouth, etc.

Oral Assessment and Care

Oral assessment and care are an essential part of nursing care. Poor oral health has cumulative negative effects on health, and good oral health is very much a part of general health and wellbeing (Public Health England, 2017) (Table 16.1). Benefits of oral hygiene include improving self-esteem and comfort, improving appetite and enjoyment of food and drink, preventing halitosis and reducing the risk of hospital-acquired pneumonia. An oral assessment provides baseline information about the patient's mouth, assists with monitoring the progress of oral care and treatments and identifies if the patient wears dentures or a dental appliance.

KEY POINTS

- Oral health reduces the risk of infection and improves comfort and patient experience.
- In the acute setting mouth care is often seen as low priority.
- Teeth should be brushed at least twice a day with a fluoride toothpaste (Public Health England, 2017; National Institute for Health and Care Excellence, 2016). They should always be brushed last thing at night.

EQUIPMENT

Pen torch
Receiver

TABLE 16.1 ■ Reasons for Poor Oral Hygiene

There are many reasons people may have poor oral hygiene, including:
- Inability to carry out oral care, e.g., due to stroke, arthritis, arm injury, head injury, surgery
- Lack of knowledge or motivation
- Lack of access to dental services
- Lack of money to afford oral care equipment
- Medicines, such as anticholinergic drugs and oxygen therapy, that cause a dry mouth or an unpleasant taste
- Poor diet or reduced fluid intake
- Nil by mouth due to surgery or dysphagia
- Xerostomia—sensation of a dry mouth—which frequently affects older people
- Surgery, radiotherapy and/or trauma to the head and neck

Modified from Dougherty and Lister (2015), Bakhtiari et al. (2018), Otukoya and Shepherd (2018), Davis et al. (2019).

Tissues

Tongue depressor

Non-sterile disposable gloves and plastic apron

Toothbrush—this is the most effective means of removing plaque and debris. A paediatric soft toothbrush can be used for patients who have a sore mouth

Toothpaste

Assessment and recording tools

PROCEDURE

1. Raise bed to safe working height.
2. Observe the patient's lips, noting whether they are normal or dry and whether there is any evidence of ulcers, sores, cracks or bleeding.
3. Position the patient in an upright position. If the patient is unable to sit up, the procedure should be undertaken with the patient's head turned to the side to prevent choking and suction equipment should be available.
4. Decontaminate hands again, and put on non-sterile gloves and a plastic apron.
5. Select an appropriate toothbrush and wet it's head. Apply a pea-sized amount of toothpaste to a gloved finger and rub it into the toothbrush—this will prevent a large amount of toothpaste from dropping into the patient's mouth. Non-foaming toothpaste should be used for patients with dysphagia (swallowing problems) (Doshi, 2016).
6. Use a gentle, rotating movement to clean the inner, outer and biting surfaces of the teeth (Fig. 16.1). You can also gently brush the surface of the tongue and the gums. Brushing should take approximately two minutes, or 30 seconds per quarter of the mouth.
7. Allow the patient to spit out excess toothpaste. They should not rinse their mouth with water as this dilutes the fluoride in the toothpaste, which protects teeth from decay (Public Health England (PHE), 2017).
8. Offer the patient tissues to wipe their mouth.
9. Apply moisturiser to the patient's lips if required. Dry-mouth gel can be used to alleviate oral dryness.
10. Check that the patient is comfortable.
11. Clean the toothbrush and allow it to air dry.
12. Remove gloves and apron, and dispose of equipment according to local policy.
13. Decontaminate hands.
14. Document care given and any observations of the patient's mouth.

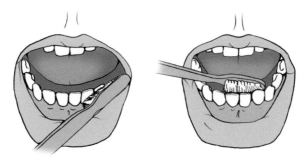

Fig. 16.1 Brushing the teeth. (Williams, P. (2022). *Fundamental Concepts and Skills for Nursing*, 6th ed. Elsevier Inc.)

Denture Care

Patients with dentures may require assistance with denture care as food and debris can collect under dentures, potentially leading to discomfort or oral thrush (Otukoya and Shepherd, 2018). In hospitals, loss of dentures affects patients' ability to eat and communicate and may also affect their psychological wellbeing (Binks et al., 2017). In addition, obtaining new dentures is expensive, and causes inconvenience for patients and poor nutritional intake.

KEY POINTS

- Dentures should be cleaned at least twice daily; ideally, after meals with a denture brush or toothbrush over a bowl filled with water.
- At night, dentures are usually removed and stored in water and placed in a labelled denture pot.
- Unconscious patients should not wear their dentures, as these may obstruct the airway. The dentures should be cleaned and stored in water in a labelled denture pot.

EQUIPMENT

Small torch
Plastic cup
Mouthwash
Denture cleaner
Denture brush
Non-sterile disposable gloves and apron
Denture pot
Tissues

PROCEDURE

1. Explain the procedure to the patient and gain their consent.
2. Decontaminate hands.
3. Assemble equipment.
4. Fill a disposable bowl with water.

5. Wash and dry your hands again, and put on non-sterile gloves and apron. Additional protective clothing may be necessary if indicated by the patient's condition.
6. Raise bed to a suitable working height. Drape a towel across the patient's chest.
7. If possible, ask the patient to remove their dentures and place it in the bowl of water. If the patient needs help to remove the denture, use a gloved finger to slide by the side of the denture to help break the seal between the mouth and the denture (Doshi, 2016). Observe the condition of the dentures: whether they are clean, stained, warped or cracked.
8. Assist the patient to rinse their mouth with water. A soft toothbrush may also be used to gently brush the gums.
9. Carry out an oral assessment using a pen torch if required.
10. Clean the dentures with a toothbrush and denture-cleaning paste. Ordinary toothpaste should not be used as this is too abrasive.
11. Rinse the denture with cold water before repositioning it in patient's mouth (avoid drying the dentures as this makes them difficult to insert) or storing it in water in a denture pot. Advise the patient to leave the denture out at night to allow the oral tissue to recover. Always use a dedicated denture container, carefully labelled with the patient's details according to local policy.
12. Use the towel to dry around the patient's mouth. If the lips are dry, a thin layer of petroleum jelly or lip balm may be applied.
13. Clean the denture brush and allow it to air dry.
14. Clear away any equipment. Remove apron and gloves and discard in the clinical waste.
15. Decontaminate hands.
16. Document the assessment in the nursing records and liaise with appropriate staff if any medication or referrals are required.

Facial Shave

Facial shaving should be performed as part of routine care, and it is important to note that male patients of any age may attach a particular importance to shaving. It is a cause for concern that this is often overlooked as a fundamental part of nursing care (Ette and Gretton, 2019).

EQUIPMENT

- Bowl of hot water
- Disposable wash clothes
- Towel
- Shaving cream or soap.
- Razor. Patient's may have their own electric razor and so will not require a wet shave.
- Aftershave/cologne according to individual preference

PROCEDURE

1. Ascertain the patient's preferences for shaving and incorporate this into the hygiene routine accordingly.
2. If possible, the patient should be sitting up.
3. Decontaminate hands.
4. Put on apron
5. Additional protective clothing may be necessary if indicated by the patient's condition (see Chapter 2).

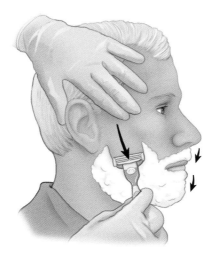

Fig. 16.2 Shaving moving towards the neck. (Sorrentino, S. A., & Remmert, L. (2021). *Mosby's Textbook for Nursing Assistants*, 10th ed. Elsevier Inc.)

6. Raise bed to a suitable working height. Drape a towel across the patient's chest.
7. Ask/assist the patient to wash their face. Inspect the face for any raised or irregular areas, such as moles or sores.
8. Apply the shaving cream or soap to the face, creating a good lather.
9. Using short strokes of the razor in the direction of the hair growth, shave the face starting with the cheeks and moving down towards the neck (Fig. 16.2). Avoid any raised area such as moles or blemishes.
10. The nurse's free hand should be used to pull the skin taut.
11. Rinse the razor after each stroke.
12. When the entire face and neck have been shaved, rinse the face in clean water and pat dry with a towel.
13. Apply aftershave or cologne if desired.
14. Lower bed and check the patient is comfortable.
15. Wash and dry the bowl and replace it in the appropriate storage area. Rinse facecloth thoroughly or discard disposable wipes in the clinical waste.
16. Replace patient's personal equipment in their locker.
17. Remove apron and decontaminate hands.
18. Document the procedure, noting how much the patient could do for themselves.

Washing Hair in Bed

The condition of a patient's hair and how it is styled is an important part of an individual's identity (Lawton and Shepherd, 2019b). Washing hair in bed will require careful planning (Peate 2015). Equipment may include inflatable basins specifically designed for hair washing, which have a gap for the neck so water is less likely to spill. Alternatively, it may be possible to use dry and no-rinse shampoos or no-rinse shampoo caps. These do not require the use of bowls or water as the hair is massaged through the cap. The cap can be warmed in a microwave before use if desired. Once the cap is removed the hair can be dried and styled as required.

Before washing the hair, the nurse should assess the condition of the scalp, noting any inflammation, dryness or redness. The condition of the hair should also be noted.

Some patients may like products applied to their hair after washing to prevent dryness and help with styling.

EQUIPMENT

- Plastic sheeting and absorbent pad or towel to protect the bed
- Shampoo and conditioner if used
- Comb and/or brush
- Flannel/disposable cloth and towels
- Two large bowls (one full of hand-hot water, the other empty) or one shaped bowl for hair washing
- Laundry skip

PROCEDURE

1. Remove the head of the bed and raise the bed to a suitable working height.
2. Place the plastic sheeting and the absorbent pad or towel over the pillows, and place the empty bowl on a chair at the top of the bed.
3. Ask/assist the patient to lie on their back at the very top of the bed, with pillows supporting the shoulders and the head positioned over the bowl. Cover the shoulders with a towel.
4. Observe the condition of the hair and scalp. Wet the patient's hair by taking warm water from the bowl into the jug and pouring it over the hair, allowing the water to run into the bowl on the chair.
5. Gently massage shampoo into the hair.
6. Rinse the hair with clean water, ensuring that the patient protects their eyes with the flannel or disposable cloth to avoid shampoo getting in. Repeat the process if the patient would like two applications of shampoo and/or conditioner.
7. If conditioner is used, comb it through the hair and leave for 2 to 3 minutes before rinsing.
8. After the final rinse, wrap the patient's hair in a towel and remove the bowl of water.
9. Assist the patient into a sitting position (if their condition allows) and towel dry the hair.
10. Lower the bed to a safe height and replace the bed head.
11. Brush or comb the hair into the desired style, using a hairdryer if one is available.
12. Leave the patient comfortable, and if no hairdryer is available, in a warm environment until the hair is dry.
13. Dispose of any wet bed linen in the linen skip.
14. Replace the bedhead and reposition the patient so that they are comfortable.
15. Style the hair according to the patient's preference.
16. Clean, dry and replace the used equipment as per local policy.
17. Remove apron and discard in clinical waste. Decontaminate hands.
18. Document the procedure.

Eye Care

Eyes assessment and care is an essential aspect of nursing care. Eyes should be assessed as a holistic patient assessment and as part of personal care (Gwenhure and Shepherd, 2019). Patients may have a long-standing eye condition that requires ongoing care; for example, glaucoma requires regular eye drops. In addition, factors affecting eyesight may complicate care; for example, poor eyesight may be associated with falls, and therefore eye assessment is a vital aspect of patient care. In addition, any sight aids such as glasses, contact lenses and a prosthetic eye should be identified. As part of good nursing care, patients should have access to these aids and nurses may need to check / assist with cleaning patient's glasses.

As part of the assessment, patients should be asked whether they have any new problems with their vision. Acute eye problems need to be assessed urgently as acute glaucoma, orbital cellulitis or retinal detachment may result in serious eye complications and/or loss of sight if treatment is delayed.

EQUIPMENT

- Sterile eye-care pack containing gallipot, gauze swabs and gloves
- Extra gauze swabs if required
- Sterile 0.9% sodium chloride (normal saline) solution
- Clinical waste bag

PROCEDURE

1. Raise bed to a suitable working height. Open the eye-care pack and arrange all equipment on a suitable work surface. Place clinical waste bag in a convenient position close to the patient.
2. Pour the saline solution into the gallipot.
3. Decontaminate hands and put on sterile gloves.
4. Fold four swabs into quarters and dip into saline solution.
5. Assess the external appearance of the eye.
6. Ask the patient to close their eyes and check for any discharge, bruising or inflammation. If the eyelids fail to close completely, report this to medical staff as it may be a sign that a lump or cyst is present (Dougherty and Lister, 2015), or there may be problems with eyelid muscles.
7. Ask the patient to open their eyes and check for signs of redness in the conjunctiva and for evidence of discharge (Dougherty and Lister, 2015). These signs may indicate the presence of infection or inflammation.
8. Explain which eye is to be cleaned first. Take a sterile swab in your hand and moisten it slightly with sterile water or saline. A very wet swab can be uncomfortable for the patient and increases the risk of contamination of the opposite eye. Always clean an infected eye last. If both eyes are infected, two separate eye-care packs should be used and the hands washed before cleaning the second eye.
9. Ask the patient to close their eyes again and swab the lower eye lid from the medial canthus outwards. Swabbing in this direction reduces the risk of introducing infection into the lacrimal punctum (Dougherty and Lister, 2015). Do not allow the swab to go above the lid, to prevent contact between the swab and cornea.
10. Repeat, using a clean swab each time to reduce the risk of infection, until the eyelid is clean.
11. Ask the patient to look down and slightly evert (turn inside out) the upper lid.
12. Moisten a swab and gently clean the upper eyelid from the medial canthus outwards.
13. Repeat with a new moistened swab until the lid is clean. Dab off any excess water/saline around the eye to ensure patient is dry and comfortable.
14. Remove gloves and put all used equipment in the waste bag.
15. Check the patient is left comfortable and lower the bed.
16. Discard the used pack in clinical waste. Because of the risk of infection, eye-care packs should not be kept for repeated use. A new pack should be used each time. Remove apron and decontaminate hands.
17. Document eye care, noting the condition of the eyes.

Caring for Fingernails and Toenails

Depending on local policies, patients may need to be referred to chiropody or podiatry services for toenail care. This is especially important in patients with diabetes and peripheral arterial disease who may have peripheral neuropathy and, therefore, be unaware of any trauma to the toes. However, if the nails are not deformed or thickened then the nurse should be able to clean and trim them.

KEY POINT

- Cut the nails straight across or follow the curve of the finger or toe, but do not cut down into the sides of the nails as this may cause trauma.

EQUIPMENT

- Bowl of warm water
- Nail clippers, nail file or emery board
- Orange stick
- Hand cream or lotion according to patient preference
- Towel

PROCEDURE

1. Explain the procedure, to gain consent and cooperation.
2. Ascertain usual nail-care habits.
3. Carry out this procedure following a bath if possible, as soaking may soften the nails.
4. Decontaminate hands.
5. Put on plastic apron. Additional protective clothing may be necessary if indicated by the patient's condition (see Chapter 2).

Fingernails

6. Inspect the hands, fingers and nails, for any signs of dryness and assess the condition of the nails and cuticles.
7. If patient has not recently had a bath, wash the hands in a bowl of warm soapy water. Avoid soaking the nails as this increases the likelihood of trauma when clipping or filing the nails.
8. Clean under the fingernails with an orange stick or nail file while washing the hands. Dry the hands.
9. If nail clippers are available, clip the nails. Clip small sections of the nail. After clipping, file the fingernails until they are level with the top of the finger. The nails can then be smoothed to the shape of the finger. If nail clippers are not available, file the nails; do not use scissors.
10. Push the cuticles back gently with an orange stick and apply hand cream or lotion as appropriate.

Toenails

11. Sit in a comfortable position so that the patient's feet can rest on a towel on your lap.
12. Inspect the feet and toenails, noting any dryness, inflammation or cracking. Also note any calluses or ulcerated areas and the colour and temperature of the feet to assess adequacy of circulation.
13. If the patient has not recently had a bath, wash the feet in a bowl of warm soapy water.

14. If clippers are available, clip the toenails. Clean and file the toenails as for fingernails, but do not file the corners as this may encourage ingrowing nails.
15. Apply moisturising lotion as required.

Finger and toenails

16. After cleaning, clipping and filing the nails leave the patient comfortable.
17. Clean any reusable equipment as per local policy and discard waste in clinical waste.
18. Remove apron and decontaminate hands.
19. Document care, noting the condition of the nails, and report any abnormal findings. Refer to chiropodist if required.

Last Offices

After death, the body is usually left for an hour before last offices are commenced, during which time a doctor or senior nurse will have certified the death. A pillow may be used to support the jaw, to prevent the mouth falling open, and the eyes closed with wet gauze swabs if necessary. The limbs should be straightened if necessary. It is important that any religious/cultural preferences must be ascertained prior to last offices (e.g. who can touch the body, non-removal of religious objects or jewelry).

KEY POINTS

- Death has to have been confirmed before starting last offices.
- Relatives will have been informed and given the opportunity to see the deceased and may wish to participate in the last offices.
- Attention must be paid to the beliefs and wishes of deceased patients and their relatives. Religious requirements should be observed. Advice from religious personnel may be required.
- Maintain privacy and dignity.
- The labels used to identify the body are found in the 'deceased patients' or 'death notice' book according to local policy. In some units, the labels are provided with other items (e.g., shroud) in a 'last offices' pack.

EQUIPMENT

- Prepare the bed area to ensure sufficient space is available
- Equipment for bed bath (see p. 240)
- Cotton wool, gauze or padding if there are any leaking wounds
- Clean sheet and shroud
- Tape for securing the sheet
- Two name bands
- Two labels from the 'deceased patients book'
- Property book
- Linen bag and clinical waste bag
- Cadaver bag (if required)

PROCEDURE

1. Take the equipment to the bedside and secure the screens, to prevent accidental opening. Raise the bed to a suitable working height.

2. Wash the front of the patient. If the patient is male, the second nurse could shave the patient whilst the first nurse washes. Leave/replace dentures if they fit. Care should be taken when shaving a dead person, as doing so when they are still warm can cause bruising or marking which does not appear until a few days later.

3. Spigot any tubes, catheters and infusions unless otherwise indicated, for example, post-mortem (autopsy) requirements. It is important to prevent leakage from the body, as this is unpleasant and potentially dangerous for porters and mortuary technicians. Refer to local policy regarding removal of drains/catheters/tubing and packing the body to prevent leakage. This should not be performed if a post-mortem examination (autopsy) is required. The medical team will advise on the need for a post-mortem examination.

4. If leakage is apparent from wounds or orifices, use packing or padding, according to local policy. It may be necessary to express urine from the bladder into a receiver.

5. With the second nurse as a witness, remove all jewellery from the body unless advised otherwise (e.g., Sikhs—leave bracelet (kara)). If jewellery is left, this should be covered with adhesive tape or tied in position to prevent loss. Document removal and add to property list.

6. Place the shroud on the patient, with the fastening at the back. Roll the patient onto their side to wash back and fasten shroud. When rolling the patient to put in the clean sheet, a deep sigh may be heard. This is due to air being forced out of the lungs.

7. If local policy requires, pack the mouth with gauze.

8. Place a clean sheet diagonally under the patient, leaving enough sheet to fold over the head and feet.

9. Place one label on the chest, attached to the shroud with adhesive tape.

10. Check there is one name band on the wrist and place the other on one ankle or according to local policy.

11. Before wrapping the patient in the sheet, check whether the relatives wish to view the body. If the patient is to be seen by the family after last offices, leave the face uncovered. A coloured counterpane or blanket makes the bed look less clinical.

12. Wrap the body in the sheet and secure with tape.

13. Place the other label on the chest.

14. If there is a risk of infection, the body may be placed in a cadaver bag.

15. Complete the property form. Both nurses must document and sign for any valuables. Any valuables left on the body should also be noted on the death form. Store property according to local policy (e.g. in the bereavement office).

16. Clear away equipment and dispose of clinical waste safely. Remove protective clothing and wash hands.

17. Contact porters or mortuary technicians to remove the body. Ensure that the other patients are screened when the body is removed, and a calm and quiet approach is adopted.

18. Ensure all documentation has been completed according to local policy.

References

Bakhtiari, S., et al., 2018. Orofacial manifestations of adverse drug reactions: a review study. Clujul Med. 91 (1), 27–36.

Binks, C., et al., 2017. Standardising the delivery of oral health care practice in hospitals. Nurs. Times. 113 (11), 18–21.

Davis, I., et al., 2019. Improving the provision of mouth care in an acute hospital trust. Nurs. Times [online]. 115 (5), 33–36.

Dougherty, L., Lister, S., 2015. The Royal Marsden Hospital Manual of Clinical Nursing Procedures. Blackwell, Oxford.

Doshi, M., 2016. Mouth Care Matters: A Guide for Hospital Healthcare Professionals. Bit.ly/HEEMouth-CareMatters.

Ette, L., Gretton, M., 2019. The significance of facial shaving as fundamental nursing care. Nurs. Times [online]. 115 (1), 40–42.

Gwenhure, T., Shepherd, E., 2019. Principles and procedure for eye assessment and cleansing. Nurs. Times. 115 (12), 18–20.

Lawton, S., Shepherd, E., 2019a. The underlying principles and procedure for bed bathing patients. Nurs. Times [online]. 115 (5), 45–47.

Lawton, S., Shepherd, E., 2019b. Procedure for washing patients' hair in bed. Nurs. Times [online]. 115 (6), 60–62.

Loveday, H.P., et al., 2014. National evidence-based guidelines for preventing healthcare-associated infections in NHS hospitals in England. J. Hosp. Infect. 86 (S1), S1–S70.

National Institute for Health and Care Excellence, 2016. Oral Health for Adults in Care Homes.

Nursing and Midwifery Council, 2018a. The Code. www.nmc.org.uk.

Nursing and Midwifery Council, 2018b. Standards of Proficiency for Registered Nurses. www.nmc.org.uk.

Otukoya, R., Shepherd, E., 2018. Principles of effective oral and denture care in adults. Nurs. Times [online]. 114 (11), 22–24.

Peate, I., 2015. Washing a patient's hair in bed: a care fundamental. Br. J. Healthcare Assist. 9 (3), 114–118.

Public Health England, 2017. Delivering Better Oral Health: An Evidence-based Toolkit for Prevention. https://assets.publishing.service.gov.uk/government/uploads/system/uploads/attachment_data/file/605266/Delivering_better_oral_health.pdf.

Royal College of Nursing, 2018. Tools of the Trade: Guidance for Health Care Staff on Glove Use and the Prevention of Contact Dermatitis. www.rcn.org.uk.

World Health Organization, 2009. WHO Guidelines on Hand Hygiene in Health Care. www.who.int.

CHAPTER 17

Elimination

Urinalysis

Urinalysis is an important screening and diagnostic tool which when used in conjunction with other tests, can help diagnose some diseases and infections through identifying pathological changes in the urine (Yates, 2016). Chemical reagent strips are used to analyse the urine sample, however, nurses need to be aware these may vary between manufacturers, so always check the instructions prior to use. Depending on the test strips used, the results can be used to indicate abnormalities.

Recent evidence and professional guidance suggest urinalysis should not be performed in adults over 65 years with a suspected urinary tract infection (UTI), because urinalysis becomes more unreliable with increasing age. Because many will have bacteria present in the bladder/urine without an symptoms of infection. This "asymptomatic bacteriuria" is not harmful, and although it causes a positive urine dipstick, antibiotics are not beneficial and may cause harm (Royal College of General Practitioners, 2020).

KEY POINTS

- Urinary dipstick reagent strips are a quick, effective screening aid to urinalysis.
- The urine should be examined for colour, clarity and odour before undertaking dipstick analysis.
- Urine can be collected in different ways depending on the test requested (Table 17.1).

EQUIPMENT

- Non-latex gloves
- Apron
- Urine jug/sterile pot
- Urinalysis test strips
- Watch with second hand

PROCEDURE

1. Decontaminate hands and wear appropriate personal protective equipment (PPE) (Chapter 2).
2. Check the expiry date of the reagent sticks and make sure that you are familiar with the manufacturer's instructions for use.
3. Remove a stick, making sure that you do not touch the coloured reagent pads with your hands. Replace the lid. The lid of the reagent-sticks pot must always be replaced immediately after use to prevent moisture getting in.
4. Dip the stick into the urine so that the reagent pads are completely covered. Remove straight away and slowly draw the edge of the stick across the top of the container/jug to remove excess urine. Removing excess urine from the testing stick will prevent it dripping and prevent the coloured reagent pads running into each other, which could give inaccurate readings.

TABLE 17.1 ▪ Urine Reagent Sticks Commonly Test for the Following

Specific gravity (SG: normal range 1001–1035).	A raised SG may indicate concentrated urine due to dehydration; a low SG may indicate renal disease or diabetes insipidus
pH (normal range 4.5–8.0).	Normal urine is slightly acidic; a low pH may indicate respiratory or metabolic acidosis and a high pH may indicate respiratory or metabolic alkalosis. Some drugs can affect the urinary pH: ascorbic acid can make the urine more acidic and sodium bicarbonate, potassium citrate and sodium citrate can make the urine more alkaline
Protein, glucose, ketones, blood and bilirubin.	All of these are negative in normal urine. The presence of these abnormalities might indicate the following: • Protein (proteinuria) – urinary tract infection, pyelonephritis, pre-eclampsia, congestive cardiac failure. • Glucose (glycosuria) – diabetes mellitus, acute pancreatitis, Cushing's syndrome or sometimes in pregnancy. • Ketones (ketonuria) – excessive fat metabolism due to diabetic ketoacidosis, vomiting or severe dieting/starvation. • Blood (haematuria) – kidney disorders (e.g. glomerulonephritis), disorders of the urinary tract (e.g. kidney stones, tumours, infection), trauma or menstruation. • Bilirubin – liver disease (e.g. hepatitis) or biliary tract obstruction (e.g. gall stones, carcinoma of the head of pancreas).
Nitrite and leucocytes	These are both negative in normal urine. Urinary tract infection causes a rise in measured nitrite and leucocytes

Modified from Yates (2016).

5. Accurate timing according to the manufacturer's instructions is crucial, therefore, note note the time on your watch.
6. When the correct period of time has elapsed, read off the results by holding the stick alongside (but not touching) the pot and comparing the colour of each reagent pad with those displayed on the side (Fig. 17.1). Document the results, however, avoid taking the patient's charts into the sluice/dirty utility room to prevent contamination or splashing with water.
7. Discard the used stick in the clinical waste and clean or dispose of the container/jug according to local policy.
8. Remove gloves and apron and decontaminate hands.
9. After documenting the urinalysis report any abnormalities. Discuss the results with the patient as appropriate (see Table 17.1).

Midstream Specimen of Urine

Midstream specimen of urine (MSU) involves obtaining a specimen of urine for laboratory or near-patient testing, for example urinalysis (see above) to assist with determining a diagnosis and treatment (Shepherd, 2017a)). The procedure must be obtained correctly to prevent the risk of introducing error, leading to inaccurate results and inappropriate treatment. Table 17.2 outlines the types of urine specimens.

KEY POINTS

• MSUs must be appropriate to the patient's clinical presentation, collected at the right time, in the correct way to reduce the risk of contamination.

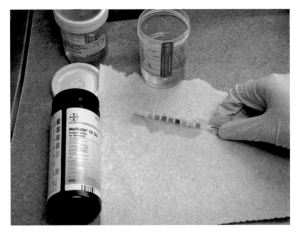

Fig. 17.1   Performing urinalysis. (Chabner, D.E. (2021). *The Language of Medicine*, 12th ed. Elsevier Inc.)

TABLE 17.2 ▪ **Types of Urine Analysis**

First-morning specimen	First urine void of the morning (or eight hours after recumbent position). May be used for cytology, TB or pregnancy.
Fasting specimen	The second voided specimen after a period of fasting.
Mid-stream urine (MSU)	Used to obtain bacterial culture. First and last part of urine stream is voided to avoid contaminating the specimen with organisms present on the skin.
Random specimen	For chemical or microscopic examination, a randomly collected specimen suitable for most screening purposes.

Yates (2016).

EQUIPMENT

- Disposable gloves and apron – additional personal protective equipment (gown, mask/respirator, visor) may be required depending on the specimen
- Protective tray to carry equipment
- Sterile container appropriate for the specimen (consult local policies)
- Gauze swabs, soap and water
- Toilet, urinal or bedpan
- Laboratory specimen form and label.
- Polythene transportation bag; biohazard (high-risk) label indicating the danger of infection

PROCEDURE

1. Explain the procedure,
2. Maintain privacy and dignity
3. Decontaminate hands and wear appropriate PPE.

Male Patient

1. Instruct/assist the patient to retract the foreskin and clean the skin surrounding the urethral meatus with soap and water, using each gauze swab only once. Dry with paper towels.

2. Ask the patient to start urinating into the urinal/toilet then stop, pass the middle part of the stream into the specimen pot (10 mL is sufficient) and then finish urinating into the urinal/toilet.
3. Remove the funnel part of the pot and close the lid securely.

Female Patient

1. Instruct/assist the patient to clean the urethral meatus with soap and water, using each gauze swab only once. Swab from front to back. Dry with paper towels.
2. Ask the patient to start urinating into the bed pan/toilet then stop, pass the middle part of the stream into the specimen pot (10 mL is sufficient) and then finish urinating into the urinal/toilet.
3. Remove the funnel part of the pot and close the lid securely.

Male and Female Patients

1. Discard all clinical waste safely and offer the patient hand washing facilities.
2. Remove gloves and apron and decontaminate hands.
3. Complete patient details on the label. Place in a plastic specimen bag with the pathology request form.
4. Place the specimen in the refrigerator for dispatch to the laboratory as soon as possible.
5. Document the date and time of the MSU according to local policy.

Catheter Specimen of Urine

Catheter specimen of urine (CSU) is often collected for bacteriological examination if the patient's symptoms suggest the presence of a UTI (Yates, 2016). CSU are usually collected for microscopy, culture and sensitivity (MC&S) testing when an infection has been suspected. The urine is tested to identify the organisms causing the infection as well as their sensitivities to antibiotics (Shepherd, 2017b).

KEY POINTS

- CSU may be taken from a sampling port or a catheter with a valve.
- The collection of a CSU must be performed as part of a holistic assessment and must be considered alongside the presenting signs and symptoms.
- A CSU should only be collected when a patient has clinical signs of a catheter-associated urinary tract infection (CAUTI) (Box 17.1).

EQUIPMENT

Clean tray to hold equipment
Non-sterile gloves

BOX 17.1 ■ Clinical Signs of CAUTI

■ Fever	■ Lethargy with no other identified cause
■ Rigor, shivering, shaking	■ Back pain/pelvic pain
■ New onset or worsening confusion/ delirium	■ Acute haematuria

Modified from SIGN (2015).

Apron
Sterile 10 mL syringe (not required if taking a specimen from a catheter valve)
Non-traumatic clamp (not required if taking a specimen from a catheter valve)
Specimen container
Alcohol-impregnated swabs (2% chlorhexidine in 70% isopropyl alcohol)
Sterile jug (if taking a CSU from a catheter valve)
Documentation and forms

COLLECTING FROM A SAMPLING PORT

1. Explain the procedure to the patient, gain consent and confirm patient details against the pathology request and label.
2. An aseptic non-touch technique (ANTT) (see chapter 2) must be used to obtain a CSU as this reduces the risk of cross infection.
3. Decontaminate hands and prepare the equipment.
4. Check the patient is comfortable and that their privacy and dignity is maintained throughout the procedure.
5. Decontaminate hands and put on an apron.
6. If taking a specimen from a sampling port (Fig. 17.2), check first whether there is urine in the catheter tubing. If the tubing is empty apply a clamp below the level of the sampling port. This allows urine to collect above the clamp so that a sample can be obtained.
7. Decontaminate your hands and apply non-sterile gloves. Clean the sampling port with an alcohol-impregnated swab according to local policy and allow to dry. This reduces the risk of cross infection or contamination of the specimen.
8. Stabilise the tubing by holding it below the level of the sampling port.
9. Insert the syringe tip into the sampling port (following manufacturer's instructions) (Fig. 17.3). Be careful to protect the sterile syringe tip and disinfected sample port from contamination.
10. Aspirate at least 10 mL of urine and withdraw the syringe (Fig. 17.4).
11. Put the urine into a sterile universal container, avoiding contact between the syringe and the pot (Fig. 17.5). Check the top of the specimen container is secured to prevent leakage and contamination of the specimen.

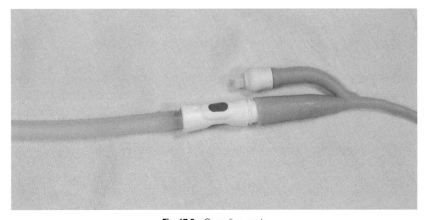

Fig. 17.2 Sampling port.

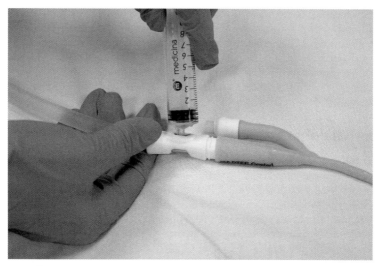

Fig. 17.3 Attaching syringe to catheter draining bag port to take sample.

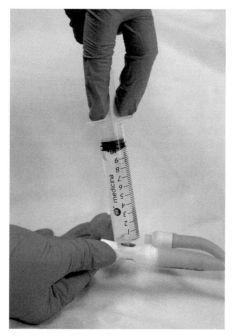

Fig. 17.4 Aspirating urine for catheter specimen of urine.

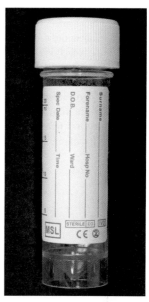

Fig. 17.5 Specimen pot.

12. Wipe the sampling port with an alcohol-impregnated swab and allow to dry. This reduces the risk of cross infection and contamination.

13. If a clamp was used, release it to allow urine drainage freely. Failure to do this will cause the bladder to fill and can result in discomfort and bypassing of urine around the catheter, which can be distressing for the patient.

14. Remove and dispose of gloves and apron, and decontaminate hands.
15. Complete the request form, label the specimen and place in a specimen bag following local policies.
16. Send the sample to the laboratory immediately or refrigerate until it can be transported to ensure accurate results are obtained.
17. Document the date and time the sample was collected in the patient's notes.

COLLECTING FROM A CATHETER VALVE

1. First, follow steps 1 to 4 above and then:
2. Confirm the patient has a full bladder.
3. Apply non-sterile gloves and clean the catheter valve port with an alcohol-impregnated swab according to local policy and allow to dry. This reduces the risk of cross infection.
4. Open the valve and release a small amount of urine to flush the valve.
5. Open the valve again and empty the remaining urine into a sterile jug, ensuring the valve does not come into direct contact with the jug.
6. Put a sample of urine in a sterile universal container. Ensure the top of the specimen container is secured to prevent leakage and any contamination of the specimen.
7. Close off the valve and wipe the port with an alcohol-impregnated swab.
8. Dispose of any remaining urine according to local policy.
9. Follow steps 13 to 16 above to complete the procedure.

24-Hour Urine Collection

24-hour collection is the collection of all urine over a 24-hour period, as the body's chemistry alters constantly. It is used to measure substances such as steroids, white cells, electrolytes, or urine osmolality (Yates, 2016). Urine collection bottles may contain either hydrochloric acid or nitric acid, the collection is to test for: catecholamines (VMA), creatinine, calcium, phosphate, oxalate, citrate and magnesium. Plain bottles are usually required for: sodium, potassium, urea, creatinine, urate, albumin, Bence Jones Protein, and urine free cortisol, histamine. The volume of acid will need to be deducted from the total volume depending on local policy.

KEY POINTS

- Should a sample of urine become contaminated or accidentally be discarded, the collection must be terminated and restarted.
- The collection of a 24-hour urine collection must be performed as part of a holistic assessment and must be considered alongside the presenting signs and symptoms.

EQUIPMENT

Urinal/bedpan as required and jug
Bed/door sign indicating 24-hour urine collection is in progress, time started and completion time
A 24-hour urine collection container (more than one may be required)
Apron and gloves should be worn
Additional protective clothing may be necessary if indicated by the patient's condition (see Chapter 2)

PROCEDURE

1. Explain the procedure and assess the patient's ability to participate in obtaining the collection.
2. Label the container clearly with the patient's name, hospital number and ward.
3. Either ask the patient to void urine or empty the catheter bag prior to starting the 24 hour collection. The 24-hour period begins at this point; write this time on the container.
4. Every time the patient passes urine, it is collected and placed in the container, which is stored in the sluice/dirty utility room.
5. If the patient is undertaking collection independently, check compliance and continued understanding.
6. Ask/assist the patient to empty their bladder at the end of the 24-hour collection period and write the time on the container.
7. Transfer the 24-hour urine collection and laboratory request form to the laboratory as soon as possible.
8. Clean or discard the jug according to local policy and remove sign from the bed/door.
9. Document the 24-hour urine collection according to local policy.

Female Catheterisation

Urinary catheterisation is the insertion of a tube into the bladder using an aseptic non-touch technique. Indications for urinary catheterisation are outlined in Box 17.2.

KEY POINTS

- An appropriately sized catheter should be chosen.
- The external diameter of the catheter shaft is measured in Charrière (ch), also known as French gauge (Fg) units. For most women a 12 ch/Fg or 14 ch/Fg will be adequate, although a larger size may be necessary if there is blood or sediment in the urine.
- Female length catheters are 23 to 26 cm. They reduce the risk of kinking and looping, and so allow more efficient drainage, and can also be more easily concealed if being used with a leg bag. However, they are not suitable for all women and male standard length catheters are recommended for women postoperatively, in those who are critically ill, immobile or clinically obese.

BOX 17.2 ■ Indications for Urinary Catheterisation

- Address acute or chronic urinary retention
- Empty the bladder, for example before pelvic surgery
- Accurately measure urinary output in patients who are acutely ill
- Irrigate the bladder, for example following surgery
- Bypass an obstruction such as a urethral stricture
- Administer drugs directly into the bladder
- Carry out bladder function tests
- Improve comfort for patients receiving end-of-life care
- Relieve incontinence and maintain skin integrity when all other conservative continence management strategies have been attempted

Dougherty and Lister (2015), Royal College of Nursing (2019a).

- The volume of water required will be indicated on the catheter. A balloon size of 10 mL is recommended for the routine drainage of clear urine, as this is usually sufficient to retain the catheter. Larger balloon sizes may irritate the bladder and cause bladder spasm and bypassing of urine. 30 to 80 mL balloons are used in specialised catheters in urology units and should not be used for routine catheterisation. It is important to use the exact amount of water as indicated on the catheter.
- Anaesthetic gel is recommended for use in female catheterisation to prevent urethral trauma and to reduce discomfort for the patient (Yates, 2016).

EQUIPMENT

- A catheterisation pack usually contains the following sterile items: kidney dish/receiver, dressing towels, gloves, and gallipot and gauze swabs. If a catheterisation pack is not available, a sterile dressing pack containing gloves can be used and the other items added as required.
- Anaesthetic gel
- Sterile gloves
- Cleansing fluid
- Syringe and sterile water for non-prefilled catheters
- Sterile individual antiseptic/lubricating gel
- Disposable apron
- Appropriate catheter
- Drainage system/catheter valve

PROCEDURE

1. Take the prepared trolley to the patient's bedside and position it on the right or left depending on the nurse's dominant hand (Fig. 17.6).
2. Raise the bed to a safe working height and ensure a good light source.
3. Ask/assist the patient to adopt a supine position with knees flexed and thighs relaxed to externally rotate the hip joints. If the patient is unable to adopt this position, assist her onto her side with her upper leg flexed at the hip and knee.
4. Arrange the bedclothes to expose the genital area and place the disposable pad beneath the buttocks.
5. Decontaminate hands.
6. Maintaining asepsis, open the catheterisation pack and any additional packs and equipment (Fig. 17.7).
7. Open the catheter, but do not remove it from its internal wrapping, and place it in the sterile receiver on the trolley. Expose the tip of the catheter by pulling off the top of the wrapper at the serrated edge.
8. Pour the sachet of 0.9% sodium chloride into the gallipot.
9. Open the catheter bag and arrange it at the side of the bed, ensuring that the catheter connection is easily accessible and remains sterile.
10. If not pre-filled draw up the amount of sterile water required to inflate the balloon.
11. Attach the nozzle to the anaesthetic lubricating gel.
12. Decontaminate hands and put on the sterile gloves.
13. Place sterile dressing towels onto the bed area between the patient's legs and over the patient's thighs.

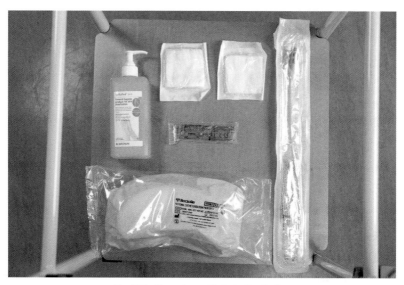

Fig. 17.6 Preparing catheterisation trolley.

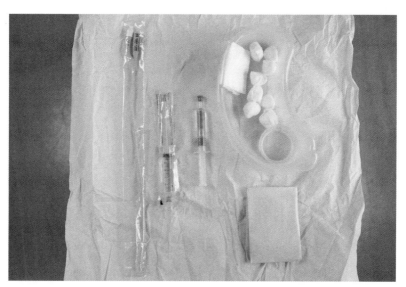

Fig. 17.7 Catheterisation equipment.

14. Using a gauze swab and your non-dominant hand, retract the labia minora to expose the urethral meatus. This hand should be used to maintain labial separation until catheterisation has been completed.
15. Clean the perineal area with 0.9% sodium chloride, using a new gauze swab for each stroke and cleaning from the front towards the anus.
16. Gently insert the nozzle of the anaesthetic gel into the urethra. Squeeze the gel into the urethra, remove and discard the tube. Leave for approximately 5 minutes (Fig. 17.8).

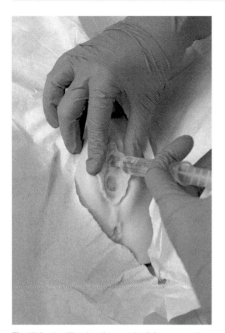

Fig. 17.8 Instilling local anaestheticin preparation for female catheterisation.

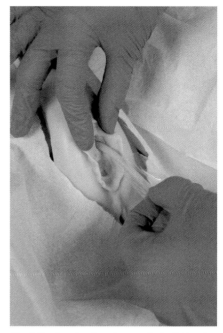

Fig. 17.9 Passing the urinary catheter in female.

17. Place the receiver holding the catheter on the sterile towel between the patient's legs.
18. Holding the catheter so that the distal end remains in the receiver and gradually advancing it out of its wrapper, introduce the catheter into the urethra in an upward and backward direction for approximately 5 to 7 cm or until urine flows out of the catheter end. Advance the catheter a further 5 cm (Fig. 17.9). Do not force the catheter. If the catheter is accidentally inserted into the vagina, leave it in place to prevent it happening again, and use a new catheter. Once this is successfully in place, remove the first catheter.
19. Attach the syringe of water to the balloon port and inflate the balloon with the correct amount of water (see Fig. 17.11 – in male catheterisation).
20. Gently withdraw the catheter until resistance is felt; the inflated balloon will hold it in place in the bladder
21. Maintaining asepsis, attach the catheter drainage bag and position it so that there is no pulling on the catheter. In some instances, a patient may have a catheter valve fitted instead of a drainage bag. This allows the bladder to fill up and is emptied intermittently (e.g. 4-hourly). They are most suitable for patients requiring long-term catheterisation who have good bladder capacity, good cognitive function and the dexterity to manage the valve. They should not be used for patients who have poor bladder sensation, urgency or who are cognitively impaired. The catheter can be secured by using a securement device or by taping it to the patient's leg.
22. Remove the sterile towel by tearing it on one side.
23. Check the catheter drainage bag is positioned below the patient's bladder. Positioning the catheter drainage bag below the level of the patient's bladder aids gravity flow and prevents reflux of urine. Ensure the bag is not touching the floor as this is an infection risk.

24. Cover the patient and replace the bedclothes. Make sure the patient is dry and comfortable.
25. Urine from the sterile receiver or contained within the plastic wrapper can be tipped into the specimen pot. Place a small amount of urine (10 to 20 mL) into the specimen pot.
26. Dispose of equipment and clinical waste appropriately.
27. Measure and record the amount of urine contained in the receiver.
28. Remove gloves and apron and decontaminate hands.
29. Document catheterisation in the patient's records. Record of the catheterisation should include: the reason for catheterisation, the date and time of catheterisation, the type of catheter (size, length and gauge), the batch number and manufacturer of the catheter (an adhesive label showing the batch number is often provided with the catheter), the size of balloon and the amount of water used to inflate it. A plan of care including review/ assessment date should be documented.
30. Send the specimen, with the request form, to the laboratory as soon as possible, for culture and sensitivity
31. If the patient's condition allows, encourage oral fluids. Document urine output on a fluid balance chart.

Male Catheterisation

Urinary catheterisation is the insertion of a tube into the bladder using an aseptic non-touch technique. Indications for urinary catheterisation are outlined in Box 17.2.

KEY POINTS

- An appropriately sized catheter should be chosen.
- The external diameter of the catheter shaft is measured in Charrière (ch), also known as French gauge (Fg) units. For most men a 12 ch/Fg or 14 ch/Fg will be adequate, although a larger size may be necessary if there is blood or sediment in the urine.
- The volume of water required will be indicated on the catheter. A balloon size of 10 mL is recommended for the routine drainage of clear urine, as this is usually sufficient to retain the catheter. Larger balloon sizes may irritate the bladder and cause bladder spasm and bypassing of urine. 30–80 mL balloons are used in specialised catheters in urology units and should not be used for routine catheterisation. It is important to use the exact amount of water as indicated on the catheter.

EQUIPMENT

- Sterile pack suitable for catheterisation (receiver, low-linting swabs, gallipots, disposable towels)
- Sterile gloves
- Cleansing fluid
- Syringe and sterile water for non-prefilled catheters
- Sterile individual antiseptic/lubricating gel
- Disposable apron
- Appropriate catheter
- Drainage system/catheter valve.

PROCEDURE

1. Explain the procedure with the patient, explaining any associated risks or benefits and gain valid consent.
2. Take the prepared trolley to the patient's bedside and position it on the right or left depending on the nurse's dominant hand.
3. Raise the bed to a safe working height and ensure a good light source.
4. Decontaminate hands.
5. Maintaining asepsis, open the catheterisation pack and any additional packs and equipment.
6. Open the catheter, but do not remove it from its inner wrapper, and place it in the sterile receiver on the trolley. Expose the tip of the catheter by pulling off the top of the wrapper at the serrated edge. Replace it in the sterile receiver.
7. If not using a pre-filled syringe draw up the amount of sterile water required to inflate the balloon.
8. Pour the sachet of 0.9% sodium chloride into the gallipot.
9. Open the catheter drainage bag and arrange it at the side of the bed, ensuring the attachment tip is easily accessible and remains sterile.
10. Arrange the bedclothes to expose the genital area and place the absorbent pad underneath the buttocks.
11. Ask/assist the patient to adopt a supine position with the legs extended.
12. Decontaminate hands. Put on one or two pairs of sterile gloves. Concerns about contamination of the hands during urethral cleansing and instillation of gel can be overcome by using two pairs of sterile gloves (one on top of the other) at the start of the procedure. The outer pair can then be removed after cleansing, prior to catheter insertion.
13. Tear a hole in the centre of the sterile towel. Cover the patient's abdomen and thighs with the towel, with the penis protruding through the hole.
14. Attach the nozzle to the anaesthetic lubricating gel.
15. With your non-dominant hand and using sterile gauze, grasp the shaft of the penis and retract the foreskin.
16. Clean the glans penis with the sterile 0.9% sodium chloride, ensuring the tips of the fingers remain sterile.
17. Still holding the penis, gently insert the nozzle of the anaesthetic lubricating gel into the urethra and instil the gel into the urethra.
18. Massage the gel along the urethra and wait 5 minutes for it to act.
19. Put on a new pair of sterile gloves or remove the top pair revealing the second pair underneath.
20. Place the receiver containing the catheter between the patient's thighs.
21. Grasp the shaft of the penis with your non-dominant hand and hold the penis upwards, to extend the peno-scrotal flexure. If difficulties are encountered force or pressure must not be used. Asking a male patient to cough may allow the catheter to pass the prostate more easily.
22. With your dominant hand holding and gradually withdrawing the wrapper, insert the catheter 15 to 25 cm into the urethra until urine flows (Fig. 17.10). If resistance is met at the external sphincter, extend the penis further towards the abdomen. Ask the patient to cough or strain gently as if passing urine. If resistance continues, do not force the catheter: stop the procedure and seek medical advice.
23. When urine is flowing, advance the catheter further, to ensure the catheter is in the bladder.
24. Inflate the balloon with the correct amount of sterile water (Fig. 17.11).

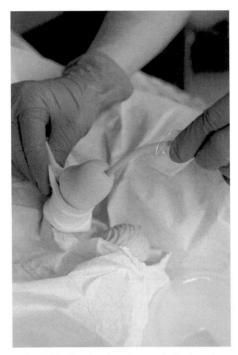

Fig. 17.10   Passing the urinary catheter in male.

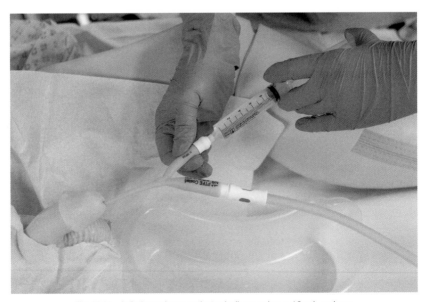

Fig. 17.11   Inflating urinary catheter balloon using a 10 mL syringe.

25. Gently withdraw the catheter until resistance is felt; the inflated balloon will hold it in place in the bladder.
26. Maintaining asepsis, attach the catheter drainage bag and position it so that there is no pulling on the catheter. The catheter can be secured by using a securement device or by taping the catheter to the patient's leg. Ensure the catheter drainage bag is positioned below the patient's bladder. Positioning the catheter drainage bag below the level of the patient's bladder aids gravity flow and prevents reflux of urine. Ensure the bag is not touching the floor as this is an infection risk.
27. Check that any residual anaesthetic gel is removed and that the glans penis is clean. Where applicable, gently push the foreskin back over the glans penis.
28. Remove the sterile towel by tearing it on one side.
29. Replace the patient's bedclothes and check he is dry and comfortable.
30. Urine from the sterile receiver or contained within the plastic wrapper can be tipped into the specimen pot. Place a small amount of urine (10 to 20 mL) into the specimen pot and send it and the request form to the laboratory as soon as possible, for culture and sensitivity testing.
31. Dispose of equipment and clinical waste appropriately. Remove gloves, apron and decontaminate hands.
32. If the patient's condition allows, encourage oral fluids.
33. Measure and document the amount of urine contained in the receiver.
34. Document catheterisation in the patient's records. Ideal records of catheterisation should include: the reason for catheterisation, patient consent, the date and time of catheterisation, the type of catheter (size, length, gauge), the batch number and manufacturer of the catheter (an adhesive label showing the batch number may be available), the size of balloon and the amount of water used to inflate it. A plan of care including review/assessment date must be documented.

Continuous Bladder Irrigation

Continuous bladder irrigation is often performed following urological surgery to remove clots and debris post-surgery. Continuous irrigation of the bladder is undertaken via a three-way catheter. This method of irrigation is normally used for short periods and only within an acute ward setting (Royal College of Nursing, 2019a).

Irrigation fluid should be suspended from a separate infusion stand from that used for intravenous infusions. 3 L bags of irrigation solution are preferable, as they require less frequent changing and interruption of the closed system. Using larger volumes of fluid reduces the risk of infection, as it reduces the frequency of the sterile closed draining system having to be broken.

EQUIPMENT

Clean trolley or other appropriate surface
Sterile dressing towel
Antiseptic skin-cleansing solution according to local policy
Non-toothed clamp
Sterile jug
Sterile 'Y'-shaped irrigation set and fluid as prescribed (usually 0.9% sodium chloride) at room temperature
Infusion stand
Large catheter drainage bag
Sterile dressing pack containing gloves
Alcohol hand-rub

PROCEDURE

1. Take the trolley and equipment to the bedside.
2. Open the irrigation fluid bags and hang on the infusion stand.
3. Maintaining asepsis, attach and prime the irrigation set to expel all air. Close the flow control clamp of the irrigation set. When priming the irrigation set, make sure that only one clamp is open. This will prevent irrigation fluid running from one bottle to the other.
4. Ask/assist the patient to adopt a supine position and expose the catheter and catheter drainage tube (Fig. 17.12).
5. Clamp the catheter using a non-toothed clamp or the clamp on the catheter-bag tubing. It is important to use a non-toothed clamp to prevent damage to the tubing.
6. Decontaminate hands.
7. Maintaining asepsis, open the dressing pack and other equipment, attach the disposal bag to the side of the trolley and pour antiseptic solution into the gallipot.
8. Decontaminate hands and put on the sterile gloves.
9. Place the sterile towel underneath the irrigation inlet of the catheter.
10. Cover both the catheter and spigot with sterile gauze, and touching only the gauze, remove the spigot from the irrigation port of the catheter and discard.
11. Thoroughly clean around the irrigation port with antiseptic solution, using each swab only once and wiping in the same direction.
12. Maintaining asepsis, attach the irrigation set to the irrigation port, but do not open the flow control clamp.
13. Release the clamp on the catheter and allow accumulated urine to drain. Empty the contents of the catheter bag into the sterile jug.
14. Discard gloves.

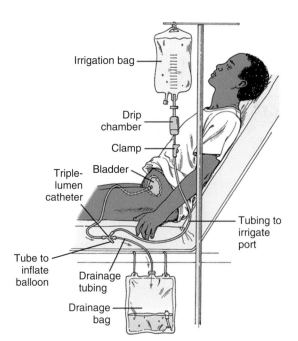

Fig. 17.12 Continuous Bladder Irrigation Bladder irrigation. (Perry, A. G., Potter, P. A., Ostendorf, W., & Laplante, N. (2022). *Clinical Nursing Skills and Techniques*. Elsevier Inc.)

15. Open the flow control clamp and set irrigation at the prescribed rate, checking that fluid/urine is draining freely into the catheter bag. The rate of infusion will vary according to the degree of haematuria (blood in the urine). The aim is to obtain drainage fluid that is rosé in colour. Haematuria will be greatest in the first 12 hours following surgery and 6 to 9 L of irrigation fluid is likely to be required. This should fall to 3 to 6 L in the second 12 hours. Irrigation is usually discontinued on the morning following surgery. Only one bag of irrigation fluid is used at a time. When the first bag is empty the second bag can be commenced immediately ensuring continuous flow. In the meantime, the empty bag can be replaced.

16. Assist the patient into a comfortable position and advise him to report any bladder distension, pain or discomfort. If clot retention is suspected (the output stops, there is evidence of abdominal distension and the patient complains of pain and discomfort) irrigation should be stopped immediately and the problem reported. Deflation and re-inflation of the catheter balloon or a bladder washout may be required.

17. Dispose of equipment and waste appropriately.

18. Measure the volume of urine and discard.

19. Remove apron and decontaminate hands.

20. Document the time of commencement and the volume of irrigation fluid being infused on the fluid balance chart.

21. Check the volume in the catheter drainage bag at least every hour for the first 24 hours, empty as necessary and document on fluid balance chart. The volume of irrigation fluid being infused and the amount of drainage in the catheter bag should be recorded on a fluid balance chart. The difference between the two figures is the urine output.

Bladder Washout

Bladder washouts involve flushing the bladder with sterile normal saline to remove clots, debris or mucus. This is a high risk of infection due to the breaking of the closed drainage system every time an administration is performed (RCN, 2019a).

KEY POINTS

- There should be a clear, documented clinical rationale for using bladder washouts with evidence of effectiveness.
- The administration should be via a pre-filled administration set.
- Bladder washouts should be administered, where possible, using gravity rather than direct pressure to avoid tissue trauma.
- Patients with a surgically augmented bladder (where bowel tissue has been used to enlarge the bladder capacity), a sterile 50 mL syringe to administer the washout due to the high level of mucus present may be required.
- Consider using an irrigation connection device (inserted into the needle-free sample port of the catheter bag) to minimise the risk of infection caused by breaking the closed drainage system.

EQUIPMENT

Sterile dressing pack containing gloves
Gloves
Bladder wash out bag (Fig. 17.13)

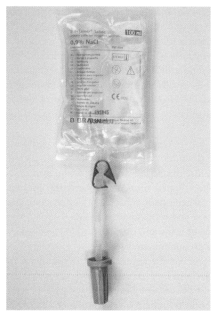

Fig. 17.13 Bladder irrigation for flushing a urinary catheter.

PROCEDURE

1. Take the prepared trolley to the patient's bedside and position it on the right or left depending on the nurse's dominant hand.
2. Maintaining asepsis, open the sterile dressing pack and additional equipment including the sterile jug, bladder syringe and sterile bowls/receivers. Pour antiseptic solution into the gallipot. Pour washout solution into the jug.
3. Open the catheter drainage bag and place it in an accessible position, leaving the cover on the catheter connector to maintain sterility.
4. Arrange the bedclothes to expose the genital area and check the absorbent pad is under the buttocks.
5. Decontaminate hands and put on the sterile gloves.
6. Place the sterile towel between the patient's legs, creating a sterile field.
7. Remove the urine drainage bag and attach the bladder wash out to the urinary catheter. Allow gravity for the fluid to run into the bladder.
8. Clamp the catheter.
9. Allow the solution to drain out naturally into the second sterile receiver. If the solution does not drain, aspirate gently using the bladder syringe. Repeat the process, using 30 to 40 mL of solution each time, until the urine is clear and flowing freely.
10. Connect the new drainage bag.
11. Check the patient is comfortable and is not experiencing bladder discomfort.
12. Dispose of equipment and waste appropriately
13. Remove gloves, apron and decontaminate hands.
14. Encourage fluids and mobilisation if condition allows.
15. Measure the input (amount of washout solution inserted) and output (drainage or aspirate) to calculate any urine output.
16. Document bladder washout and report any abnormalities.

Emptying a Catheter Bag

Urine drains from urinary catheters into a catheter bag. The drainage bag can either be one that is used at the bedside, or it can be smaller and strapped to the patient's leg. The container used to collect the drained urine will vary according to local policy; it may be disposable or one that is disinfected after each use. If using a disinfected jug it should be one that is only used for urine. This should differ in colour and design from those used for drinking water. The cleaning of the jug will vary according to local policy. If disposable, it will be discarded. If not disposable, it must be disinfected, and either placed in a bedpan washer or returned to the sterile supplies department for decontamination.

EQUIPMENT

Measuring jug and paper towel to cover
Two alcohol-impregnated swabs
PPE

PROCEDURE

1. Explain the procedure to the patient, although it should not cause any discomfort.
2. To maintain patient dignity, draw screens around the bed area. Patients with a leg bag who are mobile can empty the bag into the toilet.
3. Decontaminate hands.
4. Gloves and an apron should be worn and additional protective clothing may be necessary if indicated by the patient's condition.
5. Take the covered jug and other equipment to the bedside.
6. If the drainage bag is on a floor stand, it does not need to be removed from the stand for emptying. If the bag is hanging on the side of the bed, it may need to be removed from its holder. Hold the bag over the jug, making sure that the drainage port does not touch the jug (Fig. 17.14).

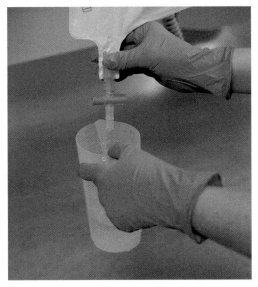

Fig. 17.14   Emptying a urinary catheter bag into a jug.

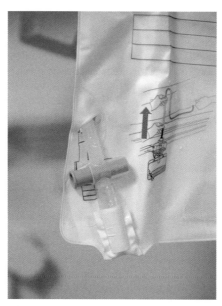

Fig. 17.15   Drainage port not touching the floor.

7. Clean the drainage port with an alcohol impregnated swab.
8. Open the drainage port and allow the urine to flow into the jug. Close the drainage port and wipe the outlet tap with the second alcohol-impregnated swab.
9. Reposition the catheter bag as necessary ensuring that the drainage port is not touching the floor and the tubing is not kinked, to allow free drainage into the bag (Fig. 17.15).
10. Cover the jug and take it to the sluice/dirty utility room. Measure the amount of urine and discard. Clean or discard the urine jug according to local policy.
11. Remove gloves, apron and decontaminate hands.
12. Record the amount on fluid balance chart.
13. If the patient's condition allows, encourage oral fluids.

Removing a Urinary Catheter (Trial Without Catheter)

Routine removal of catheters is normally undertaken in the morning, so if there are any complications such as urinary retention they can be dealt with during the day by appropriately trained staff (Yates, 2017). Potential complications post catheter removal include urinary retention, dysuria (pain when passing urine), frequency and urgency, haematuria or incontinence (Yates, 2017).

The RCN (2021) identifies three types of TWOC:

- Early daytime, with an increased fluid intake
- Daytime extended overnight with next day review. This may be appropriate for patients with likely residual urine volume.
- Night-time TWOC which may be appropriate for inpatients and those with nocturnal polyuria.

If problems are encountered when deflating the balloon or withdrawing the catheter, medical advice should be sought. Avoid pulling back on the syringe when removing the water as this may create a vacuum and cause the balloon to 'cuff', making removal difficult (RCN, 2021). It is essential that the catheter is withdrawn slowly and gently in order to reduce the trauma to the urethra caused by the creases and ridges in the balloon. Rotating the catheter as it is slowly withdrawn may also make removal easier.

The patient may well experience feelings of wanting to pass urine following removal of the catheter. Male patients should be discouraged from placing a urinal in position 'just in case', as this may encourage frequent small volumes to be passed or 'dribbling'. A frequency chart may be requested for the first 24 hours. Haematuria (blood in the urine) may be the result of trauma following catheter removal and dysuria (pain when passing urine) may be due to inflammation of the urethra.

KEY POINTS

- Urinary catheters should be removed as soon as clinically appropriate.
- It is important to understand the reason for removal, whether this is permanent or unplanned due to a complication (e.g. a blocked catheter).
- The patient may be frightened of catheter removal and imagine it to be extremely painful.
- The size of syringe required will depend on the amount of water in the catheter balloon; this is written on the catheter itself or can be obtained from the patient's records.

EQUIPMENT

Dressing pack containing paper towel, swabs and gallipot
Kidney dish to receive the catheter
Syringe for deflating the balloon (usually a 10 mL syringe)
Disposable gloves and apron
Cleansing solution, for example 0.9% sodium chloride.

PROCEDURE

1. Take the equipment to the bedside and position the clinical waste bag for easy access.
2. Decontaminate hands and apply appropriate PPE.
3. Take a catheter specimen of urine.
4. Empty the catheter bag.
5. Clean the urinary meatus if necessary.
6. Place the absorbent pad under the buttocks.
7. Check the volume of water in the balloon (usually written on the catheter or obtain from patient records), attach the syringe to the balloon port on the catheter and withdraw the water to deflate the balloon. Make sure you withdraw the full amount from the balloon.
8. Place the receiver between the patient's thighs.
9. Ask the patient to breathe in and out and on exhalation gently but firmly withdraw the catheter into the receiver.
10. Detach the catheter bag from the catheter stand (if applicable) and place it in the clinical waste bag with the receiver containing the catheter and the absorbent pad.
11. Assist the patient into a comfortable position and ensure a toilet/urinal/commode is nearby. Ask the patient to inform the nurse when urine has been passed.
12. Advise the patient regarding the possibility of frequency, urgency, haematuria and dysuria.
13. Advise the patient to increase oral fluid intake (2 to 2.5 L in 24 hours).
14. Dispose of equipment and clinical waste appropriately.
15. Remove gloves, apron and decontaminate hands.
16. Record the amount of urine obtained from the catheter drainage bag on the fluid balance chart.

17. Document the time of catheter removal and when the patient subsequently passes urine. This includes the length of time the catheter was in situ; if the balloon deflated properly and the catheter tip and balloon were intact on removal; if encrustation was evident; if the part of the catheter that was in the bladder was clean/dirty or if there is evidence of debris; if removal was painful and if there was any blood present. Any inflammation or discharge at the meatus should be reported and urine should be observed for signs of infection (e.g. cloudy, debris, colour, odour) (RCN, 2019a).

18. Label the catheter specimen and send it to the laboratory with the request form or refrigerate it as soon as possible.

Care of a Suprapubic Catheter

A suprapubic catheter is inserted through the abdominal wall into the bladder, where a water-filled balloon holds it in place. The insertion site must be treated as a surgical wound. Patients should be encouraged to care for their own catheters where possible, to encourage independence. The weight of a full urine bag may pull on the catheter. Observe the urine; if soon after insertion, haematuria is common. Encourage increased oral intake if condition allows. A 'keyhole' type dressing the catheter will be used until discharge around the catheter ceases. If a keyhole dressing is not available, use sterile scissors to cut a 'Y' shape in the centre of a self-adhesive dressing, to fit around the catheter.

PROCEDURE

1. Clean the trolley or other appropriate surface according to local policy and prepare a new length of adhesive strapping.
2. Take the trolley to the bed/chair area. Adjust the bed to a safe working height or sit down to avoid stooping.
3. Remove the dressing pack from its outer packaging; place it on the clean trolley/surface.
4. Using your fingertips and touching the edges of the paper only, open the pack and lay it flat to create a sterile field.
5. Remove the yellow waste bag and place it to one side. Touching only the edge of the glove pack (or wrist part of the gloves if loose) move them to the edge of the sterile field.
6. Taking care not to contaminate the sterile field, carefully pour the cleansing solution into the tray. Open the dressing and sterile scissors (if required), onto the sterile field.
7. Adjust any remaining bedclothes to expose the catheter and then loosen the adhesive strapping. If a dressing is in place, loosen it but do not remove it.
8. Decontaminate hands.
9. Open the yellow waste bag and put your hand inside so that the bag acts as a glove. Use this to remove the adhesive strapping and/or soiled dressing.
10. Inspect the dressing to note the type and amount of exudate. Observe the skin around the catheter for signs of infection or cellulitis.
11. Turn the bag inside out so that the dressing is contained within it, and using the self-adhesive strip, attach the bag to the side of the trolley or other convenient place close to the wound.
12. Taking care not to touch the outside of the gloves, put on the sterile gloves (chapter 2).
13. Use your non-dominant hand to hold up the catheter. In your dominant hand, use gauze swabs soaked in cleansing solution (but not dripping) to clean around the catheter to remove any encrustations. Use each swab once only (Fig. 17.16).
14. Use fresh gauze swabs to dry around the catheter and apply the new dressing.

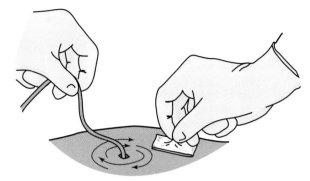

Fig. 17.16 Cleaning around a suprapubic catheter in a circular pattern. (Perry, A. G., Potter, P. A., & Ostendorf, W. (2020). *Nursing Interventions & Clinical Skills*, 7th ed. Elsevier Inc.)

15. Place all waste in the clinical waste bag.
16. Remove gloves and discard into waste bag.
17. Replace clothing and check the patient is comfortable. Use adhesive strapping to fix the catheter to the skin to prevent pulling.
18. Discard clinical waste. Remove apron and decontaminate hands.
19. Document the dressing and condition of suprapubic catheter and surrounding skin according to local policy.

Urinary Catheter Care

Where possible, patients should be taught to attend to their own meatal and perineal hygiene, thus reducing the risk of cross-infection. Powders or lotions should not be used after cleansing as these trap organisms in the area. The main aim of cleansing is to remove secretions and encrustation. Cleansing with soap and water has been shown to be as effective as any other method. Cleaning in addition to normal hygiene practice is not necessary and daily bathing or showering is sufficient to maintain meatal hygiene unless there is excessive exudate or encrustation (RCN, 2021).

GENERAL CARE

Patients should be advised to:
1. Wash their hands before and after handling their catheter
2. Bathe or shower daily to maintain meatal hygiene (Loveday et al., 2014)
3. Drink at least eight cups of fluid a day and avoid caffeine where possible
4. Avoid constipation, as pressure from a full rectum can prevent urine drainage
5. Avoid kinking the catheter tubing so urine can drain freely
6. Empty the drainage system when it is three-quarters full
7. Keep a closed system of drainage.

Female Patients

1. Clean the vulval area from above downward using warm soapy water.
2. Clean the catheter by gently wiping in one direction away from the catheter–meatal junction. Rinse well.
3. Dry the area by patting with a towel.

Male Patients

1. Retract the foreskin before cleaning.
2. Clean the shaft of the catheter away from the catheter–meatal junction and rinse well.
3. Dry the area by patting with a towel.
4. Reposition the foreskin on completion of cleaning.
5. Check the patient is dry and comfortable
6. Dispose of all waste appropriately
7. Remove gloves and apron and decontaminate hands
8. Record catheter care and report any abnormalities and/or changes.

Emptying a Urinary Catheter Bag

A urinary catheter bag depends on the reason and duration of catheterisation, patient preference and infection prevention issues (Dougherty and Lister, 2015). Types of urinary catheter bags are outlined in Table 17.3.

KEY POINTS

- Catheters must be attached to an appropriate draining device or catheter valve.
- The connection between the catheter and urinary draining system must not be broken.
- Bags should be positioned below the level of the bladder.
- Urinary drainage bags should not be allowed to fill beyond 3/4 full.

EQUIPMENT

Disposable gloves
Clean container for single patient use
Paper towels

PROCEDURE

1. Take the covered jug and other equipment to the bedside.
2. If the drainage bag is on a floor stand, it does not need to be removed from the stand for emptying. If the bag is hanging on the side of the bed, it may need to be removed from its

---

TABLE 17.3 ■ **Types of Catheter Bags**

Two-litre bags	Used for non-ambulatory patients and overnight drainage
Leg Bags	Can be worn under clothes, thereby encouraging mobility and rehabilitation as patients do not have to carry a bag attached to a catheter stand. Leg bags can also have a positive effect on patients' dignity as they are not visible to others
Urometer bags	Used to closely monitor urinary output. Urine is normally recorded hourly; a special drainage bag is used. This incorporates a small reservoir that can be emptied into the drainage bag without opening the 'closed' system (see Fig. 17.14).

Yates (2016).

holder. Hold the bag over the jug, making sure that the drainage port does not touch the jug (see Fig. 17.14).

3. Decontaminate hands and apply appropriate PPE.
4. Clean the drainage port with an alcohol impregnated swab.
5. Open the drainage port and allow the urine to flow into the jug. Close the drainage port and wipe the outlet tap with the second alcohol-impregnated swab.
6. Reposition the catheter bag as necessary ensuring that the drainage port is not touching the floor and the tubing is not kinked, to allow free drainage into the bag (see Fig. 17.15).
7. Cover the jug and take it to the sluice/dirty utility room. Measure the amount of urine and discard. Clean or discard the urine jug according to local policy.
8. Remove gloves and apron and decontaminate hands.
9. Record the amount on fluid balance chart if appropriate.
10. If the patient's condition allows, encourage oral fluids.

Observation of Faeces and Bristol Stool Chart

RATIONALE

Bowel care includes the assessment and observation of a patient's faeces (also known as a 'stool'). Normal faeces is described as brown, soft and formed; it has an odour, but should not be offensive smelling. The Bristol Stool Chart is used as an assessment tool and to evaluate the effectiveness of treatments. In addition, stools should be observed if any 'red-flag' warning symptoms are noted (RCN, 2019b).

KEY POINTS

- Red flags include rectal bleeding; change in bowel habit for six weeks; pain before, during or after defaecation; faecal mucous present on defaecation; faecal leakage or urgency; or unexplained weight loss (RCN, 2019b).

When observing faeces, the following should be noted and any abnormality reported. The classifications of the Bristol stool chart (Fig. 17.17) are used in many clinical areas.

- Amount – particularly if diarrhoea, as patients may lose a lot of fluid this way.
- Frequency – the 'normal' frequency will vary from patient to patient.
- Consistency – the normal consistency is soft and formed using the Bristol Stool Chart. The following should be noted: hard faeces (constipation); liquid (diarrhoea); mucus evident (ulcerative colitis or Crohn disease); fatty, offensive smelling and floats (steatorrhoea, seen in biliary disease); whether parasites are present.
- Colour – a pale, putty colour suggests the absence of bile pigments. The presence of bright-red blood may indicate bleeding from haemorrhoids or rectal bleeding. If the stool appears black and tarry in consistency (melaena), this indicates digested blood from the stomach or small intestine. If the stool is black and hard in consistency, this may be the result of iron medication.
- Pain/discomfort associated with a bowel action.
- Flatus – the presence of this indicates gut motility and is an important observation following abdominal surgery.

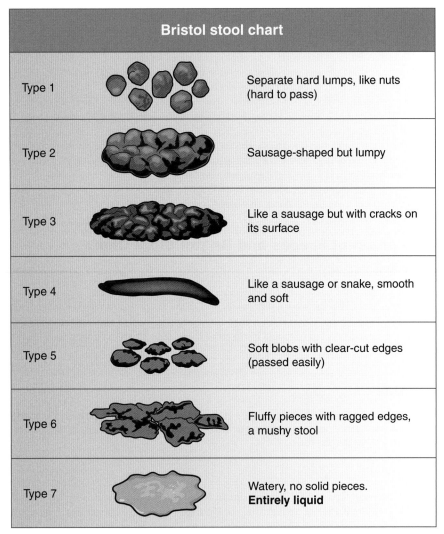

Fig. 17.17   Bristol Stool Classification. (Smith, M., Kauffman, T.L. & O'Hanlon S. (2022). *A Comprehensive Guide to Rehabilitation of the Older Patient*, 14th ed. Elsevier (Singapore) Pte Ltd.)

Obtaining a Specimen of Faeces

A stool specimen may be required to guide diagnosis and help guide the management of a patient's condition. Tests vary, therefore, you need to check the procedure to be carried out and the correct instructions followed. It has to be noted that stool specimens are obtained when patients have infections (e.g. diarrhoea). Infectious agents that may require a faecal specimen are outlined in Table 17.4. In consequence, strict infection control principles must be taken when taking samples and patients may also need to be isolated or cohort nursed until the results are available (Shepherd, 2017c).

TABLE 17.4 ▪ Infectious Agents Requiring a Faecal Specimen

Bacterial	*Salmonella, Campylobacter, Helicobacter, Shigella, Escherichia coli, Clostridium difficile*
Viral	Norovirus, retrovirus
Parasites	Protozoa, tapeworm, entamoeba

Dougherty and Lister (2015).

KEY POINTS

- Collection of a faecal specimen should be considered as part of a holistic nursing assessment.
- A comprehensive A–E assessment should be conducted to assess for associated symptoms e.g. fever, vomiting and abdominal pain, recent foreign travel, antibiotics or concerns about food poisoning,
- The stool should be assessed using the Bristol Stool Chart.
- Specimens should be collected within 48 hours of the onset of symptoms.
- Ideally, specimens should be obtained before antimicrobial therapy is commenced.

EQUIPMENT

- Non-latex gloves
- Apron
- Specimen bag
- Stool specimen pot
- Pathology request form and label
- Laboratory request form.

PROCEDURE

1. Explain the procedure, to gain consent and cooperation. Confirm patient's details.
2. Decontaminate hands and apply appropriate personal protective equipment (PPE).
3. Ask/assist the patient to use a bedpan or commode. Offer/assist with hand washing.
4. Open the sterile specimen container with attached spoon-shaped spatula (usually attached to the lid) (Fig. 17.18).
5. Use the spatula to remove a small quantity of faeces from the bedpan. Place the faeces and the spatula into the container and secure the lid (Fig. 17.19).
6. Complete the patient's details on the label of the container.
7. Place the specimen container in the specimen bag, seal it and insert the pathology request form into the pocket.
8. Dispose of faeces and place bedpan in the washer or disposal system as appropriate. If used, clean the commode according to local policy.
9. Remove gloves, apron and decontaminate hands.
10. Place specimen in the designated area to await transport to the laboratory.
11. Document that specimen has been collected.

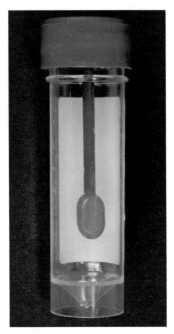

Fig. 17.18   Faecal specimen pot with spatula attached to lid.

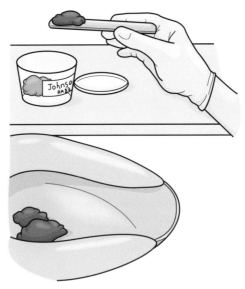

Fig. 17.19   Taking a stool specimen from a bedpan. (Scott, K., Webb, M., & Sorrentino, S. (2018). *Long-Term caring: Residential, home and community aged care*. Elsevier Australia.)

Administration of an Enema

An enema is the administration of a substance in liquid form into the rectum. If the enema is for drug administration (retention enema), this must be prescribed and checked as described on p. 195–196.

KEY POINTS

- It is necessary for the patient to be in the left lateral position because of the position of the rectum.
- Some enemas may need to be warmed before administration. Do this by placing it in a bowl of warm water. Test a little on your forearm before administration to check it is not too hot.

EQUIPMENT

- Prescription chart
- Enema as prescribed
- Cardboard tray/receiver
- Gauze swabs/tissues
- Lubricant
- Bedpan or commode, plus toilet paper.

PROCEDURE

1. Explain the procedure, to gain consent and cooperation. Draw screens to ensure privacy.
2. Decontaminate hands, put on gloves and apron. Additional protective clothing may be necessary if indicated by the patient's condition.
3. Place an absorbent pad under the buttocks. Ask/assist the patient to remove clothing below the waist and lie in the left lateral position.
4. Check the anal area for soreness, haemorrhoids or skin tags. If present seek advice before proceeding.
5. Remove the cover or removable tip from the nozzle and lubricate the tip.
6. Ask the patient to relax and take deep breaths.
7. Part the buttocks with the left hand. With the right hand, hold the nozzle of the enema and gently insert it through the anus and into the anal canal (Fig. 17.20). Because the patient needs to be in the left lateral position even left-handed nurses must use their right hand to insert the nozzle of the enema
8. Squeeze the bag/pack until all the contents have been deposited – some packs may be rolled (like a tube of toothpaste) to expel the last of the contents.
9. While still squeezing gently withdraw the nozzle. Keeping the bag rolled/squeezed while removing the nozzle prevents fluid running back into the bag.
10. Wipe away any residual lubricant and leave the patient dry. Cover the patient. Be aware that the patient may feel faint and/or nauseous.
11. Evacuant enema: ask the patient to hold the enema for as long as possible but the effect is likely to be rapid. Assist the patient onto the bedpan or commode as necessary.
12. Retention enema (drug administration): the patient should be instructed to stay in the left lateral position for at least 30 minutes to aid retention and absorption of the fluid. Raising the foot of the bed may also help.

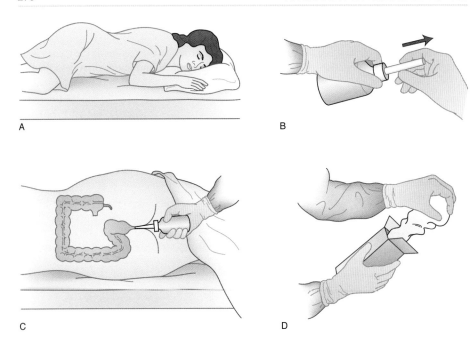

Fig. 17.20 Administering a disposable enema. (A) Place the patient in a left lateral position, unless a knee-chest position has been specified. (B) Remove the protective covering from the end of the enema and lubricate the end. (C) Insert the lubricated end into the patient's rectum and dispense the solution by compressing the plastic container. (D) Replace the used container in its original wrapping for disposal. (Willihnganz, M., Gurevitz, S. L., & Clayton, B. D. (2020). *Clayton's Basic Pharmacology for Nurses*. Elsevier Inc.)

13. After the patient has opened their bowels, observe the nature of the faeces (see p. 278).
14. Dispose of faeces and place bedpan in the washer or disposal system as appropriate. If used, clean the commode according to local policy. Offer/assist with hand washing.
15. Remove gloves and apron and decontaminate hands.
16. Document/report the result of the enema.

Changing a Stoma Bag

There is an extensive range of stoma appliances (terms bags or pouches) available that are grouped into one-piece or two-piece, which are either closed or drainable (Smith and Samways, 2020) (Fig. 17.21).

Some patients may have a urostomy or ileal conduit for urine drainage. For these patients, there are specially designed appliances.

Type of Stoma	*Colostomy*	*Ileostomy*	*Urostomy/Ileal Conduit*
Location	Usually on left side of abdomen	Usually on right side of abdomen	Usually on right side of abdomen
Appearance	Flush with skin	Stoma has a 'spout'	Stoma has a 'spout'

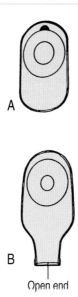

A

B

Open end

Fig. 17.21 Examples of disposable stoma bags. (A) Closed pouch. (B) Open lower end to permit emptying of the contents. (Renton, S., McGuinness, C. & Strachan, E. (2020). *Clinical Nursing Practices*, 6th ed. Elsevier Ltd.)

Type of Stoma	*Colostomy*	*Ileostomy*	*Urostomy/Ileal Conduit*
Output	Formed faeces	Loose faeces	Urine
Frequency of pouch changes	1–2 times per day	Drainable pouches used.	Pouch has a tap
Type of Stoma Bag	Closed pouch	Empty pouch approximately 5–6 times a day. Output between 400 and 1000 mL/day.	Bag emptied several times throughout day. Night bag used.

One-piece appliances have the flange and pouch as one unit whilst two piece appliances, are designed with two parts, the first part stays on the abdomen and the second part is detachable bag. (Smith and Samways, 2020). Hospitals tend to use transparent/clear bags that facilitate observation of the stoma and the contents. Once the patient comfortable with managing their applicance, they can choose an opaque or clean bag (Williams, 2012). Some appliances require the nurse to cut the flange to fit the size of the stoma, this is particularly useful when the stoma is irregular in shape and immediately post surgery (Smith and Samways, 2020).

When cutting the flange, a template needs to be used, to check the bag fits snugly around the stoma. If the aperture is too small it will cause friction on the delicate blood vessels of the stoma, causing bruising or bleeding. If, on the other hand, the aperture is too big, the contents of the bowel will leak from the stoma onto the surrounding skin, causing excoriation and soreness (Williams, 2012).

KEY POINTS

- Patients are usually taught to care for their own stomas and so should be encouraged to participate in their care, as soon as possible after surgery.
- Removal of the bag should be careful, to prevent the skin being pulled and damaged. It may be useful to use counter-pressure with one hand.
- The skin and stoma should be cleaned whenever the bag is changed, to prevent skin soreness. A barrier cream may be advocated if there are skin problems at the stoma site or to protect the skin around the stoma site. Make sure the skin surrounding the stome is dry before attaching a new bag.
- If a one-piece appliance is being used it should be applied from the bottom up. For a two-piece appliance, the flange should be placed directly over the stoma and then the pouch attached.
- If the bag drainable, there is a special 'roll-up' clip at the bottom. Take care not to discard this when emptying the bag.

EQUIPMENT

Clean stoma appliance/bag and flange
Scissors to cut the flange or aperture of the bag to size
Stoma template
Disposable wipes
Jug to dispose of the contents of the used bag (if applicable)
Disposable protective pad
Clinical waste bag
Soap and water for cleansing the skin
Barrier cream if advised

PROCEDURE

1. Put on a disposable plastic apron.
2. Decontaminate your hands and apply non-sterile gloves.
3. Place the disposable protective pad next to the stoma to protect the patient's clothing. Place the clinical waste bag in an easily accessible position.
4. If the stoma bag is drainable, empty the contents into the jug.
5. Gently peel the adhesive off the skin, using the other hand to apply counter-pressure to prevent damage to the skin.
6. Remove the bag and place into the clinical waste bag.
7. Wipe the skin free of faeces and secretions using disposable wipes.
8. Clean the skin and stoma with warm water, taking care around the sutures if the stoma is newly formed. It is common and normal for stomas to bleed a little during cleaning because they are highly vascular (Smith and Samways, 2020). However, ensure the cleaning is not too rough. Gently pat the skin until thoroughly dry.
9. Check the condition of the stoma and the surrounding skin (peristomal skin) for any soreness, redness, ulceration or other abnormalities. If the stoma appears ulcerated and/or black or-brown inform the doctor and stoma nurse specialist immediately.
10. If you know the correct stoma measurements, you can cut a hole to the correct size, otherwise you will need to measure using a circular size guide (Fig. 17.22). This is placed over the stoma to gauge the shape and size. Alternatively a paper ruler can be used to measure it from side to side and top to bottom.

11. Using clean scissors cut a hole to the correct size in the bag or flange having measured the stoma or using the stoma template as a guide. Check there is a 1 to 2 mm clearance from the stoma.

12. Place the flange and/or the bag over the stoma so that the aperture fits snugly and is well attached (Fig. 17.23).

13. If drainable type is used, attach the clip to the base of the bag.

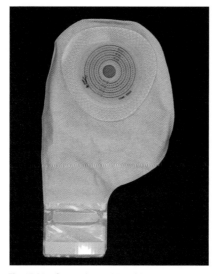

Fig. 17.22 Stoma bag with guide to cut around.

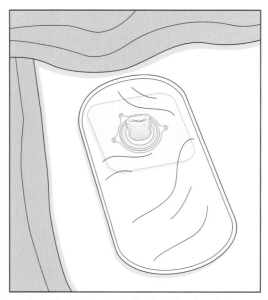

Fig. 17.23 Stoma bag in position. (Nicol, M., Bavin, C., Cronin, P., Rawlings-Anderson, K., Cole, E., & Hunter, J. (2008). *Essential Nursing Skills*, 3rd ed. Elsevier ltd.)

14. Remove the protective pad (use gloves if this is soiled) and discard into clinical waste bag.
15. Check the patient is comfortable and offer the patient hand washing facilities, if they have participated in the procedure.
16. Dispose of any excreta, the soiled bag and other clinical waste appropriately.
17. Remove apron and decontaminate hands.
18. Document the stoma bag change and the condition of the peristomal skin. Report any abnormalities.

References

Dougherty, L., Lister, S., 2015. The Royal Marsden Manual of Clinical Nursing Procedures. Wiley-Blackwell, Oxford.

Loveday, H.P., et al., 2014. National evidence-based guidelines for preventing healthcare-associated infections in NHS hospitals in England. J. Hosp. Infect. 86 (S1), S1–S70.

Royal College of Nursing, 2021. Catheter Care: RCN Guidance for Nurses. www.rcn.org.uk.

Royal College of Nursing, 2019a. Catheter Care: RCN Guidance for Health Care Professionals. www.rcn.org.uk.

Royal College of Nursing, 2019b. Bowel Care Management of Lower Bowel Dysfunction, including Digital Rectal Examination and Digital Removal of Faeces. Publication code: 007 522. www.rcn.org.uk.

Royal College of General Practitioners, 2020. UTI Resource Suite. https://www.rcgp.org.uk/clinical-and-research/resources/toolkits/amr/target-antibiotics-toolkit/uti-resource-suite.aspx.

Shepherd, E., 2017a. Specimen collection 1: general principles and procedure for obtaining a midstream urine specimen. Nurs. Times [online] 113 (7), 45–47.

Shepherd, E., 2017b. Specimen collection 2: obtaining a catheter specimen of urine. Nurs. Times [online] 113 (8), 29–31.

Shepherd E (2017c) Specimen collection 3: faecal specimen from a patient with diarrhoea. Nurs. Times [online] 113 (8), 27–29.

Smith, D., Samways, N., 2020. How to change a stoma bag. Nurs. Stand.. doi:10.7748/ns.2020.e11484.

Williams, J., 2012. Caring for the stoma patient in the community: part two. Nurs. Pract. https://www.nursinginpractice.com/caring-stoma-patient-community-part-two.

Yates, A., 2017. Urinary catheters 3: catheter drainage and support systems. Nurs. Times [online] 113 (3), 41–43.

Yates, A., 2016. Urinalysis: how to interpret results. Nurs. Times [Online issue] 2, 1–3.

CHAPTER 18

Patients With Reduced Mobility

Rationale

Although fewer and fewer patients are now confined to bed for long periods, many patients will be on partial or complete bed rest or sitting in chairs for considerable periods of time. This may be for a variety of reasons:

- To reduce cardiac effort (e.g., following a heart attack)
- To reduce respiratory effort (e.g., asthma or pneumonia)
- If the patient has a pyrexia (fever increases oxygen demand)
- To reduce pain (e.g., after an operation or arthritis)
- To prevent weight-bearing
- Treatment of back pain or following surgery to relieve back pain
- To prevent miscarriage during pregnancy or in the event of pre-eclampsia
- To rest the patient (e.g. after extensive abdominal surgery).

Although bed rest may be beneficial, there are a number of physical complications that can arise. Psychological complications such as depression and musculoskeletal complications such as contractures and muscular atrophy may also occur (Li et al., 2019).

> **KEY POINTS**
>
> - The four most common physical complications will be addressed here:
>   - Chest infection
>   - Pressure ulcers
>   - Deep vein thrombosis (DVT)
>   - Constipation.

Chest Infection

Patients confined to bed are at risk of chest infections due to a reduction in chest expansion. When lying down, the pressure of abdominal contents against the diaphragm reduces lung volume, where coughing is painful or difficult, it can lead to accumulation of secretions in the lungs hence the risk of a chest infection developing.

PREVENTION OF CHEST INFECTION

Positioning the patient upright (Fig. 18.1) will help lung expansion, and turning the patient from side-to-side helps expansion of the lung that is uppermost. Encouraging deep breathing and coughing and administering analgesics to control pain will help to clear the secretions. If the patient is receiving oxygen, humidification (see p. 45–46) will make it easier for the patient to expectorate secretions.

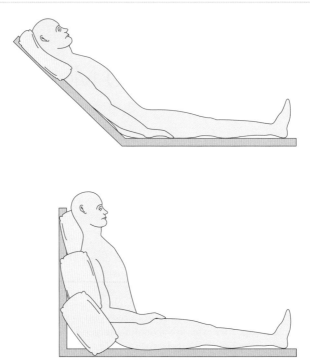

Fig. 18.1 Sitting positions. (A) Semi-upright, or semi-Fowler's. (B) Upright, or high Fowler's position may also be adapted to the orthopnoeic position if the person leans onto an over-bed table. (Koutoukidis, G., Hughson, J., Funnell, R., & Lawrence, K. (2021). *Tabbner's Nursing Care: Theory and Practice*. Elsevier Inc.)

Pressure Ulcers

There are many risk factors that make patients with reduced mobility more likely to develop pressure ulcers (e.g., incontinence, malnutrition; see chapter 11) but there are three causes: pressure, shearing and friction.

Pressure: a pressure ulcer will develop when there is localised pressure that is unrelieved, causing ischaemia (lack of blood supply) to an area of tissue. This occurs when the tissues become compressed between the bone and the surface of the bed or chair. The areas most at risk are the bony prominences such as the hips, shoulders, sacrum and heels.

Shearing: this is the damage to tissues caused when the skin 'sticks' to the surface of the bed or chair, but the skeleton moves forward, for example when sliding down the bed. This causes stretching of the tissues and kinking or rupture of the capillaries leading to ischaemia.

Friction: rubbing the skin vigorously or constantly sliding down the bed or chair causes friction. Friction is increased when the skin is wet, and this in turn causes shearing as the skin cannot slide easily over the bedclothes.

PRESSURE ULCER PREVENTION

Regular changes of position are vital to prevent pressure ulcers. Patients confined to bed will require a pressure ulcer risk assessment (see p. 298), and those on long-term bed rest may require a pressure-relieving mattress and/or other aids such as special cushions when sitting in a chair. In most clinical settings, these are obtained by contacting the tissue viability nurse.

Regular inspection (at least every 4 hours) of the patient's skin to assess the areas most at risk of pressure ulcers is crucial in order to detect any changes at an early stage (National Institute for Health and Care Excellence [NICE], 2014). Almost all pressure ulcers are preventable; poor moving and handling techniques can increase the risk, as can poor nutritional status. Nurses have a duty to protect their patients and check that risk assessment and regular position changes are carried out. Avoid leaving patients sitting in chairs for long periods of time; regular rests lying in the bed will distribute the pressure over a larger area. Teach patients who spend long periods in a chair/wheelchair to use their arms to raise themselves at regular intervals to relieve pressure and improve circulation.

PREVENTION OF PRESSURE ULCERS

NICE (2015 and 2014) recommends a pressure risk assessment be completed within 6 hours of admission or episode of care this includes skin assessment, individualised care plans, repositioning, high-specification foam mattresses and training and education.

Risk Assessments

This includes clinical judgement and the use of a validated scale such as the Braden Scare, Waterlow Score or Norton Risk assessment scale for adults. Prevention of pressure ulcers will not be achieved unless the predisposing factors are controlled or alleviated for each patient. There are general principles to follow when planning preventative strategies. Pressure ulcer risk assessment needs to be re-assessed if there is a change in clinical status.

Skin Assessment

Skin assessment includes taking into account any pain or discomfort, skin integrity of pressure areas, colour changes or discolouration, variations in heat, firmness and moisture. Potential areas for pressure damage are identified in Fig. 18.2. To assess skin, finger palpation should be used to

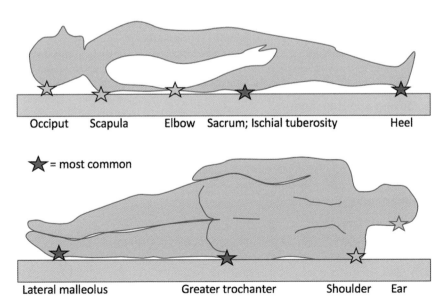

Fig. 18.2 Potential areas for pressure ulcer damage. (Mervis, J. S., & Phillips, T. J. (2019). Pressure ulcers: Pathophysiology, epidemiology, risk factors, and presentation. *Journal of the American Academy of Dermatology*, 81(4), 881-890.)

assess if the skin blanches and if there is any erythema or discolouration. Skin massage or rubbing of pressure area sites is not recommended (NICE, 2014).

Careful Positioning

Careful positioning when in bed and sitting in a chair is crucial. All patients who are vulnerable to pressure ulcers should, as a minimum, be placed on high-specification (low tech) foam mattresses as they aim to redistribute pressure over a large contact area (NICE, 2014). High-tech pressure-relieving systems are more effective than low-tech devices and should be considered for those patients who are identified as high risk of developing pressure ulcers, a history of pressure damage or a clinical condition that indicates their use. It is important to remember that friction and shear can be difficult to eliminate on alternating pressure-relieving mattresses, and therefore, additional preventative strategies need to be used (e.g., sliding sheets).

Regular Repositioning

Frequent repositioning is essential whether the patient is in bed or in a chair. Patients who have been assessed as high risk of developing a pressure ulcer should be encouraged to change their position every 2 to 4 hours, although this should be adjusted for the individual patient's need. Some patients, particularly those who are elderly, may need to be repositioned more regularly (NICE, 2014). The repositioning regimen must be rigorously implemented and, a repositioning chart (e.g. a 24-hour turning chart) may support compliance.

The use of a pressure-relieving mattress does not remove the need to regularly adjust the patient's position. The 30-degree tilt position is recommended to help evenly distribute the body weight. Using the right side, back, left side regime also prevents any direct pressure on the sacrum or trochanter (European Pressure Ulcer Advisory Panel/ National Pressure Ulcer Advisor Panel [EPUAP/NPUAP], 2014). However, it is important to discuss and agree on any repositioning regime with the patient to maximise compliance and comfort. Bedclothes should be loose and sheets not wrinkled. Pillows can be used to support patients in the desired positions to prevent further deterioration from incorrect positioning of limbs.

When seated in chairs, patients should not be left for more than 2 hours regardless of the device being used. The chair must be of appropriate dimensions to promote good posture. There is little evidence that cushions are clinically effective for acutely ill patients but may have some benefit for those who are wheelchair bound or have a chronic risk of developing pressure ulcers. Self-repositioning is equally important for patients who sit for a prolonged time in a wheelchair.

Safe Moving and Handling

When moving and handling patients, it is essential that appropriate manual handling equipment is used to prevent shear or friction (e.g. sliding sheet, hoist). Positioning patients to prevent them from sliding down the bed is important in preventing shear. Chairs are one of the main culprits in causing shearing if they fail to promote and maintain a good posture. Therefore, it is essential that nurses complete mandatory training and are competent to use manual handling equipment within their workplace.

Nutrition and Hydration

As outlined in chapter 11, consideration of patients' nutrition and hydration status are essential for the mainteance healthy skin. It is important to provide assistance with eating and drinking where necessary, a food and fluid balance chart may be useful.

Skin Care

Continuous assessment of the skin is vital and can be carried our while attending to the patient's hygiene needs. Skin should be inspected for persistent erythema, non-blanching hyperaemia, blisters, localised heat, oedema, induration, purplish/bluish localised areas and localised coolness if tissue death occurs. The skin should be kept clean and dry, and check regularly if the patient is incontinent, has a high temperature or is sweating excessively. However, caution should be exercised in the overuse of soap and detergents as they are the commonest cause of stripping of the epidermal protective barrier. Consider the use of non-soap skin cleansers. Emollients in the bath or creams are useful for dry skin, and a barrier cream for moist skin may be useful. These do, however, interfere with the use of adhesives on the skin and may also affect the absorptive properties of dressings and continence products. However, barrier creams may be appropriate in high-risk patients who are at risk of developing a moisture lesion or incontinence-associated dermatitis (NICE, 2014).

Grading Pressure Ulcers

If the patient develops a pressure ulcer, it should be graded so that appropriate treatment can be given, and this should include measuring/tracing the surface area using a validated measurement tool and estimating the depth (NICE, 2014). The National Pressure Ulcer Advisory panel classification of pressure ulcers (Fig. 18.3) provides a tool to assess the severity of pressure ulcer. A Stage I: non-blanchable erythema of intact skin. This lesion is the heralding sign of impending skin ulceration. For darker-skinned individuals, other signs may be indicators and include

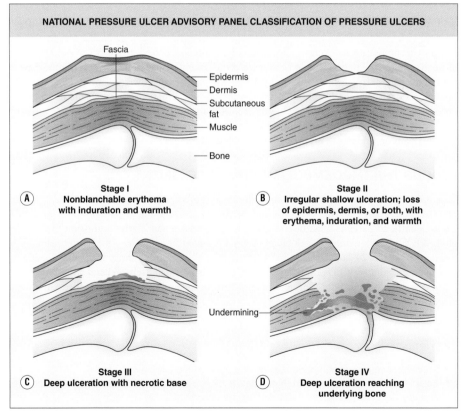

Fig. 18.3 National Pressure Ulcer Advisory Panel classification of pressure ulcers. (Bolognia, J.L., Schaffer, J.V. & Cerroni L. (2018). *Dermatology*, 4th ed. Elsevier Ltd.)

warmth, oedema, discoloration of the skin, and induration. B Stage II: partial-thickness skin loss involving the epidermis, dermis or both. This superficial lesion presents as an abrasion, blister or shallow crater. C Stage III: full-thickness skin loss, in which subcutaneous tissue is damaged or necrotic and may extend down into, but not including, the underlying fascia. This deep lesion presents as a crater and sometimes involves adjacent tissue. D Stage IV: full-thickness skin loss and extensive tissue necrosis, destruction to muscle, bone, or supporting structures such as a tendon or joint capsule, there may also be a sinus track (Bolognia et al., 2018).

Venous Thromboembolism

Venous thromboembolism (VTE) refers to DVT, which is a clot (thrombus) in the deep veins of the leg and can lead to pulmonary embolus. Immobility leads to venous stasis (slowing of blood flow) in the legs. Because the muscles, which normally help to 'pump' blood back to the heart, are not active when lying in bed or immobile in a chair. Venous stasis is made worse if the patient is not able to breathe deeply and cough (see Chest Infection, p. 287) because the negative pressure that is created in the chest during inspiration also helps venous return to the heart. Venous stasis means that clotting factors, which are normally quickly cleared from the circulation, remain active for longer and increasing the risk of clot formation (thrombosis) . If part of the clot breaks off, it can be the cause of a pulmonary embolus, which can be fatal.

Prevention of Venous Thromboembolism

VTE risk assessment is now part of most admission procedures, and early mobilisation will reduce the risk of VTE. Prophylactic measures such as subcutaneous low molecular weight heparin and anti-thrombolism stockings or a pneumatic compression device (see p. 296–297) will be prescribed, and dehydration should be avoided if the patient's condition allows. It is important to remind the patient to exercise their legs by flexing the foot towards the knee and rotating the foot; this activates the calf muscles 'pump' to increase blood flow. If patients are unable to do this (e.g., unconscious patients), the nurse or physiotherapist will perform passive leg exercises to promote circulation and maintain muscle tone. Observe and teach patients to observe for signs of DVT: swelling, pain or tenderness, erythema and discolouration.

VENOUS THROMBOEMBOLISM RISK ASSESSMENT

VTE is an umbrella term for DVT and pulmonary embolism (Greenall, 2016). It is a major cause of potentially preventable death and morbidity in hospitalised patients (NICE, 2018). Consequently, all patients must be risk assessed as soon as possible after admission to the hospital (NICE, 2018). Common risk factors for VTE are outlined in Box 18.1. Patient should be re-assessed within 24 hours of admission for risk of VTE and bleeding. In addition, patients may require extended VTE prophylaxis following their hospital discharge, and appropriate verbal and written patient education and information must be provided as part of the discharge process (Fig. 18.4).

KEY POINTS

- Prevention of venous thromboembolism is a patient safety issue.
- Early identification of deep vein thrombosis is essential so that treatment can be started, and any potential pulmonary embolism can be prevented.
- Assessment includes balancing the individuals VTE risk and their risk of bleeding.
- Hospitalisation increases the risk of VTE due to immobility and venous trauma.

> **BOX 18.1 ■ Common Risk Factors for Venous Thromboembolism**
>
> - Active cancer or being treated for cancer
> - Aged over 60 years
> - Critical care admission
> - Dehydration
> - Known thrombophilia (abnormal tendency to develop blood clots)
> - Obesity
> - One or more significant comorbidities (for example, heart disease, acute infectious diseases, inflammatory conditions)
> - Personal history or first-degree relative with a history of venous thromboembolism
> - Use of hormone replacement therapy
> - Use of oestrogen-containing contraceptive therapy
> - Varicose veins with phlebitis (inflammation of the vein walls)
>
> ---
> Greenall (2016).

FITTING ANTIEMBOLISM STOCKINGS TO PREVENT VENOUS THROMBOEMBOLISM

Antiembolism stockings (AES) and intermittent pneumatic compression (IPC) devices can be used to reduce the risk of VTE (Gee, 2019). AES reduce apply graduated circumferential pressure, which increased velocity and promotes venous return. Stockings can be either knee or thigh length. Thigh-length stocking increase blood flow velocity in the femoral vein and may provide more protection than knee-length AES. However, it has to be noted that NICE does not specify which length should be used (NICE, 2018; Gee 2019).

EQUIPMENT

- Tape measure
- Appropriate size and length AES.

PROCEDURE

1. Decontaminate hands.
2. Explain the procedure to the patient and discuss VTE risk
3. Assess for contraindications to AES (see Box 18.1).
4. Measure the patient's legs to find the correct size (Fig. 18.5), noting that different sizes may be needed for each leg. Legs can be measured while the patient is standing up or lying in bed.
5. For thigh-length stockings:
   - Measure the circumference of both thighs at their widest point;
   - Measure the circumference of both calves at their widest point;
   - Measure the distance from the gluteal furrow (buttock fold) to the heel.
6. For knee-length stockings:
   - Measure the circumference of both calves at their widest point.
   - Measure the distance from the popliteal fold to the heel.
   - Select the correct stockings using the manufacturer's measurement table.
7. Fit the stockings to the patient's legs. Turn the stocking inside out by inserting your hand into the stocking as far as the heel.

RISK ASSESSMENT FOR VENOUS THROMBOEMBOLISM (VTE)

All patients should be risk assessed on admission to hospital. Patients should be reassessed within 24 hours of admission and whenever the clinical situation changes.

STEP ONE

Assess all patients admitted to hospital for level of mobility (tick one box). All surgical patients, and all medical patients with significantly reduced mobility, should be considered for further risk assessment.

STEP TWO

Review the patient-related factors shown on the assessment sheet against **thrombosis** risk, ticking each box that applies (more than one box can be ticked).

Any tick for thrombosis risk should prompt thromboprophylaxis according to NICE guidance.

The risk factors identified are not exhaustive. Clinicians may consider additional risks in individual patients and offer thromboprophylaxis as appropriate.

STEP THREE

Review the patient-related factors shown against bleeding risk and tick each box that applies (more than one box can be ticked).

Any tick should prompt clinical staff to consider if bleeding risk is sufficient to preclude pharmacological intervention.

Guidance on thromboprophylaxis is available at:

National Institute for Health and Clinical Excellence (2010) Venous thromboembolism: reducing the risk of venous thromboembolism (deep vein thrombosis and pulmonary embolism) in patients admitted to hospital. NICE clinical guideline 92. London: National Institute for Health and Clinical Excellence.

http://www.nice.org.uk/guidance/CG92

This document has been authorised by the Department of Health
Gateway reference no: 10278

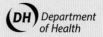

Fig. 18.4   Risk assessment for venous thromboembolism (VTE). (Reproduced with the permission of the Department of Health and Social Care under the Open Government Licence, https://www.nice.org.uk/re-using-our-content/uk-open-content-licence.)

RISK ASSESSMENT FOR VENOUS THROMBOEMBOLISM (VTE)

Mobility – all patients (tick one box)	Tick		Tick		Tick
Surgical patient		Medical patient expected to have ongoing reduced mobility relative to normal state		Medical patient NOT expected to have significantly reduced mobility relative to normal state	
Assess for thrombosis and bleeding risk below				Risk assessment now complete	

Thrombosis risk			
Patient-related	**Tick**	**Admission-related**	**Tick**
Active cancer or cancer treatment		Significantly reduced mobility for 3 days or more	
Age > 60		Hip or knee replacement	
Dehydration		Hip fracture	
Known thrombophilias		Total anaesthetic + surgical time > 90 minutes	
Obesity (BMI >30 kg/m^2)		Surgery involving pelvis or lower limb with a total anaesthetic + surgical time > 60 minutes	
One or more significant medical comorbidities (e.g., heart disease;metabolic,endocrine or respiratory pathologies;acute infectious diseases; inflammatory conditions)		Acute surgical admission with inflammatory or intra-abdominal condition	
Personal history or first-degree relative with a history of VTE		Critical care admission	
Use of hormone replacement therapy		Surgery with significant reduction in mobility	
Use of oestrogen-containing contraceptive therapy			
Varicose veins with phlebitis			
Pregnancy or < 6 weeks post partum (see NICE guidance for specific risk factors)			

Bleeding risk			
Patient-related	**Tick**	**Admission-related**	**Tick**
Active bleeding		Neurosurgery, spinal surgery or eye surgery	
Acquired bleeding disorders (such as acute liver failure)		Other procedure with high bleeding risk	
Concurrent use of anticoagulants known to increase the risk of bleeding (such as warfarin with INR >2)		Lumbar puncture/epidural/spinal anaesthesia expected within the next 12 hours	
Acute stroke		Lumbar puncture/epidural/spinal anaesthesia within the previous 4 hours	
Thrombocytopaenia (platelets< 75x10^9/l)			
Uncontrolled systolic hypertension (230/120 mmHg or higher)			
Untreated inherited bleeding disorders (such as haemophilia and von Willebrand's disease)			

Fig. 18.4, Cont'd

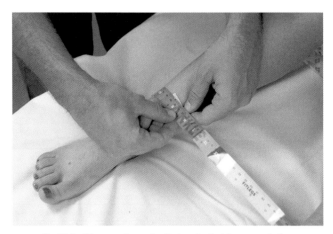

Fig. 18.5 Measure the patient's legs to find the correct size.

8. Position the stocking over the foot and heel.
9. Gently and carefully move the stocking around the patient's ankle and up the leg (Figs 18.6 and 18.7).
10. Assess the patient to ascertain if they feel any discomfort, numbness, tingling or pain associated with the AES.
11. Explain to the patient how to apply and remove the stockings.
12. Decontaminate hands and document your actions.
13. Stockings should be removed daily for washing and to inspect the condition of the patient's skin, particularly over the heels and bony prominences. Patients who have significantly reduced mobility, poor skin integrity or sensory loss—for example, diabetic neuropathy— should have their skin checked two to three times per day.

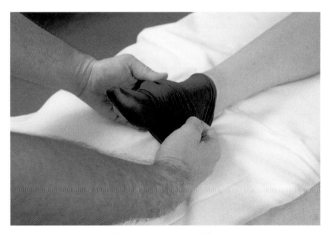

Fig. 18.6 Applying AES.

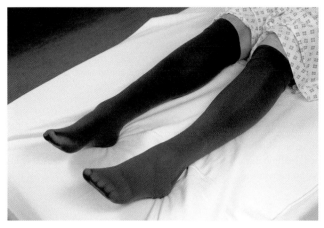

Fig. 18.7 Knee-high AES.

Contraindications for Antiembolism Stockings

Do not offer antiembolism stockings to a patient with:
- Suspected or proven peripheral arterial disease
- Peripheral arterial bypass grafting
- Peripheral neuropathy or other causes of sensory impairment
- Any conditions in which stockings may cause damage, for example fragile skin, dermatitis, gangrene or recent skin graft
- Known allergy to the stocking fabric
- Cardiac failure
- Severe leg oedema or pulmonary oedema from congestive heart failure
- Unusual leg size or shape or deformity preventing correct fit

NICE (2018) and Gee (2019).

Constipation

Immobility leads to the slowing of peristalsis in the large intestine, meaning that faeces takes longer to pass through, allowing more water to be re-absorbed. This leads to drying and hardening of the faeces, making them more difficult to pass. When accompanied by dehydration and a diet low in fibre, the risk of constipation in the immobile patient is even greater. Lack of fibre and fluid reduces the bulk of the faeces, meaning that the bowel may not be sufficiently distended to stimulate the defaecation reflex. If the patient is also embarrassed about using the commode or bedpan and 'busy' nurses do not respond quickly to requests to go to the toilet, patients may well ignore the urge to defaecate and become constipated.

PREVENTION AND TREATMENT OF CONSTIPATION

Monitor the bowel actions, and if the patient's condition allows, increase oral fluids (2 litres a day if possible) and include fruit juices and vegetable soups to add fibre. If the patient is not on any fluid restriction or at risk of bowel obstruction, encourage them to choose foods that are high in dietary fibre (fruit, vegetables, wholemeal bread and wholegrain cereals). Encourage increased mobility where possible, as this will increase peristalsis and ensure privacy and dignity when using the commode or bed pan. Review all medications to see if there are any alternatives to medications known to cause constipation (e.g., codeine-based analgesics). Consider the use of laxatives if these measures are unsuccessful.

Lying and Standing Blood Pressure

Lying and standing blood pressure involves taking three blood pressures over a period of 5 minutes, with the patient initially lying and then standing, preferably using a manual sphygmomanometer to give a more accurate reading.

KEY FACTS

A manual sphygmomanometer should be used to record blood pressure.
A positive result includes:
- Drop in systolic blood pressure (BP) of 20 mmHg or more (with or without symptoms).
- Drop to <90 mmHg on standing even if the drop is less than 20 mmHg (with or without symptoms).
- Drop in diastolic BP of 10 mmHg with symptoms (although clinically less significant than a drop in systolic BP).

Royal College of Physicians (2017).

EQUIPMENT REQUIRED

- Personal protective equipment
- Manual sphygmomanometer
- Stethoscope
- Vital signs chart

PROCEDURE

1. Review the patient's manual handling assessment and assess if you need assistance to help the patient to stand and simultaneously take the BP.
2. Explain the procedure to the patient and gain consent.
3. Measure the BP lying down.
4. Ask/ assist the patient to stand and measure the BP after standing for one minute.
5. Measure the BP again after the patient has been standing for 3 minutes.
6. Repeat the BP measurement if BP is still dropping and assess the patient.
7. Check for symptoms (e.g., dizziness, light headiness, vagueness, pallor, visual disturbances, feelings of weakness and/ or unsteadiness) occur, stop the procedure and assess the patient.
8. Document your findings and discuss with the medical team.
9. In the event of a positive result:
   - Explain the results to the patient.
   - Discuss with the medical and nursing team.
   - Take immediate actions to prevent falls.

Royal College of Physicians (2017).

References

Age UK, 2013. Expert Series: Falls Prevention Exercise—Following the Evidence. https://www.ageuk.org. uk/globalassets/age-uk/documents/reports-and-publications/reports-and-briefings/health—wellbeing/ rb_2013_falls_prevention_guide.pdf,

Age UK. 2022. I want to be active but I find exercise difficulthttps://www.ageuk.org.uk/information-advice/ health-wellbeing/exercise/simple-exercises-inactive-adults/

Bolognia, J.L., Schaffer, J.V., Cerroni, L., 2018. Dermatology, fourth ed. Elsevier Ltd.

European Pressure Ulcer Advisory Panel/ National Pressure Ulcer Advisor Panel (EPUAP/NPUAP), 2014. Prevention and Treatment of Pressure Ulcers: Quick Reference Guide. https://www.epuap.org.

Gee, E., 2019. How to apply anti-embolism stockings to prevent venous thromboembolism. Nurs. Times [online]. 115 (4), 24–26.

Gillespie, L.D., Robertson, M.C., Gillespie, W.J., et al., 2012. Interventions for preventing falls in older people living in the community. Cochrane Database Syst. Rev. 9, CD007146.

Greenall, R., 2016. Using patient education to reduce risk of VTE. Nurs. Times. 12 (online issue 3), 5–8.

Li, J, Wu, X, Li, Z, et al. (2019). Nursing resources and major immobility complications among bedridden patients: A multicenter descriptive study in China. J Nurs Manag. 27: 930–938.

Royal College of Nursing (RCN), 2020. Falls. https://www.rcn.org.uk/clinical-topics/older-people/falls.

Royal College of Physicians, 2017. How to measure a lying and standing blood pressure (BP) as part of a falls assessment. Falls and Fragility Fracture Audit Programme.

National Institute for Health and Care Excellence (NICE), 2013. Falls in older people: assessing risk and prevention. Clinical Guideline CG161. www.nice.org.uk.

National Institute for Health and Care Excellence (NICE), 2014. Pressure ulcers: prevention and management. Clinical Guideline 179. https://www.nice.org.uk/guidance/cg179/chapter/1-Recommendations#prevention-adults.

National Institute for Health and Care Excellence (NICE), 2015. Pressure Ulcers. Quality statement1: pressure ulcer risk assessment in hospitals and care homes with nursing. https://www.nice.org.uk/guidance/ qs89/chapter/quality-statement-1-pressure-ulcer-risk-assessment-in-hospitals-and-care-homes-with-nursing.

National Institute for health and Care Excellence (NICE), 2018. Venous thromboembolism in over 16s: reducing the risk of hospital-acquired deep vein thrombosis or pulmonary embolism. NICE guideline [NG89]. https://www.nice.org.uk/guidance/ng89/chapter/Recommendations#risk-assessment.

Yip, J.L., Khawaja, A.P., Broadway, D., et al., 2014. Visual acuity, self-reported vision and falls in the EPIC-Norfolk Eye study. Br. J. Ophthalmol. 98 (3), 377–382. doi:10.1136/bjophthalmol-2013-304179.

CHAPTER 19

Emergency Procedures

Emergency Equipment

Clinical settings must provide staff with immediate access to appropriate emergency resuscitation equipment. The Resuscitation Council (UK) has developed recommendations for immediate and accessible emergency equipment and drugs (Resuscitation Council [UK], 2020). These include a requirement that all resuscitation equipment is checked regularly in accordance with local policy. (Gwinnutt et al., 2019). Nurses are often the first healthcare professional involved in an emergency and therefore must know the location of the emergency equipment, emergency numbers, layout of equipment and its uses. Also, nurses must make sure that the equipment is regularly checked in accordance with local and national policies (Davies et al., 2014, Resuscitation Council (UK), 2022)

KEY FACTS

- Equipment used for resuscitation and the layout of equipment and drugs should be standardised in all clinical settings.
- Equipment must be checked regularly in accordance with local policy.
- All staff must know location of equipment equipment, how to activate the emergency teams and what to do in an emergency.

EMERGENCY EQUIPMENT

Pocket mask with oxygen port
Non re-breath mask with oxygen tubing
Self-inflating bag with reservoir also termed bag, valve mask (BVM)
Clear face masks, sizes 3, 4, 5
Oropharyngeal airways size 2, 3, 4 (Fig. 19.1)
Nasopharyngeal airways, sizes 6, 7 (and lubrication) (Fig. 19.2)

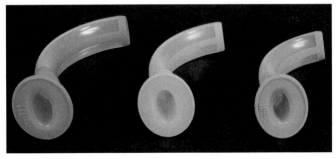

Fig. 19.1 Oropharyngeal airways.

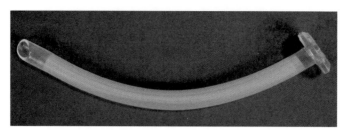

Fig. 19.2   Nasopharyngeal airway.

Portable suction (battery or manual) with Yankauer sucker and soft suction catheters

Supraglottic airway device with syringes, lubrication and ties/tapes/scissors as appropriate (e.g., laryngeal mask airway), i-gel® (Figs 19.3 and 19.4)

Oxygen cylinder (with key where necessary)

Oxygen tubing

Magill forceps

Stethoscope

Tracheal tubes, cuffed, sizes 6, 7, 8 (Fig. 19.5)

Tracheal tube introducer (stylet)

Laryngoscope handles (×2) and blades (size 3 and 4) (Fig. 19.6). Spare batteries for laryngoscope and spare bulbs (if applicable).

Syringes, lubrication and ties/tapes/scissors for tracheal tube

Waveform capnograph

Defibrillator (manual and/or automated external defibrillator). Pacing/cardioversion function depending on clinical area.

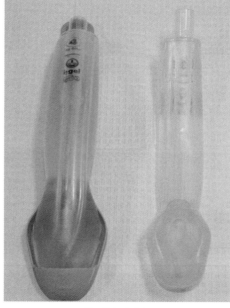

Fig. 19.3   I-Gel.

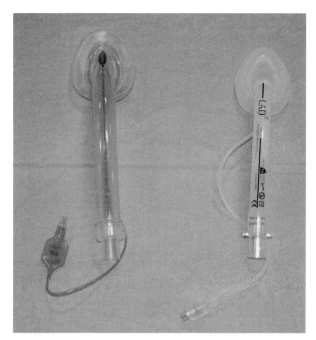

Fig. 19.4. Laryngeal mask airway.

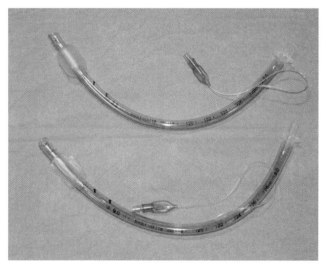

Fig. 19.5 Endotracheal tubes.

Adhesive defibrillator pads – there is currently no international standard for defibrillator pad attachments. Therefore, check that the correct defibrillator pads are appropriate for the defibrillator used and that a spare set of pads are available.

Razor to remove any chest hair prior to defibrillator pad placement.

ECG electrodes

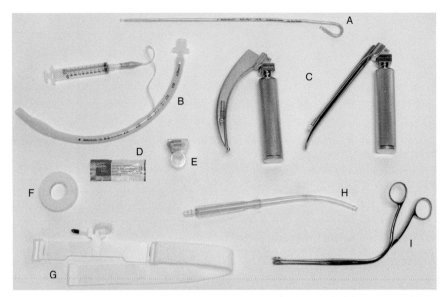

Fig. 19.6 Selection of intubation equipment: rigid suction catheter (Yankeur sucker), laryngoscope blade, endotracheal tubes, introducer (stylet), 10 mL syringe to inflate endotracheal tube cuff, Magills forceps, catheter mount, soft suction catheter and endotracheal ties. (Sole, M. L., Klein, D. G., & Moseley, M. J. (2017). *Introduction to Critical Care Nursing*. Elsevier Inc.)

Intravenous cannula and equipment for insertion
Adhesive tape
Intravenous fluids and giving sets
Selection of needles and syringes
Intra-osseous access device
Central venous access – Seldinger kit, full barrier precautions (hat, mask, sterile gloves, gown) and skin preparation (2% chlorhexidine/alcohol). Placed with ultrasound guidance, where possible
Ultrasound / echocardiography
Clock/timer
Gloves, aprons, eye protection
Nasogastric tube
Sharps container and clinical waste bag
Large scissors
Pressure bags for infusion
Blood gas syringe
Drug labels
Manual handling equipment
Cardiorespiratory arrest record forms for patient records, audit forms and Do not attempt cardiopulmonary resuscitation (DNACPR) forms
Access to algorithms, emergency drug doses

CARDIAC ARREST DRUGS

Adrenaline 1 mg (= 10 mL 1:10,000) as a prefilled syringe
Amiodarone 300 mg as a prefilled syringe
Calcium chloride 10 mL 10% or calcium gluconate.

DEPENDING ON CLINICAL AREA EMERGENCY DRUGS INCLUDED MAY BE FOR

Anaphylaxis
Hypoglycaemia
Local anaesthetic overdose
Acute coronary syndrome
Life-threatening arrhythmias
Asthma/exacerbation of Chronic Obstructive Pulmonary Disease (COPD)
Therapeutic hypothermia post-cardiac arrest.

Anaphylaxis

Anaphylaxis is a severe, life-threatening, generalised hypersensitive reaction (Resuscitation Council [UK], 2021), involving the airway involving the airway (pharyngeal or laryngeal oedema, stridor or hoarse voice), breathing (bronchospasm, tachypnoea, increased work of breathing, wheeze, fatigue, cyanosis, SpO2 <94%)) and circulation (hypotension, tachycardia signs of shock, confusion or reduced level of consciousness). (NICE, 2011).

Triggers for anaphylaxis include.

- Neuromuscular blocking drugs (e.g. Suxamethonium)
- Antibiotics
- Intravenous contrast agents
- Blood products
- Plasma expanders
- Non-steroidal anti-inflammatory drugs
- Stings from insects
- Food (e.g. nuts, sea fish)
- Latex or natural rubber.

KEY FACTS

- Anaphylaxis is a sudden, severe and potentially life-threatening allergic reaction

TREATMENT

- Assess the patient's airway, breathing, circulation, disability, exposure (ABCDE).
- Call for emergency team/ambulance. Ask colleagues to bring the emergency equipment and the anaphylaxis kit.
- If possible lie the patient flat (with or without legs elevated) or a sitting position may support breathing.
- Stop/remove the likely allergen (e.g., stop antibiotic infusion or remove latex gloves).
- Give high flow oxygen (15 L/min) via a non-rebreathe mask.
- Give adrenaline intramuscularly (Box 19.1). Inject at the antero-lateral aspect of the middle third of the thigh. Some patients may have a special 'pen-like' syringe (epi-pen, anapen). IM injection must not be given over clothes.
- Give an H_1 antihistamine (e.g. chlorphenamine).
- Corticosteroids may be appropriate to prevent further reactions.
- Nebulised salbutamol 5 mg
- If severe hypotension does not respond to medication, give intravenous fluid boluses. (500-1000ml for adults/10ml/kg for children). Do not use artificial plasma expanders in fluid resuscitation; use crystalloid infusions.

BOX 19.1 ■ Intramuscular Adrenaline 1mg/ml (1:1,000) Concentration Dosage

- Adults and children over 12 years – 500 micrograms IM (0.5ml) 0.5
- Children 6–12 years – 300 micrograms (0.3mL).
- Children 6 months to 6 years: 150 micrograms IM (0.15mL)
- Child <6 months: 100-150 micrograms IM (0.1-0.15mL).

Each dose may be repeated within 5 min if there is no improvement in the patient's condition.

Resuscitation Council (UK), 2021.

- The patient may require emergency endotracheal intubation to secure and protect the patient's airway.
- Ongoing monitoring in response to treatment, patients are likely to require admission to a critical care unit for observation and mechanical ventilation.

Resuscitation Council (UK) (2021).

Adult Choking

Choking (complete foreign body airway obstruction) is usually associated with eating and drinking and may be associated with a muscle, neurological or cerebral impairment (Pavitt et al., 2017). In care settings, patients with dysphagia may require food texture modifications. A recent review of incidents highlighted misunderstanding of the problem of dysphagia and the type diets required for these patients. This has led to incidents of choking requiring an emergency response, if not treated promptly, complications may include aspiration pneumonia and deaths (NHS Improvement, 2018).

KEY FACTS

- Choking is a life-threatening emergency requiring immediate action.
- Choking often occurs when eating.
- Call for help (Emergency team 2222 or Emergency Services 999)

SIGNS AND SYMPTOMS

- Coughing
- Struggling to breath
- Unable to talk
- Gasping
- Grasping their throat

CONSCIOUS PERSON

- Encourage the patient to cough and spit out any foreign body. Do not use your fingers to help remove the obstruction.
- If the cough becomes ineffective, give up to five slaps on the back. Stand behind but beside the individual and use the heel of your hand to deliver up to five sharp blows between their shoulder blades. Between each back slap check to see if the foreign body has been removed.
- If unsuccessful, perform up to five abdominal thrusts (also termed Heimlich manoeuvre). To perform an abdominal thrust the practitioner stands behind the person and places

their hands around the patient's waist, above the umbilicus and below the rib cage. They then deliver a sharp inward and upward thrust to the abdomen below the rib cage.
- If the obstruction is not cleared, call for the emergency team or ambulance service. Continue with back slaps and abdominal thrusts until the obstruction is cleared, the individual becomes unconscious or help arrives.

NHS (2019) and Pavitt et al. (2017).

UNCONSCIOUS

- If the person loses consciousness, immediately perform cardiopulomary resuscitation (CPR) 30:2 starting with chest compressions.
- Check for signs of the obstruction being cleared, then re-assess the patient, for signs of life.

Emergency Tracheostomy Equipment

Tracheostomy emergencies can develop rapidly into life threatening situations, and being prepared with the right knowledge, equipment and support can help prevent complications. The National Tracheostomy Safety Project (2016) recommends patients with a tracheostomy should have a bed head sign detailing information on the type of tracheostomy, size of tube and any additional essential information relating to the tracheostomy, an emergency tracheostomy algorithm poster and an emergency tracheostomy box immediately available.

KEY POINTS

- All patients with a tracheostomy tube must have immediate access to emergency equipment.
- Information regarding the type and size of tracheostomy tube must be readily available in case of an emergency.
- Emergency equipment must remain at the patient's bedside for at least 48 hours following decannulation, in case of respiratory decline and the need for rapid reinsertion of a tracheostomy.

EMERGENCY EQUIPMENT

The National Tracheostomy Safety Project (2016) recommends that essential emergency tracheostomy equipment, may be stored in a portable box/pack and should include:
- Three cuffed tracheostomy tubes and inner cannula. Minimum: spare same size and type tracheostomy tube and one smaller.
- Tracheal dilators to maintain stoma opening in the event of accidental tube removal until replacement tube is inserted.
- Suture cutter for removal of a tube that is sutured in place (e.g. when surgically inserted).
- Sterile scissors to cut cotton tracheostomy tapes.
- 10 mL syringe
- Tracheostomy tapes and Velcro holder
- Tracheostomy dressing
- Aqua gel sachet or appropriate water-soluble lubricant
- Cleaning swab
- Duoderm dressing
- Gauze
- Cuff manometer

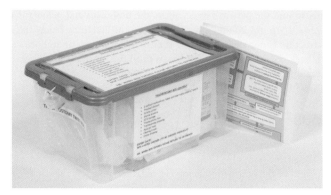

Fig. 19.7   Emergency tracheostomy equipment.

Additional emergency equipment includes:
■ Emergency airway equipment e.g. oropharyngeal airways, intubation equipment and bag, valve mask.
■ Suction equipment
■ Appropriately sized suction catheters
■ Piped oxygen with flow regulator attached

Blocked Tracheostomy Emergency

A blocked tracheostomy is a medical emergency, and expert airway help must be called immediately. A partial or completely blocked tracheostomy tube may occur due to dried secretions, blood clots, a displaced over-inflated cuff or if the tracheal tube is poorly positioned.

KEY FACTS

• Patients with a tracheostomy must have immediate access to tracheostomy emergency equipment, including oxygen, suction and appropriately sized suction catheters.
• Emergency algorithms should be displayed above the bed in case of an emergency.
• Nurses who are required to care for tracheostomy patients must be competent in recognising and responding to common airway complications including tube obstruction or displacements.

RED FLAGS/SIGNS OF A BLOCKED TRACHEOSTOMY

■ Respiratory distress
■ Increased respiratory rate
■ Increased NEWS
■ Increased oxygen requirements
■ Reduced SPO2
■ Apnoea
■ Hypotension
■ Tachycardia
■ Reduced level of consciousness
■ Noisy breathing

- Difficulty removing secretions (e.g., coughing or inability to pass suction catheter).
- Patient complaining of increased shortness of breath.
- Inability to pass a suction catheter
- Altered capnography trace
- Talking or noises heard over a cuffed tracheostomy tube
- Frequent requirement for excessive cuff inflation to prevent air leaks
- Pain or bleeding from the tracheostomy site
- Visibly displaced tracheostomy tube

PROCEDURE

1. Apply PPE.
2. Call for expert airway help immediately.
3. Check for breathing at both the mouth and tracheostomy. Depending on where you work, you may use waveform capnography, or attach the patient to a C-Circuit (Waters Circuit) that can help to assess breathing.
4. If the patient is not-breathing/no signs of life or carotid pulse: Start CPR.

If the patient is breathing:

Apply high flow oxygen to both the face and tracheostomy.

Assess the patency of the tracheostomy by:

- Removing the speaking valve or cap if in place.
- Remove the inner tube.
- Then try to pass a suction catheter.
  - Able to pass a suction catheter, this indicates a potential partial obstruction.
    - Perform tracheal suction
    - Consider ventilating the patient if apnoeic
    - Continue with your ABCDE Assessment.
  - Unable to pass the suction catheter:
    - Deflate the cuff if present.
    - Look, listen and feel at both the mouth and tracheostomy for breathing. If the patient is breathing, continue with your assessment. If the patient shows no signs of improving:
      - Remove the tracheostomy tube. Then re-assess the patient, checking for breathing at both the mouth and tracheostomy stoma.
      - If the patient is breathing, continue with the ABCDE assessment.
      - If the patient remains apnoeic:
        - Use standard airway opening manoeuvres.
        - Cover the stoma with gauze and your hand.
        - Ventilate using a bag-valve-mask.
        - Use oral and nasal airway adjuncts.
        - Use supraglottic devices.
        - Tracheostomy stoma ventilation includes covering the stoma with a paediatric oxygen mask, or a Laryngeal Mask airway (LMA) applied to the stoma.
        - When expert help arrives, oral intubation (Difficult Airway Equipment will need to be available) or intubation via the stoma may be attempted.

National Tracheostomy Safety Project (2016).

Basic Airway Opening Procedures

Early preventable deaths from a compromised airway may occur due to vomiting, altered level of consciousness, and choking on objects in the mouth such as false teeth or food (Mayo, 2017).

In addition, complications may occur if there is a failure to recognise the urgent need for intervention, selecting an inappropriate airway manoeuvre or becoming distracted by less urgent problems in an emergency situation. Therefore, nurses must be competent and confident in the recognition of airway compromise, basic airway techniques and airway adjuncts.

A reduced level of consciousness may allow the tongue to fall back and block the hypopharynx. This may cause a partial or full obstruction and should be suspected if the patient has difficulty talking, is choking, is using accessory muscles to aid breathing or breathing loudly, including stridor (high-pitched wheezing sound) or 'gurgling' (Mayo, 2017; Thim et al., 2012; Resuscitation Council [UK], 2021). Potential causes of airway compromise may be caused by a reduced level of consciousness due to head injury, poisoning, hypoglycaemia, or alcohol.

KEY POINTS

- A compromised airway is a medical emergency. Expert help must be sought immediately.
- Once the airway has been opened, you must check interventions have been effective by looking, listening and feeling for breathing / change in condition.
- To maintain a patent airway, an airway adjunct may be necessary.
- Once the airway has been opened, high flow oxygen should be administered as soon as possible.

ORAL SUCTIONING

It may be necessary to remove secretions from the airway (e.g., saliva, vomit, blood or sputum), through suctioning, prior to any airway opening procedure.

1. Turn suction machine on and check that it is working.
2. Remove suction catheter from packaging.
3. Using a rigid suction catheter (also termed Yankeur suction catheter), insert the suction catheter into the patient's mouth. Only suction what is visible and always keep the suction catheter tip in view (Fig. 19.8).
4. Once the secretions have been removed, re-assess the patient.

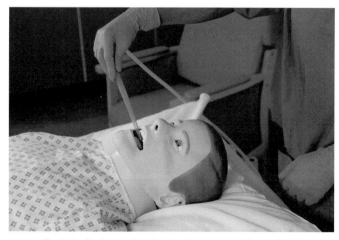

Fig. 19.8 Suctioning the airway using a rigid suction catheter.

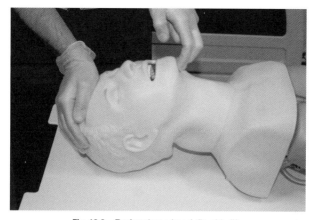

Fig. 19.9 Performing a head tilt, chin lift.

HEAD TILT CHIN LIFT

In patients who have a reduced level of consciousness it may be necessary to use airway manoeuvres to maintain a patent airway. There are two techniques which can be used.

The first technique is known as the head tilt chin lift manoeuvre:

1. One hand is placed on the patient's forehead and the head is gently tilted back.
2. The fingertips of the other hand should be placed under the chin and gently lifted (Fig. 19.9).

JAW THRUST TECHNIQUE

The alternative manoeuvre is known as the jaw thrust technique. This is suitable for use with patients who have or are suspected of having a cervical spine injury. This technique is also most easily used when facilitating bag mask valve ventilation.

1. The angle of the mandible should be located.
2. All fingers, except the thumbs, should be placed behind the angle of the mandible and gently pushed upwards (Fig. 19.10).
3. The thumbs should slightly open the mouth and push the chin downwards.

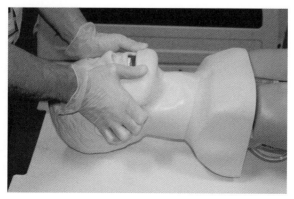

Fig. 19.10 Performing a jaw thrust.

Insertion of an Oropharyngeal Airway

An OPA is a simple airway adjunct which can be used during an emergency to help maintain airway patency. Nurses should be aware that these devices are only for use during emergencies and should be used in conjunction with airway manoeuvres such as head tilt, chin lift or a jaw thrust. A patient who tolerates an OA is critically ill, requiring advanced airway management in an intensive care unit.

PROCEDURE

1. Nurses should first check that the airway is not obstructed by foreign material before OA insertion.
2. Different sizes of OA are available. To estimate the required size, the OA should be held against the angle of the jaw and reach the patients incisors (Fig. 19.11).
3. The OA should be inserted into the patient's airway in the upside-down position and then rotated 180 degrees (Fig. 19.12).

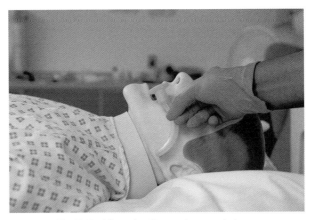

Fig. 19.11   Measuring the oropharyngeal airway.

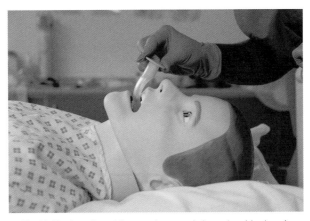

Fig. 19.12   Insertion of the oropharyngeal airway 'upside down'.

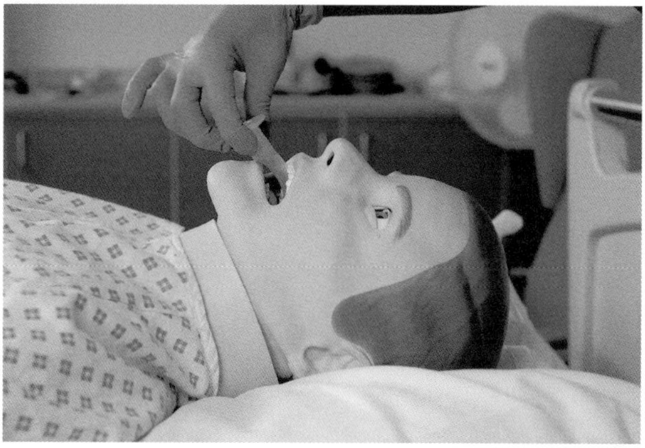

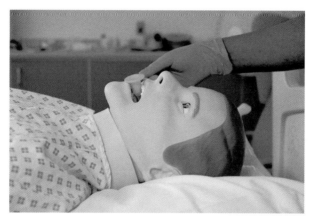

Fig. 19.13   Rotating the oropharyngeal airway into position.

Fig. 19.14   Oropharyngeal airway in position.

4. The airway should then be advanced further back into pharynx (Fig. 19.13).
5. The oval reinforced section should lie between the patients' teeth (Fig. 19.14).
6. Nurses should check that the airway is still patent after insertion by listening to breath sounds and watching for the rise and fall of the chest wall (Resuscitation Council [UK], 2021).

Insertion of a Nasopharyngeal Airway

An NPA is another useful simple airway adjunct which can be used to maintain airway patency. Generally, NPAs are easier to tolerate and can be used in cases where an OA cannot be inserted, such as jaw spasms or some maxillofacial injuries.

The NPA is made from soft flexible plastic and can be inserted directly into the nasal cavity (Fig. 19.15). There are no standard methods for measuring the correct size of an NP airway; however, sizes 6 and 7mm are suitable for adults. NP airways are not suitable for those patients

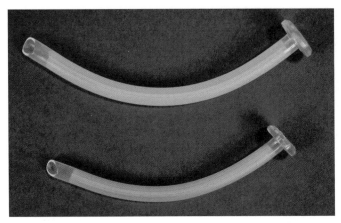

Fig. 19.15   Nasopharyngeal airways.

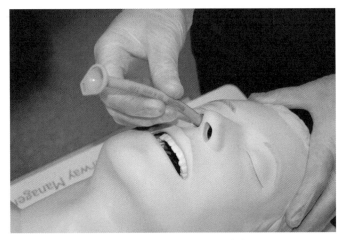

Fig. 19.16   Inserting nasopharyngeal airway.

who have, or are suspected to have a basal skull fracture. Nurses should also be aware that insertion of any similar airway adjunct could stimulate laryngospasm or vomiting (Resuscitation Council [UK], 2021).

Procedure for insertion:

1. Water based lubricant can be applied to the NPA to aid insertion.
2. The bevelled end is inserted into the patient's nostril (Fig. 19.16).
3. The NP is then gently lowered down until the flat large end is near the nostril. If there is any resistance, the procedure should be terminated immediately.
4. Care should be taken to carry out this procedure gently as the mucosal lining can become damaged, causing irritation and/or bleeding.
5. Nurses should also check airway patency using the same techniques as described above (Fig. 19.17). Suction using a flexible catheter can also be performed via an NPA.

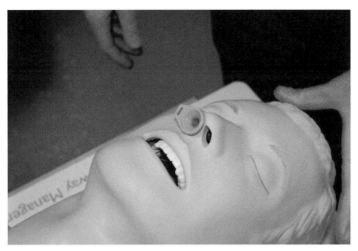

Fig. 19.17 Nasopharyngeal airway in place.

Use of Bag Valve Mask Technique

The bag valve mask (BVM) (also termed self-inflating bag) device allows the delivery of higher concentrations of oxygen to facilitate ventilation during cardiac arrest. As the bag is squeezed, positive pressure forces oxygen enriched air (if attached to oxygen) into the lungs. When released, the self-inflating bag refills automatically. The advantage of a self-inflating system is that ventilation can be delivered without having a gas supply attached. An oxygen reservoir bag is normally attached, and with oxygen flow rate of 15L/min, an inspired oxygen concentration of approximately 85% can be achieved (Resuscitation Council [UK], 2021). This technique should be used in the short term only, as there is a high risk of aspiration of stomach contents into the lungs.

A two-person technique is recommended, as it may be difficult to achieve a seal, maintain an open airway and squeeze the bag alone; one person should open the airway and maintain a good seal with the mask, while the other squeezes the bag.

KEY POINTS

- Use of a bag-valve mask is normally part of a medical emergency.
- A two-person technique is recommended.
- The bag-valve mask should be attached to 15 L/min oxygen.

EQUIPMENT

PPE
Bag, valve mask and suitably sized mask
Oxygen source and flow meter

PROCEDURE

1. Safely move the patient into the supine position.
2. Move the bed away from the wall and remove the backrest if applicable. Check that the brakes of the bed are on, and if the height of the bed should be adjusted.
3. Stand at the top of the bed.
4. Select an appropriately sized mask—one that comfortably covers the mouth and nose but does not cover the eyes or override the chin.
5. Check that oxygen is connected to the bag-valve mask (BVM) at a flow rate of 15 L/min (Fig. 19.18).
6. First nurse: Tilt the head back, apply the mask to the face, pressing down on it with the thumbs, while performing a jaw thrust technique (Fig. 19.19). It is important to ensure

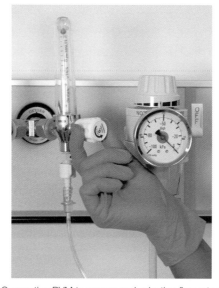

Fig. 19.18   Connecting BVM to oxygen and selecting flow rate of 15 L/min.

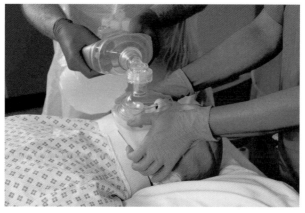

Fig. 19.19   Two person technique, creating air tight seal.

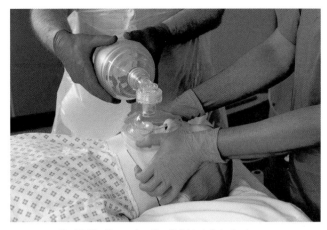

Fig. 19.20 Squeezing the BVM to inflate the lungs.

that the mask has a good seal to deliver adequate ventilation and to ensure that gas is not being forced into the stomach. A pillow under the patient's head and shoulders can help to maintain this position.

7. Second nurse (positioned beside the bed): Squeeze the mask bag (not the oxygen reservoir bag) sufficiently to cause visible chest rise (Fig. 19.20). Each ventilation should be delivered over one second. Hyperventilation should be avoided.

An airway adjunct such as an oropharyngeal airway (OPA) or a nasopharyngeal airway (NPA) can be used to maintain a patent airway. The insertion of an airway adjunct may make it easier to ventilate a patient.

Observe for chest rise and fall. If the chest does not rise, re-check the patency of the airway; slight readjustment may be all that is required.

To attach the self-inflating bag to a laryngeal mask airway, tracheostomy tube or endotracheal tube, the mask is removed. A catheter mount can also be attached.

Basic Life Support and Use of an Automated External Defibrillator

Nurses are expected to be are able to recognise and appropriately respond to emergencies. This includes being able recognise and respond to a cardiac arrest and continue basic life support until skilled help and equipment are available.

KEY FACTS

- All nurses must be able to recognise and respond to a cardiac arrest and safely use an automated external defibrillator (AED).

DANGER

Approach the person/surroundings carefully to exclude any risk of danger to yourself. You should also apply PPE as appropriate.

RESPONSE

Assess the person's conscious state. Shake their shoulders (unless there is a possibility of a cervical spine injury) and shout (in both ears) to see if they respond.

SHOUT FOR HELP

If the patient is unconscious:
- In a clinical setting, pull the emergency buzzer to alert colleagues to an emergency situation, and request an emergency call (2222) is made; this must include the location and type of emergency team needed (e.g., adult cardiac arrest).
- In the pre-hospital setting, call for help from a bystander. Ask the bystander to wait while you complete your assessment. If you are completely alone do not go for help yourself until you have checked the airway and breathing.

AIRWAY

Look for any obvious obstruction in the mouth. With one hand tip back the forehead (unless there is neck injury) and with two fingers of your other hand lift the chin to raise the tongue from the back of the throat to open the airway. Maintain head tilt chin lift.

BREATHING AND CIRCULATION OR SIGNS OF LIFE

Place your cheek near the person's nostrils to feel for any breathing. Look for chest movement and listen for breath sounds. Observe for no more than 10 seconds.

Feel for the carotid pulse if you have been trained to do so, as this pulse is nearest to the heart. If no pulse can be felt here, there is no cardiac output. Alternatively, look for signs of life, be aware gasping is an abnormal sign and sometimes observed in the early stages of cardiac arrest.

If no breathing, pulse (signs of life)
- Call the emergency team (2222). This must include clearly stating the location and type of emergency team needed (e.g., adult cardiac arrest).
- Depending on location, call 999 for an ambulance.

BEGIN CARDIO-PULMONARY RESUSCITATION (CPR)

With the person lying flat on their back, commence external cardiac compressions.

Identify the middle of the sternum (breastbone) and place the heel of one hand in the middle of the lower half of the sternum. Place your other hand on top and interlock the fingers (Fig. 19.21).

Keeping your arms straight and your shoulders in line with your elbows and heels of your hands, give 30 compressions at a rate of 100 to 120 per minute. You should press hard enough to compress the chest wall by 5 to 6 cm (Resuscitation Council [UK], 2021).

Give two ventilations using a BVM. Confirming the chest rises with every breath/ventilation. If it does not, re-check the mouth for visible obstruction and the airway is open. Do not over ventilate as this may inflate the stomach and cause vomiting. Wait for the chest to fall after each breath before giving another breath. Each breath should take 1 second and the two breaths no more than 5 seconds in total.

Continue giving cycles of 30 compressions and two breaths until the AED arrives.

When the AED arrives, switch it on and follow the voice prompts. Continue cardiac compressions if another person is present to attach the AED.

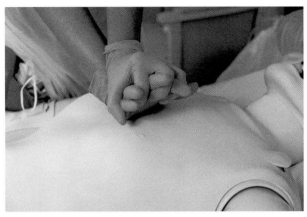

Fig. 19.21   Hand position for chest compressions.

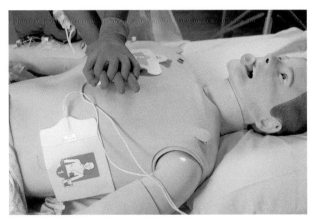

Fig. 19.22   Hand position with defibrillator pads attached.

Expose the chest fully and apply the pads to the patient's bare chest and plug-in pad connector. If there is poor contact, consider shaving the sites before applying the pads (a razor is supplied with the AED). Check that the chest is dry. Remove any metal objects (e.g. neck chains and under-wire bras). Remove any medication patches (e.g. nicotine patch) on the front of the torso. If in doubt, remove it.

Firmly apply the pads, as indicated in the diagram on the pad. Chest compressions should continue during this process (Fig. 19.22).

The machine will prompt you when it is about to 'analyse'. Instruct everyone to stand back while the machine analyses the heart rhythm. A trace will be stored in the memory for later retrieval.

If the machine detects either Ventricular Fibrillation (VF) or Ventricular Tachycardia (VT), it will prompt 'Shock advised' and 'Charging'. Depending on the type of AED used, compressions may continue while the machine is charging (Fig. 19.23).

When the machine is charged, it will prompt 'Stand clear' and 'Press to shock now'. Before the shock is delivered, the operator MUST ensure that all personnel are clear and that any oxygen being administered is removed (Fig. 19.24). The patient may jump or flinch as the shock discharges.

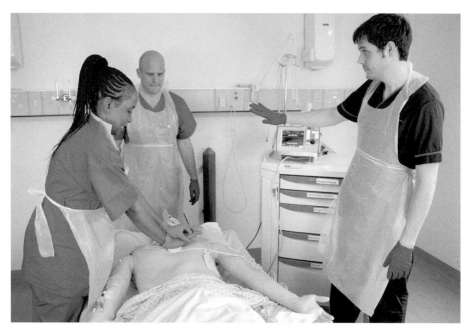

Fig. 19.23 Continuing chest compressions during charging.

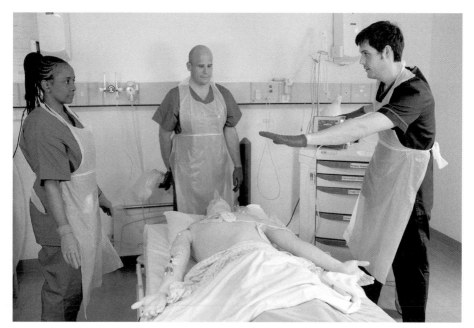

Fig. 19.24 Delivering safe shock.

Re-commence CPR as soon as the shock has been delivered. It may take several seconds for the heart to begin to function again. Unless there are signs of return spontaneous circulation, continue CPR. The machine will run another cycle after 2 minutes, analysing and, if required, charging for a shock. Repeat the process until either the patient recovers or expert help arrives.

If the outcome is successful, the patient will be transferred to a critical care unit. If unsuccessful, tidy away any equipment and prepare the patient to be seen by their family. Despite your best efforts, the patient may not survive.

Document all activities, the timing of events and, if resuscitation was unsuccessful, whether circulation was restored at any point during the resuscitation.

Replenish equipment and return the AED. Team debriefing should take place.

References

Bethel, J., 2013. Anaphylaxis: diagnosis and treatment. Nurs. Stand. 27 (41), 49–56.

Davies, M., Couper, K., Bradley, J., et al., 2014. A simple solution for improving the reliability of cardiac arrest equipment provision in hospital. Resuscitation. 85: 1523–1526.

Gwinnutt, C., Davies, R., Soar, J., 2019. In-Hospital Resuscitation. https://www.resus.org.uk/resuscitation-guidelines/in-hospital-resuscitation/

National Institute for Health and Clinical Excellence (NICE), 2011. Anaphylaxis: assessment to confirm an anaphylactic episode and the decision to refer after emergency treatment for a suspected anaphylactic episode. NICE Clinical Guideline 134.

National Tracheostomy Safety Project, 2016. Emergency Tracheostomy Management: Patent Upper Airway. http://www.tracheostomy.org.uk/healthcare-staff/emergency-care/emergency-algorithm-tracheostomy.

NHS, 2019. What Should I Do If Someone Is Choking? https://www.nhs.uk/common-health-questions/accidents-first-aid-and-treatments/what-should-i-do-if-someone-is-choking/

NHS Improvement, 2018. Patient Safety Alert: Resources to Support Safer Modification of Food and Drink. NHS/PSA/RE/2018/004 https://improvement.nhs.uk/documents/2955/Patient_Safety_Alert_Resources_to_support_safer_modification_of_food_and_drink_v2.pdf.

Mayo, P., 2017. Undertaking an accurate and comprehensive assessment of the acutely ill adult. Nurs. Stand. 32 (8), 53–61. doi:10.7748/ns.2017.e10968.

Pavitt, M.J., Nevett, J., Swanton, L.L., et al., 2017. London ambulance source data on choking incidence for the calendar year 2016: an observational study. BMJ Open Respir. Res. 4:e000215. doi:10.1136/bmjresp-2017-000215.

Resuscitation Council (UK), 2016. Advanced Life Support Manual. London.

Resuscitation Council (UK). (2021). Emergency treatment of anaphylactic reactions: Guidelines for healthcare provider. https://www.resus.org.uk/library/additional-guidance/guidance-anaphylaxis/emergency-treatment

Resuscitation Council (UK). (2022). Quality standards: acute care equipment and drug lists. https://www.resus.org.uk/library/quality-standards-cpr/acute-care-equipment-and-drug-lists

Thim, T., Krarup, N.H.V., Grove, E.L., et al., 2012. Initial assessment and treatment with the Airway, Breathing, Circulation, Disability, Exposure (ABCDE) approach. Int. J. Gen. Med. 5, 117–121

Walker, S.T., Brett, S.J., McKay, A., et al., 2012. The "Resus: Station": the use of clinical simulations in a randomised crossover study to evaluate a novel resuscitation trolley. Resuscitation. 83, 1374–1380.

CHAPTER 20

Adult Blood Tests

The values below represent an 'average' reference range, in adults, for blood. These ranges should be used as a guide only. Reference ranges vary between individual laboratories, and readers should consult their own laboratory for those used locally. This is especially important where reference values depend upon the analytical equipment and temperatures used.

Haematology Bloods Tests

Test	Reference Range
Activated partial thromboplastin time (APTT)	26–37 s
Erythrocyte sedimentation rate (ESR)	<10 mm/h
Eosinophils	0.02–0.5 10^9/L
Fibrinogen	1.5–4.0 g/L
Folate (serum)	1.5–20.6 μg/L
Haematocrit	
▪ Female	0.33–0.47 L/L
▪ Male	0.35–0.53 L/L
Haemoglobin	
▪ Female	118–148 g/L
▪ Male	133–167 g/L
International normalised ratio	2–3 or 3–4
Leucocytes	4.0 × 11.0 × 10^9/L
Lymphocytes	1.0–3.0 10^9/L
Mean cell haemoglobin (MCH)	26–33 pg
Mean cell haemoglobin concentration	330–370 pg/L
Mean cell volume (MCV)	77–98 fL
Monocytes	0.2–1.0 10^9/L
Neutrophils	2.0–7.0 10^9/L
Partial thromboplastin time	24–34 s
Platelets (thrombocytes)	143–400 10^9/L
Prothrombin time	11–14 s
Red cells (erythrocytes)	
▪ Female	3.9–5.0 10^{12}/L
▪ Male	4.3–5.7 10^{12}/L
White cells total	
▪ Neutrophil granulocytes	2.0–7.5 × 10^9/L
▪ Lymphocytes	1.5–4.0 × 10^9/L
▪ Monocytes	0.2–0.8 × 10^9/L
▪ Eosinophil granulocytes	0.04–0.4 × 10^9/L
▪ Basophil granulocytes	0.01–0.1 × 10^9/L
D-dimers	<500 Units/mL

Blann (2013) and Peate et al. (2014).

Biochemistry Blood Tests

Test	Reference Range
Alanine aminotransferase (ALT)	5–42 IU/L
Albumin	35–50 g/L
Alkaline phosphatase	20–120 IU/L
Amylase	<300 IU/L
Aspartate aminotransferase (AST)	10–50 IU/L
Bicarbonate (hydrogen carbonate)	24–29 mmol/L
Bilirubin	<21 μmol/L
Calcium	2.2–2.6 mmol/L
Chloride	95–107mmol/L
Total cholesterol	<5.0 mmol/L
Low-density lipoprotein cholesterol	<3.0 mmol/L
High-density lipoprotein cholesterol	>1.2 mmol/L
C-Reactive protein	<10 mg/L
Creatine kinase (total)	
■ Male	30–200 mmol/L
■ Female	30–150 mmol/L
Creatinine	71–133 μmol/L
Estimated glomerular filtration rate (eGFR)	>90 mL/min/1.73 m^2
Ferritin	
■ Female	17–300 μg/L
■ Male	14–150 μg/L
Gamma-glutamyl-transferase (GGT)	5–55 IU/L
Glucose (venous blood, fasting)	3.5–5.5 mmol/L
Lactate venous whole blood	0.7–1.9 mmol/L
Lactate dehydrogenase (total)	240–480 IU/L
Magnesium	0.8–1.2 mmol/L
Phosphate	0.8–1.4 mmol/L
Potassium (serum)	3.8–5.0 mmol/L
Protein	60–80 g/L
Sodium	135–145 mmol/L
Transferrin	
■ Thyroid stimulating hormone	0.2–3.5 mU/L
■ Triglycerides (fasting)	<1.7 mmol/L
■ Urea	3.3–6.7 mmol/L

Blann (2013) and Peate et al. (2014).

Arterial Blood Gases

Test	Reference Range
pH	7.35–7.45
PaO$_2$	>10 kPa
	80–100 mm Hg
PaCO$_2$	4.5–6 kPa
	35–45 mm Hg
Bicarbonate (HCO$_3$)	22–26 mmol/L
Base Excess	−2 to +2 mmol/L

Blann (2013) and Peate et al. (2014).

References

Blann, A., 2013. Routine Blood Results Explained. M&K Update Ltd. UK
Peate, I., Wild, K., Nair, M. (Eds.), 2014. Nursing Practice: Knowledge and Care. John Wiley and Sons. USA